Winston & Kuhn's Herbal Therapy & Supplements

A Scientific & Traditional Approach

2nd edition

Merrily A. Kuhn, RN, PhD, ND
President, Educational Services, Inc.
Hamburg, New York
Associate Professor, D'Youville College
  and Daemen College
Buffalo and Amherst, New York

David Winston, RH (AHG)
Registered Herbalist and Ethnobotanist
Herbal Therapeutics Research Library
Washington, New Jersey

*with a Foreword to this edition by
Tieraona Low Dog, MD*

Wolters Kluwer | Lippincott Williams & Wilkins
Health
Philadelphia · Baltimore · New York · London
Buenos Aires · Hong Kong · Sydney · Tokyo

Senior Acquisitions Editor: Margaret Zuccarini
Editorial Consultant: Susan Rainey
Editorial Assistant: Season Evans
Production Project Manager: Cynthia Rudy
Director of Nursing Production: Helen Ewan

Senior Managing Editor/Production: Erika Kors
Design Coordinator: Joan Wendt
Manufacturing Coordinator: Karin Duffield
Production Services/Compositor: Aptara, Inc.

2nd edition

9 8 7 6 5 4 3 2 1

Library of Congress Cataloging-in-Publication Data

Kuhn, Merrily A., 1945–
    Winston & Kuhn's herbal therapy & supplements : a scientific & traditional approach /
Merrily A. Kuhn, David Winston ; with a foreword to this edition by Tieraona Low Dog. —
2nd ed.
        p. ; cm.
    Rev. ed. of: Herbal therapy & supplements / Merrily A. Kuhn, David Winston. c2000.
    Includes bibliographical references and index.
    ISBN-13: 978-1-58255-462-4 (alk. paper)
    ISBN-10: 1-58255-462-5 (alk. paper)
    1. Herbs—Therapeutic use—Handbooks, manuals, etc. 2. Dietary supplements—
Handbooks, manuals, etc. I. Winston, David, 1956– II. Kuhn, Merrily A., 1945–
Herbal therapy & supplements. III. Title. IV. Title: Winston and Kuhn's herbal therapy
and supplements V. Title: Herbal therapy & supplements.
    [DNLM: 1. Medicine, Herbal—Handbooks. 2. Phytotherapy—Handbooks.
3. Plants, Medicinal—Handbooks. WB 39 K96h 2008]
    RM666.H33K84 2008
    615'.321—dc22

                                                            2007031762

CD102023

at it has
e with a
the best
well-bal-
ration-
ic items
s a wel-
ring on
d possi-
riod of
offers a
hy new
tion of
health

o
h and
Cl
ucts
ct
ative
ns
he
a

To my parents, Audrey and Norbert Kuhn, who taught me perseverance;

To my husband, James, the love of my life, for his devotion, care, and daily concern;

To Martha Kulwicki, a loving and beautiful person, who taught me to laugh and appreciate life day to day;

To Debbie Pleskow, my administrative assistant, for her organization and typing of this manuscript; and

To all readers who are willing to take a step beyond their comfort zone into complementary medicine!

Merrily A. Kuhn, RN, PhD, ND

I would like to dedicate this book to the generations of herbalists who, by practicing their craft, have left us the legacy of traditional herbal medicine. Specifically, I sincerely thank my teachers, colleagues, patients, and students for all they have taught me.

David Winston, RH (AHG)

Lisa Bedner, RN, RH, AHG
Director, Pipsissewa Herbs
Teacher, Lecturer
Practice of Herbal Medicine
Medicine Woman
Teehahnahmah Nation, Tennessee

Janice E. Benjamin, RN
Healthcare and Private Practice in Acupuncture
   and Alternative Medicine
Durham, North Carolina

Steve Blake, DSc, MH
Researcher
Haiku, Hawaii

Patricia Bratianu, PhD, RN
Owner, Simply Health
Palm Bay, Florida

Carol A. Buttz, MS, RN, CEN
Nursing Instructor
Dakota County Technical College
Rosemount, Minnesota

T. Sean Diesel, DOM, RH (AHG)
Private Practice
Albuquerque, New Mexico

Keturah R. Faurot, PA, MPH
Research Associate
Program on Integrative Medicine
Department of Physical Medicine & Rehabilitation
School of Medicine
University of North Carolina at Chapel Hill
Chapel Hill, North Carolina

Foreword to the Second Edition

While herbal medicine has its roots in the past, it remains a valuable and popular therapy today. Recent surveys indicate that roughly 10% to 19% of Americans use herbal medicines for health conditions, especially for upper respiratory infections, arthritis, depression, musculoskeletal pain, menopause, and for improving their memory. With unprecedented access to information online 24 hours a day, consumers likely will continue to explore the use of botanicals and other dietary supplements as they seek ways to improve their health and well-being. But because of the potential for both benefit and harm with the use of herbal medicines, it is important that health care practitioners feel confident counseling patients about their use. We must consider what level of evidence of effectiveness is acceptable to support the use of any particular medicinal plant within the context of safety, the condition being treated, and the beliefs and preferences of our patients—a task that seems daunting to the busy practitioner who is not formally trained in herbal medicine.

Overall, most herbs commonly used in the United States have a relatively good safety profile, and incidences of herb-related adverse events are infrequent. However, the excellent safety record of a traditional oral preparation may have limited relevance to the same herb taken as a highly concentrated extract, at a high dose, for an extended period of time. Moreover, herbs that are apparently safe under normal conditions may be more hazardous in certain patients (eg, pregnant women, or people with impaired renal or liver function); under special circumstances (eg, during the perioperative period); or when combined with particular conventional drugs. Indeed, the interactions between pharmaceutical drugs and herbal remedies are an area of major concern for many practitioners, because as many as 27 million Americans are using herbal supplements in conjunction with other over-the-counter medications or prescription drugs—and most are not sharing that information with their primary care providers.

Winston & Kuhn's Herbal Therapy & Supplements is designed to serve as a bridge between the worlds of conventional and herbal medicine. Like any bridge, this requires having a firm footing on both sides of the span. Hence, one author of this book is a nurse with a PhD in physiology, and the other is one of America's most highly respected clinical herbalists. Quick and easy to use, their book provides important, clinically relevant information for the practitioner, such as dose, dosage form, traditional and modern uses, contraindications, side effects, long-term safety, and herb–drug interactions, as well as use in children and during pregnancy and lactation. I highly recommend this valuable resource, and thank Merrily Kuhn and David Winston for their contribution to the field.

Tieraona Low Dog, MD
Director of Education
Program in Integrative Medicine
Clinical Assistant Professor
Department of Medicine
University of Arizona College
    of Medicine

Preface

Herbal therapy has its roots in history and folk medicine. In this new millennium, herbal therapy is reaching a turning point. It is becoming a field of science with its own research and data base. Socrates once said, "There is only one good: knowledge; and one evil: ignorance." Certainly this statement should guide us as health care professionals to learn as much as we can from both worlds of herbal therapy: the traditional use passed on from eclectic physicians and folk practitioners, and now the scientific evidence that supports the traditional approach.

I have had the distinct pleasure to coauthor this book with a noted herbalist, David Winston, RH (AHG). We have both learned much in the process! Together, we have combined the traditional and scientific worlds so that we can educate today's practitioners in the use of herbal products. Often, patients know more (or think they do) about herbal products than their health care providers do. This text attempts to enlighten the orthodox health care provider about both traditional and mounting scientific evidence available on herbal products.

As an RN with a PhD in physiology and as an author of two pharmacology texts, a critical care handbook, and a laboratory pocket guide, my roots are securely in the traditional and scientific medical world. Since beginning to study herbal therapies, I have come to appreciate the power of herbs to improve and heal simple conditions such as the common cold, flu, and nail fungus, as well as more complex problems such as hypertension and menopausal changes, and, finally, serious health problems such as cancer. I have also obtained an ND (Naturopathic Doctor) degree and have a practice in holistic health. Seeing and experiencing the effects of herbal and supplemental therapy is believing!

ORGANIZATION

This handbook is organized into three parts: an introductory section; the main section, which presents herbal monographs; and the third section, which presents monographs of supplements that are commonly used singly or in combination with herbal or traditional medicinal products.

Part I. The introductory chapter reviews the concept of herbal therapy. What is an herb? How have herbs been used in traditional systems of medicine (ie, Chinese, Indian, Cherokee, and Ayurvedic)? What is the research process for evaluating herbs? How are herbs used to treat various conditions, and what types of products are available? The chapter also addresses the issue of standardization—is it appropriate?

Part II. This part of the text presents the most up-to-date information on herbal therapies. The format for each herb monograph includes its common names; scientific names; plant family; description; medicinal part; constituents; nutritional ingredients; traditional use; current use; available forms, dosage, and administration guidelines; pharmacokinetics; toxicity; contraindications; side effects; long-term safety; use in pregnancy/lactation/children; drug/herb interactions; special notes; and a bibliography.

The most common herbs available in the United States and Canada are reviewed. Many herbs have demonstrated scientific value; however, some herbs that do not yet have scientific research support are discussed because they are commonly sold.

Part III. The section about supplements includes products that are very popular, such as glucosamine, chondroitin, and coenzyme Q10. The information given for each supplement includes its scientific name; common name; biologic activity; nutritional sources; current use; available forms, dosage, and administration guidelines; pharmacokinetics; toxicity; contraindications; side effects; long-term safety; use in pregnancy/lactation/children; drug/herb interactions; and bibliography.

Some supplements, like herbs, have a scientific basis for use, but some do not. We have chosen to include some supplements even though research study results on them are not yet available.

APPENDICES AND GLOSSARY

Several appendices present important reference material and resources.

Appendix A reviews herbs contraindicated during pregnancy and breast-feeding.

Appendix B is a listing of medical disorders and their appropriate herbal or supplemental therapy. People should be encouraged not to self-diagnose and treat, but to consult with a clinical herbalist, naturopathic physician, or medical doctor well-versed in herbal practice. As pointed out in Part I, two people with the same diagnosis seen by an herbalist/naturopath may be treated with different herbal protocols.

Appendix C is an annotated guide to recommended references for further study.

In addition to the appendices, we include a glossary of herbal/medical terms that may not appear in current medical dictionaries. Also, an explanation of medical abbreviations used in the text appears on the inside front cover of the book.

Let us all enhance our own healing and health, and share our knowledge with our patients. The ultimate goal of this book is to place health and healing within the grasp of all people.

Enjoy maximal health and longevity!

Merrily A. Kuhn, RN, PhD
David Winston, RH (AHG)

Acknowledgments

This book would never have come to be without the foresight of Margaret Zuccarini, Senior Acquisitions Editor at Lippincott Williams & Wilkins. Our thanks to Susan Rainey, Editorial Consultant, who integrated all of the updates and prepared the manuscript for production; and to Season Evans, Editorial Assistant, who managed multiple tasks and ensured that no details were overlooked in this revision. Also, our thanks to all the production staff at Lippincott Williams & Wilkins, particularly Cynthia Rudy, Production Project Manager.

Our thanks also go out to the reviewers of this book for their knowledge and encouraging comments. All of the reviewers with whom we worked were willing to share their knowledge and expertise with us and the medical community.

Contents

PART I

An Introduction to Herbal Medicine

David Winston, RH (AHG)

Herbs: Panaceas or Poisons?

Certain herbs have become popular during the past 25 years, but herbal medicine is still poorly understood by the public, medical practitioners, and the media. After a brief honeymoon where herbs were portrayed as "wonder drugs," we are now seeing article after article on the dangers of herbs. As in most situations, the truth lies hidden under the media hype, bad or poorly understood science, exaggerated claims, and our natural resistance to new ideas.

Seeing herbal medicines as either panaceas or as poisons blinds us to the reality that in most cases they are neither. Lack of experience, education, and good information about herbs makes consumers easy victims of marketing exploitation and herbal myths. The same lack of experience, education, and information makes many physicians and other orthodox health care providers suspicious and uncomfortable, especially with the exaggerated claims, miracle cures, and unproven remedies that their patients are taking.

We as a culture are coming out of what I call the "Herbal Dark Ages," a period of time when the use of herbs virtually ceased to exist in the United States. A few ethnic communities continued to use herbs, but from the 1920s into the 1970s, the only herbs that mainstream Americans used were spices in cooking. Out of this almost total lack of exposure, we have seen an amazing resurgence of interest in "natural" remedies.

Along with this new interest is a profound ignorance, with many people equating "natural" with "harmless." Anyone who uses herbal products needs to understand a few basic safety rules.

The fact that something is natural does not necessarily make it safe or effective. In Cherokee medicine, we distinguish between three categories of herbs (Winston, 1992). The *food herbs* are gentle in action, have very low toxicity, and are unlikely to cause an adverse response. Examples of food herbs include lemon balm, peppermint, marshmallow, ginger, garlic, chamomile, hawthorn, rose hips, nettles, dandelion root and leaf, and fresh oat extract. These herbs can be used in substantial quantities over long periods of time without any acute or chronic toxicity. Allergic responses are possible, as are unique idiosyncratic reactions, and even common foods such as grapefruit juice, broccoli, and okra can interact with medications.

The second category is *medicine herbs*. These herbs are stronger and need to be used with greater knowledge (dosage and rationale for use), for specific conditions (with a medical diagnosis), and usually for a limited period. These herbs are not daily tonics and should not be taken just because they are "good for you." These herbs have a greater potential for adverse reactions and in some cases drug interactions. Examples of medicine herbs include andrographis, blue cohosh, cascara sagrada, celandine, ephedra, goldenseal, Jamaica dogwood, Oregon grape root, senna, and uva-ursi.

The last category is *poison herbs*. These herbs have a strong potential for either acute or chronic toxicity and should be used only by clinicians who are trained to use them and clearly understand their toxicology and appropriate use. Even though the herb industry is often portrayed as unregulated* and irresponsible, most of the herbs in this category are not available to the public and are not sold in health food or herb stores. Examples of poison herbs include aconite, arnica, belladonna, bryonia, datura, gelsemium, henbane, male fern, phytolacca, podophyllum, and veratrum.

Another example of a traditional system of medicine that categorizes herbs according to their safety or potential toxicity is traditional Chinese medicine (TCM). The Chinese materia medica is also divided into three categories. The upper-class (superior) drugs are nontoxic and are tonic remedies. The middle-class (ministerial) drugs may have some mild toxicity, and they support the superior medicines. The last category is the lower-class (inferior) remedies, which are toxic and used only for specific ailments for limited periods.

The practitioner must have a clear understanding of an herb's benefits and possible risks and a clearly defined patient diagnosis so that he or she can counsel patients about safe and effective

---

*The herb industry is regulated by the FDA and laws such as the Dietary Supplement, Health and Education Act, passed by Congress in 1994.

choices in herb use. A second problem commonly experienced with the public is the belief that if a little of an herb (or medicine) is good, then more must be better. A well-publicized example is the herb ma huang (ephedra), which has been used for weight loss or as a stimulant. Serious adverse reactions, including death, have occurred; in most cases, the people were foolishly taking two to four times the recommended dose. Many herbs are useful and safe in small, appropriate doses, but, as with any medication, overdoses can cause unwanted side effects, possible injury, and, if the statistics are correct, rare fatalities.

DANGERS AND TOXICITY OF HERBAL MEDICINES

This book is divided into two sections, one on herbal products and the other on nutritional supplements. They are not the same. A recent hysterical report claimed that herbal products could cause bovine spongiform encephalitis, also known as mad cow disease. The author failed to notice that herbs are from the vegetable kingdom and do not contain animal tissue. The author of this report was correct in noting that some supplements do contain animal glandular tissue such as liver, thymus, bone marrow, and thyroid and that the possibility of contamination by infectious proteins from these products may exist. If we are going to critique herbs and supplement products, let us do it with clear knowledge and understanding of the topic.

It is not uncommon for studies to be done on animals and the results extrapolated to humans, even though we may metabolize or digest various phytochemicals quite differently. Researchers have done studies on an herb without authenticating its identity, making results meaningless (Leung, 2000).

Sometimes information on isolated constituents is confused with the whole herb, or studies on intravenous forms of herbs are confused with oral administration. This type of misinterpretation and misunderstanding gives rise to incorrect information, which often continues to be repeated even decades after the original research has been disproven. Other studies have taken hamster oocytes and human sperm, put them into extracts of herbs (St. John's wort, saw palmetto, ginkgo, and echinacea) and found that in high concentrations, some of the herbs denatured the sperm or inhibited the sperm from penetrating the hamster oocyte (Ondrizek et al., 1999). This study was widely reported in medical journals and the popular press. One medical editor said that it was an important study showing a possible correlation between infertility and the use of herbs. The author of the study, Dr. Richard Ondrizek, was "flabbergasted" that his in vitro laboratory research is being reported as evidence that these herbs can cause infertility in humans. Dr. Ondrizek stated, "there is absolutely no parallel between this study and humans."

Another recent error is due to lack of knowledge about phytochemistry. Several reports have surfaced suggesting that echinacea may be hepatotoxic. There is no evidence of this whatsoever. The error comes from the fact that echinacea contains very small amounts of pyrrolizidine alkaloids, some forms of which are known hepatotoxins. Unfortunately, the authors of this misinformation failed to differentiate between unsaturated (hepatotoxic) alkaloids and the nontoxic saturated alkaloids found in echinacea. This is an easy error for the uninformed to make, but one that creates unnecessary fear and confusion.

According to the information gathered by acclaimed researcher and scientist James Duke, PhD, the statistics on deaths caused by herbs compared with other causes are quite revealing:

Herbs: 1 in 1 million
Supplements: 1 in 1 million
Poisonous mushrooms: 1 in 100,000
Nonsteroidal anti-inflammatories: 1 in 10,000
Murder: 1 in 10,000
Hospital surgery: 1 in 10,000
Car accident: 1 in 5,000
Improper use of medication: 1 in 2,000
Angiogram: 1 in 1,000
Alcohol: 1 in 500
Cigarettes: 1 in 500
Properly prescribed medications: 1 in 333
Medical mishap: 1 in 250
Iatrogenic hospital infection: 1 in 80
Bypass surgery: 1 in 20

If put into perspective, herbs (food herbs and medicine herbs) can cause problems, but they are substantially safer than over-the-counter and prescription medications. Will we find that some herbs can have side effects? Definitely. Will we find that some herbs interact with medications? Absolutely. We only have to look at reports that St. John's wort reduced the blood levels of cyclosporine in heart transplant patients to be aware of possible risks. At the same time, reports that followed stating that St. John's wort can interfere with birth control and would cause an epidemic of unwanted pregnancies were unfounded. Not only is there no proof of this, but millions of German women who take contraceptive pills and St. John's wort have failed, in the past 20 years, to provide any substantiation to the concerned researchers.

Recently, Merck & Co. removed the COX-2 selective non-steroidal anti-inflammatory medication rofecoxib (Vioxx) from the marketplace even though it had been through extensive testing and FDA drug approval. Any drug researcher will tell you that for most pharmaceuticals, the real test is when they are being used by the general population. This popular medication was deemed "safe" but caused increased risk of heart attack and strokes with an estimated 89,000 to 140,000 deaths in the United States (defective drugs, adrugrecall.com). One benefit of the long history of human use of most herbs is that they have hundreds or thousands of years of use in the general population and a substantial record of safety or danger and effectiveness or lack thereof.

Frequently, we hear complaints that herbs are poorly studied and, as such, are dangerous. It is true that the research on most herbs cannot compare to the 10 years of FDA clinical trials required for new drugs. Because herbs are rarely patentable, it is highly unlikely that any company is going to invest the time (approximately 10 years) and money (approximately $350 million to $500 million) to have an herbal product approved as a new drug. Herbs and supplements are sold in the United States as dietary supplements, with no research necessary before being sold. There are significant numbers of studies being performed on herbal medicines, but most are done in Germany, France, Japan, China, and India, and many are hard to access or never translated into English. It would be of tremendous benefit to consumers and clinicians if American companies would increase funding for well-designed and relevant herbal research.

The quality of this research would also benefit if clinical herbalists who understand appropriate forms of the medication, dosage, and traditional and clinical uses were part of the research team. In 1997, a study was done on the effects of the Chinese herb dong quai on menopausal symptoms (Hirata et al., 1997). This herb is frequently used in TCM formulas for female reproductive problems. Although the study clearly showed that dong quai had no estrogenic effects and did not affect menopausal symptoms, it failed to take into account why and how this herb is used in Chinese medicine. First, dong quai is never used as a simple herb. It is not used for its estrogenic effects, but for its ability to improve cardiac function, increase uterine circulation, reduce anxiety, and mildly stimulate bowel function. Someone who understood this could have helped to design a much more useful and beneficial study.

The gold standard for proof of efficacy for a medication is the controlled double-blind trial. Many herbs, probably most, have not undergone this type of study. Although these studies are very valuable and may offer proof of activity and effectiveness, we also need to understand the usefulness of other types of herbal data. In addition to controlled double-blind trials and meta-analysis, less definitive but still valuable are well-designed unblinded trials, small uncontrolled clinical trials, population (epidemiologic) studies, and some animal and phytochemical studies. The herbalist should use all of these resources while also incorporating additional information often ignored by academics. Traditional herb use, ethnobotanical use, and practical clinical experience are extremely valuable tools that stand as the basic foundation of good herbal practice. When you find three disparate groups of people using the same herb or closely related species for the exact same use, you can be fairly certain that it does indeed have the stated effect. A good example is coptis, used as an effective antibacterial and antifungal agent by Native Americans, Northern Europeans, and the Chinese.

During the 1940s and 1950s, drug companies spent millions of dollars doing random drug screenings on plants, fungi, and soil microorganisms in search of the starting materials for new drugs. There were a few notable successes, such as the Madagascar periwinkle (*Vinca rosea*), the source of vinblastine and vincristine. However, overall the programs were failures. Rarely did any new drug develop from random screenings. In the past 10 years, pharmaceutical companies have once again begun to search the plant kingdom for new bioactive phytochemicals, but now they use ethnobotanists and even old herbals to do the preliminary searching (Holland, 1996). They have realized that for hundreds or thousands of years, indigenous people depended on these herbs to treat illness. Keen observers of their world, native people used what worked. In addition to the knowledge of preliterate peoples, the accumulated folk wisdom of Europe has been printed in books since the 1500s. Some of the information is exaggerated, some fantastical, and some totally wrong, but much of this herbal wisdom is the basis for modern European phytotherapy, and we are using many of the same herbs for the same conditions as did our distant ancestors.

Traditional systems of medicine such as Ayurveda (India), TCM, Tibetan medicine, Unani-tibb (Greco-Arabic), and Kampo (Japan) have a long and impressive history of effectiveness. Modern research has confirmed the usefulness and safety of what has been used as primary medical care by much of the world's population.

In the United States, eclectic medicine was practiced widely from the 1830s until 1940. This sectarian medical system was founded by a physician, Wooster Beach, MD, who rejected the mainstream medical practice of bleeding, leeching, purging, and using toxic medicines such as arsenic and mercury (Winston & Dattner, 1999). As an alternative, Beach and his followers embraced and studied the American vegetable materia medica. Eclectic physicians during the 1890s represented 10% of the doctors in the United States. Their clinical experience of treating millions of patients over 100 years was carefully chronicled in their voluminous literature. Today, this is an extremely valuable body of experiential knowledge about the successful clinical use of herbal medicines in a time without antibiotics or the advances of technological medicine.

Modern clinical herbalists in the United States and even more so in Great Britain and Australia (where herbalists are recognized practitioners) have also begun to chronicle their clinical experience carefully and even to conduct small-scale clinical studies of herbal treatments. All of this information is valuable, and along with personal clinical experience, it gives the clinician a strong understanding of the appropriate, safe, and effective use of an herb or herbal protocol. In my clinical experience, working from this accumulated knowledge is a highly accurate way of matching effective protocols to each patient. Where this type of proof does not work well is when physicians call and want to know which herbs may be useful for a liver transplant patient, a patient undergoing dialysis, or someone who has just had a bone marrow transplant. In these instances, where there is no tradition, our only guides are careful observation and research studies.

DIFFERENCES BETWEEN ALLOPATHIC USE OF HERBS AND TRADITIONAL HERBAL MEDICINE

As I mentioned earlier, during the past 10 years, certain herbs (black cohosh, echinacea, garlic, kava, milk thistle, saw palmetto, and St. John's wort) have become very popular, but herbal medicine has not. There is a very real difference between the allopathic use of an herb and the practice of good herbal medicine. Different systems of herbal medicine have their own views and distinctive practices, but they all have three things in common.

First, they have an underlying philosophy that creates a foundation and structure for the practice of medicine. Frequently, the underlying belief focuses on what naturopathic medicine calls *Vis Medicatrix Naturae*, or the healing power of nature (Kirchfield & Boyle, 1994). This idea was a central tenet of medicine as taught by Hippocrates, Maimonides, the German physician C. W. Hufeland, and the early American physician Jacob Bigalow. In many systems of medicine, not only is the body seen as inherently self-healing, but there is an important relationship and connection between the physical, emotional, and spiritual aspects of each patient. In Chinese, Tibetan, and Cherokee medicine (Nvwoti), attention may also be given to what we perceive as external relationships and the effects of the family, community, and the environment on each patient.

The second and third aspects of traditional systems of medicine are interrelated: a system of energetics, and differential diagnosis. Energetics is a way of describing the activity and qualities of a given herb. Does it increase (stimulate) or decrease (sedate) function? Does it increase nutrition, tonify an organ, or moisten or dry tissue? Energetics is an effective way of understanding an herb, not by its constituents, which can be very problematic,* but by its activity and effects on the human body. This traditional form of pharmacology is used along with various types of differential diagnosis, so there is an understanding of the underlying imbalances or disease and the treatment is specific to the patient.

Good herbal medicine treats people, not diseases. Physicians and nurses are always surprised that the protocols are so patient-specific. Two different patients, both with rheumatoid arthritis, can have almost entirely different treatments, because clinical herbalists do not view these patients as "two cases of rheumatoid arthritis." They might see John Smith, age 68, with achlorhydria, chronic constipation, impaired circulation, and rheumatoid arthritis, and Alice Jones, age 38, with premenstrual syndrome, depression, biliary dyskinesia, and rheumatoid arthritis. The focus in good herbal, naturopathic, Chinese, or Ayurvedic medicine is affecting the terrain: strengthen the organism, improve overall function (circulation, digestion, elimination, endocrine and immune function), reduce stress, and improve sleep and nutrition.

Many diseases, especially chronic degenerative ones, respond very well to this type of treatment. Benign prostatic hyperplasia is a good example. The orthodox treatment is terazosin (Hytrin). Saw palmetto as an allopathic herbal substitute works about as well as the pharmaceuticals, costs less, and has fewer adverse effects. As an herbalist, I will probably use saw palmetto as a part of my protocol, but in addition I might add nettle root, white sage, Bidens, or collinsonia to improve the activity, effectiveness, and specificity of the formula. This combination of herbs, in my clinical experience, is far superior to the pharmaceutical agents or saw palmetto as an individual remedy.

Herbal medicine, like orthodox medical practice, is an art as well as a science. Knowing how to combine herbs to create a synergistic effect is more than random polypharmacy. Another

●

*Individual constituents can have widely diverse effects as isolates. Chinese ginseng (*Panax ginseng*) is a good example: ginsenoside Rb1 is sedating, whereas ginsenoside Rg1 is a central nervous system stimulant. Despite these opposing effects, the whole herb has an overall stimulating effect.

example of an herbal formula that has benefits over individual herbs would be my protocol for seasonal affective disorder. St. John's wort is touted as an effective herbal antidepressant, and in some cases it is, but for seasonal affective disorder, St. John's wort alone is inadequate. In this situation, combining lemon balm and lavender with St. John's wort increases its benefits while also improving digestion and sleep quality. Other dietary and lifestyle changes would be considered as well as additional herbs specific to the patient.

It is important to recognize that serious acute illnesses such as myocardial infarction, bacterial meningitis, stroke, acute asthma attacks, head trauma, and liver and kidney failure cannot be treated in this manner. For many years, both patients and practitioners have tended to view this difference in treatment paradigms as a choice: one or the other. Nothing could be further from the truth. Where Western medicine is most effective, herbal medicine is often ineffective, but where herbal medicine is most effective, orthodox medicine often has little to offer patients. Not only can botanicals be very useful in many chronic degenerative conditions or mild to moderate functional ailments, but they also can play an important role in recovery from serious illness. Once head trauma victims have been stabilized, the use of ginkgo, rosemary, St. John's wort, and bacopa has dramatically reduced recovery time and improved memory as well as cognitive and motor functions. Western medicine and herbal medicine working in concert offers the best of both worlds, and the patient is the beneficiary in this new relationship.

ADMINISTRATION OF HERBS

Herbs as medicines can be administered in many forms. Some can be taken as foods or consumed regularly in the diet, such as basil, blueberries, garlic, or ginger. Teas (infusions or decoctions) are a reliable way of administering some herbs. Drinking a hot cup of a pleasant-tasting tea can be a wonderfully relaxing and healing experience in itself. Liquids are also absorbed more quickly, especially in patients with impaired digestion. For certain herbs (green tea, slippery elm), tea is the most effective way to take them. The drawbacks to teas are that many herbs have constituents that are poorly water-soluble (boswellia, ginkgo, gum guggul, milk thistle) and are not effective as teas. Other herbs have an unpleasant taste (saw palmetto, feverfew, valerian), and having to drink cupfuls of a noxious-tasting brew will limit patient compliance. Some patients also find having to make teas too much of a bother.

Tinctures are hydroalcoholic extracts of herbs. Although tinctures are not very concentrated (1:5 wt/vol), the menstruum (alcohol and water) extracts a wide range of constituents, the alcohol increases absorption of the herb by approximately 30% (Anonymous, 1998), the doses are much smaller than with teas (so the taste factor is less of a problem), and tinctures are convenient. A patient can carry a small 1-oz dropper bottle, and the tincture can be placed in water, tea, or juice when needed. An additional benefit to tinctures is that fresh herbs that lose potency when dried (echinacea, eyebright, skullcap) can be made into fresh tinctures (1:2 wt/vol), which preserves their activity very effectively. The biggest limitation for tinctures is that they contain alcohol, and people with alcohol abuse issues or serious liver disease should avoid its consumption.

Fluid extracts, more concentrated alcohol-and-water extracts (1:1 wt/vol), offer many of the same benefits as tinctures, with greater potency and a smaller dose. True fluid extracts are not common in the American marketplace, and there is great confusion because different manufacturers use different terminology, technology, and menstruums (extracting liquids) to produce their products. The pharmaceutical definition of a fluid extract includes the use of heat in the manufacturing process, which can be useful for heat-soluble constituents or damaging for heat-sensitive constituents.

Spray-dried extracts are liquid extracts that are spray-dried onto a powdered carrier (cellulose, powdered herbs). These extracts are fairly concentrated (4:1, 5:1 wt/vol), maintain the activity of the whole herb, and are easily encapsulated, so taste is not an issue. The drawbacks of capsules in general, whether they contain ground herbs or a spray-dried extract, are that they are more difficult to digest than liquids, and patients, especially young children, who cannot swallow capsules cannot use this type of product.

Capsules containing ground, dried herbs tend to have very limited activity and digestibility. Herbs that should be taken in this form are ones containing minerals as primary constituents (alfalfa, horsetail, nettles, oat straw). As long as the patient has reasonable digestive function, capsules are a superior way to ingest mineral-rich herbs.

Gelcaps are a useful method of ingesting oily nutrients such as vitamin E or oil-based supplements such as borage seed oil, flaxseed oil, or evening primrose seed oil. Gelcaps are easier to swallow than capsules or tablets, but the ingredients are subjected to considerable heat during processing, and rancidity of the oils is a substantial problem.

Tablets are often difficult to digest, but greater amounts of herbs and herb extracts can be squeezed into this format. Uncoated tablets are harder to swallow but are more absorbable. Most tablets contain proprietary herb/supplement formulas, and their effectiveness depends on the quality of the ingredients and the validity of the formula as a therapeutic regimen.

Standardized herbal products are frequently recommended in the popular literature, especially by authors who are not herbalists. The idea that each dose of an herb has exactly the same levels of active constituents is an attractive concept and a comfortable one for practitioners used to dealing with pharmaceutical products. They need to know that 0.25 mg digoxin is exactly that. Too much can cause arrhythmias and death; too little, and the patient may die of congestive heart failure. However, most herbs are not used for life-threatening conditions, nor do they have the toxicity of digoxin, so doses do not need to be as precise. The belief that each herb has an active constituent is false: most herbs have dozens or even hundreds of constituents that may contribute to their activity. Some of the constituents may have direct activity, whereas other "inert" ingredients may increase bioavailability, reduce toxicity, or stimulate function by means of a synergistic activity. To most herbalists, the active constituent is the herb itself.

Many manufacturers and academic "herbal authorities" would have you believe that only standardized herbal products work and that all herbs should be standardized. This is disingenuous and is more a matter of marketing and belief system than fact. The reality is that fewer than 10% of the standardized products in the marketplace are standardized to known active constituents.

There are actually two types of standardization. The first is true standardization, where a definite phytochemical or group of constituents is known to have activity. Ginkgo, with its 26% ginkgo flavones and 6% terpenes, is a good example of real standardization. Other products that meet these parameters are milk thistle, curcumin from turmeric, *Coleus forskollii,* and saw palmetto (85%–95% fatty sterols). These products are highly concentrated; they no longer represent the whole herb and are now phytopharmaceuticals. In many cases, they are vastly more effective than the whole herb (*Coleus forskollii*, ginkgo, milk thistle), but some effects of the herb may be lost and the potential for adverse effects and herb/drug interactions may increase. Curcumin may have stronger anti-inflammatory activity than whole turmeric, but in large doses it acts as a gastric mucosa irritant, whereas the whole root extract has a gastroprotective effect.* The standardized saw palmetto (serenoa) is believed to be much more effective than crude extracts of the berry, but again no comparative studies have been done. The dried berries and tincture, in addition to reducing symptoms of benign prostatic hypertrophy, have beneficial effects on the immune system, lungs, and gastrointestinal tract that are lost in the standardized saw palmetto.

The other type of standardization is based on a manufacturer's guarantee of the presence of a certain percentage of a marker compound. Rarely are these known active constituents, and although they may help to identify the herb, they are not indicators of therapeutic activity. An echinacea product standardized to caffeic acid or a St. John's wort product standardized to 0.3% hypericin is virtually meaningless because neither of these compounds represents the therapeutic activity or quality of the herb.

This is not to say that no quality standards are needed; they most certainly are. First, every herb product needs to be botanically identified to ensure that the correct herb is in the product. Adulteration of scullcap with germander has resulted in liver damage in several people. Recent substitution of Aristolochia

---

*There are no studies comparing the activity of one with the other, and many additional anti-inflammatory constituents of turmeric rhizome have been discovered since the curcuminoids were deemed "the active ingredients."

species for the Chinese herb stephania has caused kidney failure and renal cancers. In addition to accurate botanical identification, it is very important that the right part of the plant is used, that it is harvested at the right time and prepared properly, and that the appropriate pharmaceutical techniques are used to make the best medicines.

Herbalists have always standardized their herbal products. St. John's wort was gathered in bud or flower, and only the tops of the plants were picked. The tincture or oil of hypericum should turn a deep burgundy red and have a strong and distinctive aroma. How much hypericin is present per dose, I do not know; how much hyperforin per dose, I do not know. What I do know is that this preparation will be active and will work because the markers that herbalists have always looked for are present. Herbalists have standardized their medicines to quality, not numbers.

As the herbal marketplace continues to grow, simply using the old organoleptic quality standards probably is not practical. I would suggest that simply applying random levels of an easy-to-test-for phytochemical is not the answer either. A synthesis of traditional herbal knowledge and modern research will benefit the herbal manufacturer, the consumer, and the practitioner. The bridge between traditional herbalism and modern phytotherapy and the interface between academia and industry must be a person who has spent his or her lifetime gaining a hands-on practical knowledge of botanical medicine: the herbalist. The combined skills of the physician, the pharmacist, the herbalist, nurses, and other clinical staff provide patients with the best of both worlds—safe, effective, and appropriate herbal medicine, as part of our health care system.

BIBLIOGRAPHY

Anonymous. (March 1998). Alcohol improves bioavailability. *Mediherb Monitor.* 252.

Defective Drugs, adrugrecall.com, 2006, www.adrugrecall.com/vioxx/death.html. Accessed August 25, 2006.

Eldin S, Dunford A. (1999). *Herbal Medicine in Primary Care.* Oxford: Butterworth-Heinemann.

Hirata JD, et al. (1997). Does dong quai have estrogenic effects in postmenopausal women? A double-blind placebo-controlled trial. *Fertility and Sterility.* 68(6):981–986.

Holland BK. [Ed.]. (1996). *Prospecting for Drugs in Ancient and Medieval European Texts.* Amsterdam: Harwood Academic Publishers.

Kirchfield F, Boyle W. (1994). *Nature Doctors.* Portland, OR: Medicina Biologica.

Leung A. (2000). Scientific studies and reports in the herbal literature: What are we studying and reporting? *HerbalGram.* 48:63–664.

McCaleb R. (1999). Research reviews: Possible shortcomings of fertility study on herbs. *HerbalGram.* 46:22.

Ondrizek PR, et al. (1999). An alternative medicine study of herbal effects on the penetration of zona-free hamster oocytes and the integrity of sperm deoxyribonucleic acid. *Fertility and Sterility.* 71(3):517–522.

Winston D. (1992). Nvwoti, Cherokee medicine and ethnobotany. In Tierra M. [Ed.]. *American Herbalism.* Freedom, CA: The Crossing Press.

Winston D, Dattner A. (1999). The American system of medicine. *Clinics in Dermatology.* 17(1):53–556.

PART II

Herb Monographs

NAME: Aloe (*Aloe vera*)

Common Names: Cape, Zanzibar, Curacao, Barbados aloes; aloe vera; burn plant (*Aloe barbadenisis* is a synonym for *Aloe vera*)

Family: *Liliaceae*

Description of Plant
- There are more than 360 species in the Aloe genus.
- Perennial succulents native to Africa, now grown throughout the world
- Short plant has 15 to 30 tapering leaves about 20" long and 5" wide.
- Leaf has three layers: outer (tough), middle (corrugate lining), and inner (a colorless mucilaginous pulp, the aloe gel). The plant contains 99% water.
- Yields both aloe gel and aloe latex. Although they share certain chemical components, the gel and latex are distinct, with different properties and uses.
  - The gel is naturally occurring. Undiluted gel is obtained by stripping away the outer layer of the leaf. It is for topical use and is famous for its wound-healing properties. It provides moisture and soothes the skin and thus is widely used in cosmetics, moisturizing creams, and lotions.
  - Aloe vera concentrate is gel from which the water has been removed. For topical use.
  - Aloe vera juice contains a minimum of 50% aloe vera gel, usually mixed with fruit juice. For internal use.
  - Aloe vera latex is the bitter yellow liquid derived from the pericyclic tubules of the rind of aloe vera. The primary constituent is aloin. It is rarely used internally because of its powerful cathartic activity.

Medicinal Part
- Aloe gel
- Latex

Constituents and Action (if known)
Latex Constituents
- Anthraquinones have antiviral, antibacterial, antitumor activity (Boik, 1996).
- Anthraquinone barbaloin: when concentrated, produces aloin, local irritants to GI tract, and soothes the skin.
- Aloinosides A and B have a strong purgative effect (Muller et al., 1996).

Aloe Gel Constituents
- Polysaccharide glucomannan (similar to guar gum) is found in aloe gel. It has an emollient effect and hinders the formation of thromboxane, a chemical that delays wound healing (Hunter & Frunkin, 1991).
- Bradykininase, a protease inhibitor, relieves pain and reduces swelling (Vazquez et al., 1996; Visuthiokosol et al., 1995).
- Magnesium lactate blocks histamine and may contribute to antipruritic effect (Schmidt & Greenspoon, 1991).
- Tannins

Nutritional Ingredients: None known

Traditional Use
- Ancient Egypt (1500 BC) and Middle East: used to heal the skin and treat wounds, hemorrhoids, and hair loss
- In US, the latex has been used as a purgative since colonists brought it from Europe in their medicine chests.

Current Use
Topical (Gel)
- Helps to heal burns and reduce burn pain. Useful for first- and second-degree burns (sunburn, radiation burns, scalds). First report of clinical use for radiation burns was in 1935 in the *American Journal of Roentgenology*. There are several negative studies using bottled aloe gel for healing burns. Many of these products contain stabilizers and preservatives, and they may not have the same effect as fresh aloe gel from the leaf.
- May help to heal venous ulcers
- Anti-inflammatory activity by inhibiting arachidonic acid
- Soothes skin and may enhance skin healing

Oral
- Aloe gel soothes gastric ulcers (Eamiamnam et al., 2006).
- Cathartic (concrete resin)
- Two studies indicate that aloe gel reduces inflammation in the GI tract and can help ulcerative colitis (Langmead et al., 2004) and possibly diarrhea that is prominent in IBS (Davis et al., 2006).

Available Forms, Dosage, and Administration Guidelines

Preparations
- *Gel:* Sunscreens, skin creams, lotions, cosmetics
- *Juice:* Available in various concentrations and as powdered dry juice. Highly concentrated products degrade quickly; check for inclusion of gums, sugars, starches, and other additives.

Typical Dosage
- *Fresh gel (topical):* Cut a leaf lengthwise, scrape out the gel, and apply externally as needed. Discontinue if burning or irritation occurs.
- *Juice (internal):* Take 1 tbsp after meals, or follow manufacturer or practitioner recommendations.

Pharmacokinetics—If Available (form or route when known): None known

Toxicity: Internal use of latex can cause severe GI cramping.

Contraindications
- *Topical:* Deep, vertical wounds; hypersensitivity to aloe products
- *Internal:* Bowel obstruction, kidney, and liver disease

Side Effects
- *Topical:* Contact dermatitis is possible but uncommon.
- *Internal (latex):* May cause fluid and electrolyte imbalances, intestinal cramping

Long-Term Safety
- *Gel:* Safe
- *Latex:* Not safe for daily long-term dosing because it is irritating to the bowel. When used for more than 1 to 2 weeks, it may cause intestinal sluggishness and laxative dependence.

Use in Pregnancy/Lactation/Children
- *Oral:* Latex contraindicated in all because of severe GI symptoms
- *Topical:* Safe in all

Drug/Herb Interactions and Rationale (if known)
- Gel, taken internally, may reduce absorption of some medications. Separate by at least 2 hours from most drugs.
- In a recent study, aloe gel taken concurrently with vitamins C and E significantly increased absorption of both nutrients (Vinson et al., 2005).
- Latex, because of its cathartic effect, causes loss of K^+ and therefore may increase the likelihood of toxicity with cardiac glycosides, antiarrhythmics, steroids, loop diuretics, and other K^+-wasting drugs. Avoid concurrent use of internal latex and these drugs.

Special Notes
- Juice is nontoxic and has been found to be ineffective for arthritis.
- Unapproved use of parenteral aloe vera for cancer has been associated with death.
- An extracted polysaccharide, acemannan, has shown immune-stimulating activity and has been approved by the USDA as an adjunctive treatment for canine and feline fibrosarcoma. This product has been used clinically and for self-treatment of cancer and HIV. As far as the authors know, no human trials have confirmed the effectiveness of this product for these conditions.
- Phytosterols isolated from aloe gel reduced hemoglobin $A1_C$ levels and fasting blood glucose levels in diabetic mice (Tanaka et al., 2006).

BIBLIOGRAPHY

Boik J. (1996). *Cancer & Natural Medicine.* Portland: Oregon Medical Press.

Davis K, et al. (2006). Randomised double-blind placebo-controlled trial of aloe vera for irritable bowel syndrome. *International Journal of Clinical Practice.* 60(9):1080–1086.

Davis RH, et al. (1989). Anti-inflammatory activity of aloe vera against a spectrum of irritants. *Journal of the American Podiatric Medicine Association.* 79(6):263–276.

Dykman KD, et al. (1998). The effects of nutritional supplements on the symptoms of fibromyalgia and chronic fatigue syndrome. *Integrative Physiological Behavioral Science.* 33(1):61–71.

Eamiamnam K, et al. (2006). Effects of aloe vera and sucraifate on gastric microcirculatory changes, cytokine levels and gastric ulcer healing in rats. *World Journal of Gastroenterology.* 12(13):2034–2039.

Hunter D, Frunkin A. (1991). Adverse reactions to vitamin E and aloe vera preparations after dermabrasion and chemical peel. *Cutis.* 47(3):193.

Langmead L, et al. (2004). Randomized, double-blind placebo-controlled trial of oral aloe vera gel for active ulcerative colitis. *Alimentary Pharmacology and Therapy.* 19(7):739–747.

Muller SO, et al. (1996). Genotoxicity of the laxative drug components emodin, aloe-emodin, and danthron in mammalian cells: Topoisomerase II-mediated. *Mutation Research.* 371:165–173.

Phillips T, et al. (1995). A randomized study of an aloe vera derivative gel dressing versus conventional treatment after shave biopsy excision. *Wounds.* 7(5):200–202.

Sato Y, et al. (1990). Studies on chemical protectors against radiation. XXXI. Protection effects of aloe arborescens on skin injury induced by X-irradiation. *Yakugaku Zasshi.* 110(11):876–884.

Schmidt JM, Greenspoon JS. (1991). Aloe vera dermal wound gel is associated with a delay in wound healing. *Obstetrics and Gynecology.* 78(1):115.

Syed TA, et al. (1996). Management of psoriasis with aloe vera extract in a hydrophilic cream: A placebo-controlled, double-blind study. *Tropical Medicine and International Health.* 1(4):505–509.

Tanaka M, et al. (2006). Identification of five phytosterols from aloe vera gel as anti-diabetic compounds. *Biological and Pharmaceutical Bulletin.* (7):1418–1422.

Vazquez B, et al. (1996). Antiinflammatory activity of extracts from aloe vera gel. *Journal of Ethnopharmacology.* 55(1):69–75.

Vinson JA, et al. (2005). Effect of aloe vera preparations on the human bioavailability of Vitamins C and E. *Phytomedicine.* 12(10):760–765.

Visuthiokosol V, et al. (1995). Effect of aloe vera gel to healing of burn wound: A clinical and histologic study. *Journal of the Medical Association of Thailand.* 78(8):403–409.

NAME: American Ginseng (*Panax quinquefolius*)

Common Names: Sang, man root

Family: *Araliaceae*

Description of Plant

- American ginseng grows from Canada to Georgia. It is considered an endangered species, so much of the ginseng crop is cultivated.
- It is a slow-growing perennial that takes 5 to 7 years to produce a marketable root.
- The herb is a small perennial with a single stem, which has three to six long petioled compound leaves at the top.

Medicinal Part: The mature root is used and is gathered in the autumn (September), when the red berries are ripe. The berries should be replanted.

Constituents and Action (if known)

- Triterpene saponins (4.3%–4.9%) protect LDL cholesterol from oxidation (Li et al., 1999).
  - Ginsenoside Rg1 stimulates vascular endothelial growth factor (Leung et al., 2006), inhibits amyloid beta peptide (Chen et al., 2006).
  - Ginsenoside Rb1 has a stimulant action on protein and RNA synthesis in animal serum and liver. It has hypotensive, anticonvulsant, analgesic, antiulcer (induced by stress), and nerve regeneration–inducing activity.
  - Ginsenoside Re inhibits amyloid beta peptide (Chen et al., 2006).
- Triterpene oligoglycosides: quinquenosides I, II, III, IV, V; quinqueginsin has anti-HIV, antifungal activity (Wang & Ng, 2000).
- American ginseng extract has antioxidant activity (Kitts et al., 2000).

Nutritional Ingredients: Used as a flavoring and tonic in beverages

Traditional Use

- Adaptogen, mild stimulant, bitter tonic
- Native Americans have used ginseng as a bitter tonic and for nervous afflictions (Cherokee), for short-windedness (Creek), as a general tonic and panacea (Delaware, Mohegan), for upset stomach and vomiting (Iroquois), and for strengthening the mind (Menominee).
- Among early Americans, a debate raged over this plant's effects. Some authorities claimed that it had great powers; others believed that it had no activity.
- Eclectic physicians used *Panax* for neurasthenia, digestive torpor, fatigue, loss of appetite, and nervous dyspepsia.
- American ginseng has been exported to China since 1716, after its "discovery" by a Jesuit priest in Canada. In TCM, American ginseng (xi yang shen) is considered much milder and less stimulating than Asian ginseng and is used to nourish the *yin* and fluids. It is used for dry coughs, hemoptysis, exhaustion after fevers, chronic thirst, and irritability (Bensky et al., 2004).

Current Use

- Mildly stimulating adaptogen appropriate for regular use by overworked, overstressed Americans (Winston & Maimes, 2007)
- A useful adjunctive therapy or tonic remedy for mild depression, postperformance immune depletion in athletes, CFS, fibromyalgia, stress-induced asthma, chronic stress, age-related memory loss (Cui & Chen, 1991), and menopausal cloudy thinking
- Concurrent with antineoplastic agents, ginseng synergistically inhibits MCF-7 breast cancer cell growth (Duda et al., 1999).
- American ginseng (3 g/day) reduced blood sugar in diabetic and nondiabetic patients (Vuksan et al., 2000).
- In two studies, taking American ginseng from 8 weeks to 4 months reduced the incidence of upper respiratory tract infections (McElhaney et al., 2004; Predy et al., 2005).
- A combination of American ginseng and gingko significantly reduced ADD symptoms in a study of 36 children aged 3 to 17 years (Lyon et al., 2001).

Available Forms, Dosage, and Administration Guidelines

- *Tea:* 1 tsp root to 12 oz water. Slowly decoct 15 to 20 minutes until liquid is reduced to 8 oz. Take 4 oz three times daily.
- *Tincture* (1:2 or 1:5, 35% alcohol): 40 to 60 gtt (2–3 mL) three times daily
- *Capsules:* Two capsules three times daily

Pharmacokinetics—If Available (form or route when known): Not known

Toxicity: None

Contraindications: None known

Side Effects: Large amounts may cause overstimulation. If insomnia, nervousness, or mild elevation of blood pressure occurs, discontinue use. Several texts caution against the use of this herb in hypertensive patients. The concern was hypothetical, and in a double-blinded control trial, American ginseng was found to have a neutral effect on the blood pressure of hypertensive patients (Stavro et al., 2005).

Long-Term Safety: Safe

Use in Pregnancy/Lactation/Children: No known contraindication. Use cautiously and in small amounts.

Drug/Herb Interactions and Rationale (if known): Some studies have suggested a possible interaction with blood-thinning medications (Yuan et al., 2004), but others show that American ginseng does not alter warfarin pharmacokinetics. Use cautiously together. In animal studies, American ginseng did not affect CYP450 isoforms—CYP2B1, CYP3A23, or CYP1AZ (Yu et al., 2005).

Special Notes: Avoid using wild-harvested plants. The best American ginseng products are made from 5- to 10-year-old, organically woods-grown roots.

BIBLIOGRAPHY

Bensky D, Clavey S, et al. (2004). *Chinese Herbal Medicine: Materia Medica* (pp. 820–822). 3rd ed. Seattle: Eastland Press.

Chen F, et al. (2006). Reductions in levels of Alzheimer's amyloid beta peptide after oral administration of ginsenosides. *FASEB Journal.* Jun;20(8):1269–1271.

Chen SE, et al. (1980). American ginseng III. Pharmacokinetics of ginsenosides in the rabbit. *European Journal of Drug Metabolism and Pharmacokinetics.* 5(3):161–168.

Chen SE, Staba EJ. (1980). American ginseng II. Analysis of ginsenosides and their sapogenins in biological fluids. *Journal of Natural Products.* 43(4):463–466.

Cui J, Chen KJ. (1991). American ginseng compound liquor on retarding-aging process. *Chung Hsi I Chieh Ho Tsa Chih.* 11(8): 457–460.

Duda RB, et al. (1999). American ginseng and breast cancer therapeutic agents synergistically inhibit MCF-7 breast cancer cell growth. *Journal of Surgical Oncology.* 72(4):230–239.

Hsu CC, et al. (2005). American ginseng supplementation attenuates creatine kinase level induced by submaximal exercise in human beings. *World Journal of Gastroenterology.* Sept 14;11(34): 5327–5331.

Kitts DD, et al. (2000). Antioxidant properties of a North American ginseng extract. *Molecular and Cellular Biochemistry.* 203(1–2): 1–10.

Leung KW, et al. (2006). Ginsenoside-Rg1 induces vascular endothelial growth factor expression through glucocorticoid receptor-related phosphatidylinositol 3-kinase/Akt and beta-catenin/TCF-dependent pathway in human endothelial cells. *Journal of Biological Chemistry.* Nov 24;281(47):36280–36288. Epub 2006 Sep 28.

Li J, et al. (1999). *Panax quinquefolius* saponins protect low-density lipoproteins from oxidation. *Life Science.* 64(1):43–62.

Lyon MR, et al. (2001). Effect of the herbal extract combination *Panax quinquefolium* and ginkgo biloba on attention-deficient hyperactivity disorder: A pilot study. *Journal of Psychiatry and Neuroscience.* May;26(3):221–228.

McElhaney JE, et al. (2004). A placebo-controlled trial of a proprietary extract of North American ginseng (CVT-E002) to prevent acute respiratory illness in institutionalized older adults. *Journal of the American Geriatric Society.* Jan;52(1):13–19.

Moerman D. (1998). *Native American Ethnobotany* (p. 376). Seattle: Timber Press.

Predy GN, et al. (2005). Efficacy of an extract of North American ginseng containing poly-furanosylpyranosyl-saccharides for preventing upper respiratory tract infections: A randomized controlled trial. *Canadian Medical Association Journal.* Oct 25;173(9):1043–1048.

Sloley BD, et al. (1999). American ginseng extract reduces scopolamine-induced amnesia in a spatial learning task. *Journal of Psychiatry and Neuroscience.* 24(5):442–452.

Stavro PM, et al. (2005). North American ginseng exerts a neutral effect on blood pressure in individuals with hypertension. *Hypertension.* Aug;46(2):406–411.

Stavro PM, et al. (2006). Long-term intake of North American ginseng has no effect on 24-hour blood pressure and renal function. *Hypertension.* Apr;47(4):791–796.

Vuksan V, et al. (2000). American ginseng (*Panax quinquefolius L.*) reduces postprandial glycemia in nondiabetic subjects and subjects with type 2 diabetes mellitus. *Archives of Internal Medicine.* 160(7):1009–1013.

Wang HX, Ng TB. (2000). Quinqueginsin, a novel protein with anti-human immunodeficiency virus, antifungal, ribonuclease and cell-free translation-inhibitory activities from American ginseng roots. *Biochemical and Biophysical Research Communications.* 269(1):203–208.

Winston D, Maimes S. (2007). *Adaptogens, Herbs for Strength, Stamina, and Stress Relief* (pp. 130–134). Rochester, VT: Inner Traditions.

Yoshikawa M, et al. (1998). Bioactive saponins and glycosides. XI. Structures of new dammarane-type triterpene oligoglycosides, quinquenosides I, II, III, IV, and V, from American ginseng, the roots of *Panax quinquefolius L. Chemical Pharmaceutical Bulletin (Tokyo).* 46(4):647–654.

Yu CT, et al. (2005). Lack of evidence for induction of CYP2B1, CYP3A23, and CYP1A2 gene expression by *Panax ginseng* and *Panax quinquefolius* extracts in adult rats and primary cultures of rat hepatocytes. *Drug Metabolism and Disposition.* Jan;33(21):19–22.

Yuan CS, et al. (1998). Modulation of American ginseng on brain stem GABA-ergic effects in rats. *Journal of Ethnopharmacology.* 62(3):215–222.

Yuan CS, et al. (2004). Brief communication: American ginseng reduces warfarin's effect in healthy patients: A randomized, controlled trial. *Annals of Internal Medicine.* Jul 6;141(1):23–27.

 NAME: Amla Fruit (*Emblica officinalis,* syn. *Phyllanthus emblica*)

Common Names: Amalaki, Emblic myrobalan, Indian gooseberry

Family: *Euphorbiaceae*

Description of Plant

- It is a small- or medium-sized tree that is widely cultivated throughout India, Myanmar, Malaya, and Sri Lanka.
- The yellow-green fruits also have a slightly reddish tinge when fully ripe.

Medicinal Part: The dried, ripe fruit

Constituents and Action (if known)

- Tannins
  - Gallic acid (methyl gallate): antioxidant, nitric oxide radical scavenging activity (Kumaran & Karunakaran, 2006)
  - Corilagin: antioxidant, nitric oxide radical scavenging activity (Kumaran & Karunakaran, 2006)
  - Furosin: antioxidant, nitric oxide radical scavenging activity (Kumaran & Karunakaran, 2006)
  - Geraniin: antioxidant, nitric oxide radical scavenging activity (Kumaran, & Karunakaran, 2006)
  - Phyllemblin: antioxidant, antibacterial, spasmolytic, adrenergic (Williamson, 2002)
- Ascorbic acid (0.4% w/w): antioxidant, nitric oxide radical scavenging activity (Scartezzini et al., 2006)

Other Actions: Hepatoprotective (Tasduq, Mondhe et al., 2005), antitussive (Nosal'ova et al., 2003), hypolipidemic agent (Mathur et al., 1996), gastroprotective (Al-Rehaily et al., 2002), radioprotective (Singh et al., 2005)

Nutritional Ingredients: Amla is used in India as a major ingredient in a nutritive and tonic paste or jam known as chyavanprash.

Traditional Use

- Anti-inflammatory, antioxidant, antitussive, aperient, astringent, diuretic, hepatoprotective, laxative, nutritive tonic, and digestive aid
- Amla has been used in Ayurvedic medicine since ancient times. It is mentioned in the earliest medicine texts, the *Charaka Samhita* and the *Sushruta Samhita*.
- It is used in Ayurvedic medicine for diarrhea, dysentery, diabetes, epistaxis, jaundice, asthma, coughs, digestive upset,

as a rejuvenating tonic, to enhance healing of fractures, and for urinary difficulties.

Current Use

- It stabilizes connective tissue and helps to prevent inflammatory damage in degenerative diseases such as rheumatoid arthritis, osteoarthritis, scleroderma, atherosclerosis, and IBS (Winston & Maimes, 2007).
- It reduces capillary fragility and is of benefit for bleeding gums, macular degeneration, allergic purpurea, and spider veins. Use it with Blueberry and Hawthorn (Winston, 2006).
- Animal studies (Mathur et al., 1996) give credence to current use of amla to reduce LDL and VLDL cholesterol levels. These studies also showed that the herb reduced existing atherosclerotic plaques. A small human study has also found that daily consumption of the raw fruits lowered total cholesterol levels (Williamson, 2002).
- Amla's strong antioxidant and anti-inflammatory effects make it useful for stabilizing mast cells, reducing histamine response and inflammation of the respiratory tract. It is useful to reduce oxidative triggers for allergic rhinitis, allergic asthma, and reactive airway disease. It also helps to stop coughing; it was less effective than codeine but more effective than dropropizine (Nosal'ova et al., 2003).
- Several animal studies also indicate that this herb can protect the liver (Tasduq, Mondhe et al., 2005; Tasduq, Kaisar et al., 2005) from damage caused by environmental toxins and medications; it also was beneficial for acute pancreatitis in dogs (Thorat, 1995).
- Herbalists use it along with ashwagandha and processed rehmannia to increase red blood cell counts (Winston, 2006).
- A combination of amla fruit, haritaki (*Terminalia chebula*), and vibhitaki (*Terminalia belerica*) is used in Ayurvedic medicine for atonic constipation and to lower cholesterol and triglyceride levels (Singh et al., 1998). This formula, known as Triphila, can be mixed with equal parts gum guggal to enhance weight loss or with shilajatu to treat diabetes and insulin resistance (Tillotson, 2001).

Available Forms, Dosage, and Administration Guidelines

Preparations: Dried fruit, tea, tablet, tincture, paste

Typical Dosage

- *Powdered dried fruit:* 3 to 6 g
- *Tea:* 1 to 2 tsp dried fruit in 8 oz water, decoct 15 to 20 minutes, steep 30 minutes. Take two to three cups a day.
- *Tablets:* Take 2 tablets three times a day.
- *Tincture* (1:5, 30% alcohol): 60 to 100 gtt (3–5 mL) three times a day
- *Paste (Chyavanprash):* 1/2 to 1 tsp two to three times a day

Pharmacokinetics—If Available (form or route when known): Not known

Toxicity: None known

Contraindications: None known

Side Effects: None known

Long-Term Safety: Its long history of use as a food and medicine suggests a lack of toxicity.

Use In Pregnancy/Lactation/Children: Its frequent use in India for both pregnant women and children suggests that it is safe for use.

Drug/Herb Interactions and Rationale (if known):
Tannins can inhibit absorption of minerals (especially iron) and alkaloidal medications. In animal studies, amla protected mice against the toxic effects of arsenic (Tillotson, 2001) and cadmium (Khandelwal et al., 2002). In vitro studies found that amla protected rat hepatocytes from damage caused by antituberculosis medications (Tasduq, Kaisar et al., 2005).

Special Notes: The regular use of amla is believed to enhance the growth and repair of the hair, nails, bones, and teeth. An Indian method of processing the fruit (cooking it in its own juice) increased the vitamin C content from 0.4% to 1.28% (Scartezzini et al., 2006).

BIBLIOGRAPHY

Al-Rehaily AJ, et al. (2002). Gastroprotective effects of "Amla" *Emblica officinalis* on in vivo test models in rats. *Phytomedicine.* Sep;9(6):515–522.

Dharmananda S. (2003). *Emblic myrobalans*: Amla. Retrieved September 15, 2006, from www.itmonline.org/arts/amla.htm.

Khandelwal S, et al. (2002). Modulation of acute cadmium toxicity by *Emblica officinalis* fruit in rats. *Indian Journal of Experimental Biology.* May;40(5):564–570.

Krishnamurthy KH. (circa 1990). *Amalaka and Bhumi Amalaka.* Delhi: Books For All.

Kumaran A, Karunakaran RH. (2006). Nitric oxide radical scavenging active components from *Phyllanthus emblica L. Plant Foods for Human Nutrition.* Mar;61(1):1–5.

Mathur R, et al. (1996). Hypolipidaemic effect of fruit juice of *Emblica officinalis* in cholesterol-fed rabbits. *Journal of Ethnopharmacology.* Feb;50(2):61–68.

Nosal'ova G, et al. (2003). Antitussive activity of the fruit extract of *Emblica officinalis Gaertn.* (Euphorbiaceae). *Phytomedicine.* 10(6–7):583–589.

Scartezzini P, et al. (2006). Vitamin C content and antioxidant activity of the fruit and of the Ayurvedic preparation of *Emblica officinalis Gaertn. Journal of Ethnopharmacology.* Mar 8;104(1–2):113–118.

Singh I, et al. (2005). Radioprotection of Swiss albino mice by *Emblica officinalis*. *Phytotherapy Research.* May;19(5):444–446.

Singh RB, et al. (1998). Hypoglycemic and antioxidant effects of fenugreek seeds and triphila as adjuncts to dietary therapy in patients with mild to moderate hypercholesterolemia. *Perfusion.* 11:124–130.

Tasduq SA, Mondhe DM, et al. (2005). Reversal of fibrogenic events in liver by *Emblica officinalis* (fruit), an Indian natural drug. *Biological and Pharmaceutical Bulletin.* Jul;28(7):1304–1306.

Tasduq SA, Kaisar P, et al. (2005). Protective effect of a 50% hydroalcoholic fruit extract of *Emblica officinalis* against anti-tuberculosis drugs induced liver toxicity. *Phytotherapy Research.* Mar;19(3):193–197.

Thorat SP, et al. (1995). *Emblica officinalis:* a novel therapy for acute pancreatitis-an experimental study. *HPB Surgery.* 9(1): 25–30.

Tillotson A. (2001). *One Earth Herbal Sourcebook* (pp. 97–99). New York: Twin Streams/Kensington.

Williamson E. (2002). *Major Herbs of Ayurveda* (pp. 210–214). Edinburgh: Churchill Livingstone.

Winston D. (2006). *Winston's Botanic Materia Medica.* Washington, NJ: DWCHS.

Winston D, Maimes S. (2007). *Adaptogens, Herbs for Strength, Stamina, and Stress Relief* (pp. 134–138). Rochester, VT: Inner Traditions.

NAME: Andrographis (*Andrographis paniculata*)

Common Names: Chiretta, kalmegh (Hindi), chuan xin lian (Chinese)

Family: *Acanthaceae*

Description of Plant: Common annual plant native to India and cultivated in China

Medicinal Part: Herb

Constituents and Action (if known)

- Diterpenoid lactones (andrographolides): greater hepatoprotective activity than silymarin (Bone, 1996); andrographolide (antipyretic, antileukemic, anticancer, immunostimulatory); neoandrographolide (immunostimulatory); and dehydroandrographolide (immunostimulatory) (Kumar et al., 2004). The whole herb extract was shown to have greater activity than andrographolide alone (You-ping Zhu, 1998) and to inhibit PAF-induced platelet aggregation (Amroyan et al., 1999).
- Flavones (oroxylin, wogonin)
- Andrographis extract mildly inhibits *Staphylococcus aureus, Pseudomonas aeruginosa, Proteus vulgaris, Shigella dysenteriae, Escherichia coli*. It also inhibits ROS, lipid peroxidation, and other oxidative compounds as well as significantly reducing inflammation (Sheeja et al., 2006).

Nutritional Ingredients: None

Traditional Use

- Anti-inflammatory, antipyretic, antifertility activity, anthelmintic, immune stimulant, bitter tonic, cholagogue, antimalarial, hepatoprotective
- Used in Ayurvedic medicine to treat diarrhea, dysentery, dyspepsia, impaired bile secretion, hepatitis, malaria, pyelonephritis, pneumonia, and tonsillitis (Kapoor, 1990).

Current Use

- Prophylaxis and treatment of colds, sinusitis, influenza, and pharyngotonsillitis, with reduction of many symptoms, including headache, fatigue, earache, sore throat, nasal and bronchial catarrh, and cough (Caceres

et al., 1999; Gabrielian et al, 2002; Kulichenko et al., 2003; Spasov et al., 2004)
- As prophylaxis, patients treated with andrographis for 3 months caught colds 2.1 times less than the placebo group (Melchior et al., 1997; Mills & Bone, 1999).
- Several Chinese studies have shown that andrographis is useful for acute bacterial dysentery and enteritis (You-ping Zhu, 1998).
- Clinical trials show that this herb is useful for leptospirosis.

Available Forms, Dosage, and Administration Guidelines
- *Dried herb:* 1.5 to 5 g/day
- *Tea:* 1/2 to 1 tsp dried herb in 8 oz hot water, steep 30 minutes, take 4 oz three times daily
- *Tincture* (1:5, 30% alcohol): 20 to 60 gtt (1–3 mL) three times daily
- *Standardized tablets:* 100-mg tablets containing 5 mg andrographolide and deoxyandrographolide, four tablets three times daily
- Kan Jang (SHA-10) is a proprietary extract derived from *Andrographis paniculata* and *Eleutherococcus senticosis*, one 350 mg tablet twice a day.

Pharmacokinetics—If Available (form or route when known): Rapidly absorbed and distributed to the gallbladder, kidney, ovary, and lung. Ninety percent is excreted in the urine and feces in 24 hours and 94% after 48 hours (Tang & Eisenbrand, 1992).

Toxicity: Low potential for toxicity

Contraindications: Pregnancy

Side Effects: Nausea, vomiting; rarely urticaria

Long-Term Safety: No serious adverse effects expected; long-term human use and animal studies have found no safety issues. There have been several reports that andrographis can decrease animal fertility. In a human trial, men taking three times the normal dose of an *andrographis/Eleutherococcus senticosis* formula (SHA-10) had no reduction in sperm count, quality, or motility. In fact, there was a positive trend in all sperm parameters (Mkrtchvan et al., 2005).

Use in Pregnancy/Lactation/Children: Possible antifertility effect; avoid use during pregnancy. Several controlled trials have used andrographis with children (4–11 years old) with colds with no adverse effects (Spasov et al., 2004).

Drug/Herb Interactions and Rationale (if known): Mice given andrographis were protected against cyclosphosphamide-induced urothelial toxicity (Sheeja, Kuttan et al., 2006).

Special Notes: Capsule or pill form will achieve the highest patient compliance because the herb is intensely bitter. The well-studied proprietary product Kan Jang is made by the Swedish Herbal Institute.

BIBLIOGRAPHY

Amroyan E, et al. (1999). Inhibitory effect of andrographolide from *Andrographis paniculata* on PAF-induced platelet aggregation. *Phytomedicine.* 6(1):27–32.

Bone K. (1996). *Clinical Applications of Ayurvedic and Chinese Herbs* (pp. 96–100). Queensland, Australia: Phytotherapy Press.

Caceres DD, et al. (1999). Use of visual analogue scale measurements (VAS) to assess the effectiveness of standardized *Andrographis paniculata* extract SHA-10 in reducing the symptoms of common cold. A randomized double-blind placebo study. *Phytomedicine.* 6(4):217–223.

Gabrielian ES, et al. (2002). A double-blind, placebo-controlled study of *Andrographis paniculata* fixed combination Kan Jang in the treatment of acute upper respiratory tract infections including sinusitis. *Phytomedicine.* Oct;9(7):489–497.

Hoyhannisyan AS, et al. (2006). The effect of Kan Jang extract on the pharmacokinetics and pharmacodynamics of warfarin in rats. *Phytomedicine.* May;13(5):318–323.

Jarukamjorn K, et al. (2006). Impact of *Andrographis paniculata* crude extract on mouse hepatic cytochrome P450 enzymes. *Journal of Ethnopharmacology.* 2006 May 24;105(3):464–467.

Kapoor LD. (1990). *CRC Handbook of Ayurvedic Medicinal Plants* (p. 39). Boca Raton, FL: CRC Press.

Kulichenko LL, et al. (2003). A randomized controlled study of Kan Jang versus amantadine in the treatment of influenza in Volgograd. *Journal of Herbal Pharmacotherapy.* 2003;3(1):77–93.

Kumar RA, et al. (2004). Anticancer and immunostimulatory compounds from *Andrographis paniculata*. *Journal of Ethnopharmacology.* Jun;92(2–3):291–295.

Madau SS, et al. (1996). Anti-inflammatory activity of andrographolide. *Fitoterapia.* 67(5):452–458.

Melchior J, et al. (1997). Controlled clinical study of standardized *Andrographis paniculata* extract in common cold: A pilot trial. *Phytomedicine*. 3(4):315–318.

Mills S, Bone K. (2000). *Principles and Practice of Phytotherapy* (pp. 262–268). Edinburgh: Churchill Livingstone.

Mkrtchvan A, et al. (2005). A phase I study of *Andrographis paniculata* fixed combination Kan Jang versus ginseng and valerian on the semen quality of healthy male subjects. *Phytomedicine*. Jun;12(6–7):403–409.

Puri A, et al. (1993). Immunostimulant agents from *Andrographis paniculata*. *Journal of Natural Products*. 56:995–999.

Sheeja K, Kuttan G. (2006). Protective effect of *Andrographis paniculata* and andrographolide on cyclophosphamide-induced urothelial toxicity. *Integrative Cancer Therapies*. Sep;5(3):244–251.

Sheeja K, et al. (2006). Antioxidant and anti-inflammatory activities of the plant *Andrographis paniculata Nees*. *Immunopharmacology and Immunotoxicology*. 28(1):129–140.

Spasov AA, et al. (2004). Comparative controlled study of *Andrographis paniculata* fixed combination, Kan Jang and an Echinacea preparation as adjuvant, in the treatment of uncomplicated respiratory disease in children. *Phytotherapy Research*. Jan;18(1):47–53.

Tang W, Eisenbrand G. (1992). *Chinese Drugs of Plant Origin* (pp. 97–103). Berlin: Springer-Verlag.

Williamson, E. (2002). *Major Herbs of Ayurveda* (pp. 40–44). Edinburgh: Elsevier.

You-ping Zhu. (1998). *Chinese Materia Medica—Chemistry, Pharmacology, and Applications* (pp. 189–191). Amsterdam: Harwood Academic Publishers.

 NAME: Angelica (*Angelica archangelica*)

Common Names: Garden angelica

Family: *Apiaceae*

Description of Plant: Commonly cultivated, aromatic biennial plant in the parsley family; numerous species occur in Europe, North America, Asia

Medicinal Part: Root, rhizome

Constituents and Action (if known)

- Angelica root oil (alpha angelica lactone) augments Ca^{++} binding in cardiac microsomes (in canines), which may increase contractility; antibacterial activity against *Mycobacterium avium*; antifungal activity against 14 types of fungi (Blumenthal et al., 2000)

- Coumarin
  - Osthol: anti-inflammatory and analgesic properties (Chen et al., 1995)
  - Umbelliferone
- Furanocoumarins (angelicin, bergapten)—photosensitizing (Wichtl & Bisset, 1994)
- Volatile oil
  - Monoterpenes: beta-phellandrene (13%–28%), alpha-pinene (14%–31%), alpha-phellandrene (2%–14%)—cytotoxic (Sigurdsson et al., 2005)
  - Sesquiterpenes: beta-bisabolene, bisabolol, beta-caryophyllene
- Resins (6%)

Nutritional Ingredients: The young leaves have been used as a cooked vegetable; the stems can be candied. Angelica root is used as an ingredient in cordials such as Benedictine.

Traditional Use

- Antibacterial, anti-inflammatory, antioxidant, antispasmodic, antiulcerogenic, bitter and digestive tonic, carminative, cholagogue, diaphoretic, diuretic, emmenagogue, hepatoprotective, sedative
- According to legend, angelica was revealed to humans by an angel as a cure for the plague, hence its name.
- A popular European herbal medicine. It has been used for dyspepsia, nausea, borborygmus, flatulence, menstrual cramps, colds, fevers, coughs, headaches, and nervous stomach.

Current Use

- GI complaints: feeling of fullness, mild intestinal spasms, flatulence, achlorhydria, nausea (Wichtl & Bisset, 1994)
- It stimulates gastric HCL and pancreatic juices, enhancing digestion and absorption. Used with orange peel, dandelion root, and artichoke leaf, it makes a superb digestive bitter (Winston, 2006).
- In India, it is used to treat anorexia nervosa and dyspepsia (Karnick, 1994).

- In animal studies, angelica was hepatoprotective against alcohol-induced liver damage (Yeh et al., 2003) and had antiulcerogenic activity (Khayval et al., 2001).

Available Forms, Dosage, and Administration Guidelines

- *Dried root and rhizome:* 1 to 2 g, three times daily
- *Infusion:* Steep 1 tsp of the fine-cut root in 8 oz boiled water for approximately 10 to 20 minutes. Take 4 oz a half-hour before meals.
- *Tincture* (1:5, 45% alcohol): 20 to 40 gtt (1–2 mL) three times daily
- *EO (Oleum angelicae):* 5 to 10 drops in a carrier oil for topical application in neuralgic and rheumatic complaints (see Side Effects)

Pharmacokinetics—If Available (form or route when known): None known

Toxicity: Generally recognized as safe

Contraindications: None known

Side Effects: Possible photosensitivity with topical application. Avoid excess sun or ultraviolet radiation exposure.

Long-Term Safety: Probably safe; long history as a medicine, tea, and in liqueurs

Use in Pregnancy/Lactation/Children: Not recommended in pregnancy. Small doses have been and are regularly used in Europe by children and breast-feeding women.

Drug/Herb Interactions and Rationale (if known): None known

Special Notes: The cut, sifted root—if properly stored in a cool, dry environment in an airtight container—has a shelf life of 12 to 18 months. The powdered root has a shelf life of 24 hours (Blumenthal et al., 2000).

BIBLIOGRAPHY

Blumenthal M, et al. (2000). *Herbal Medicine: Expanded Commission E Monographs* (pp. 3–6). Austin, TX: American Botanical Council.

Chen YF, et al. (1995). Anti-inflammatory and analgesic activities from roots of *Angelica pubescens*. *Planta Medica*. 61(1):2.

Hoffmann D. (2003). *Medical Herbalism, the Science and Practice of Herbal Medicine* (pp. 527–528). Rochester, VT: Healing Arts Press.

Karnick CR. (1994). *Pharmacopeial Standards of Herbal Plants* (pp. 11–23). Dehli: Sri Satguru Publishers.

Khayval MT, et al. (2001). Antiulcerogenic effect of some gastrointestinally acting plant extracts and their combination. *Arzneimittelforschung*. 51(7):545–553.

Sigurdsson S, et al. (2005). The cytotoxic effect of two chemotypes of essential oils from the fruits of *Angelica archangelica L. Anticancer Research*. May-Jun;25(3B):1877–1880.

Wichtl M, Bisset NG. (1994). *Herbal Drugs and Phytopharmaceuticals*. Boca Raton, FL: CRC Press.

Winston, D. (2006). *Winston's Botanic Materia Medica*. Washington, NJ: DWCHS.

Yeh ML, et al. (2003). Hepatoprotective effect of *Angelica archangelica* in chronically ethanol treated mice. *Pharmacology*. Jun;68(2):70–73.

 NAME: Arnica (*Arnica montana, A. chamissonis*)

Common Names: Leopard's bane, wolf's bane, mountain tobacco, Mexican arnica, mountain snuff, mountain arnica

Family: *Asteraceae*

Description of Plant
- Perennial; grows 1' to 2' and has bright yellow, daisy-like, aromatic flower.
- It is native to mountain regions of Europe to southern Russia.
- A new world species, *Arnica cordifolia*, grows in the Pacific Northwest up to Alaska.

Medicinal Part: Dried flower heads, rhizome

Constituents and Action (if known)
- Flavonoid glycosides (betuletol, eupafolin, flavonol glucuronides, hispidulin, luteolin, quercetin): improves circulation, reduces cholesterol, stimulates CNS (Chevallier, 1996; Wichtl & Bisset, 1994)
- Terpenoids (arnifolin, arnicolides)

- Sesquiterpene lactones (helenalin, dihydrohelenalin)
  ○ Anti-inflammatory and mild analgesic (Klaas et al., 2002)
  ○ Antibacterial effect (Schaffner, 1997)
  ○ Antifungal activity (Wichtl & Bisset, 1994)
  ○ May inhibit platelet activity (Baillargeon et al., 1993)
  ○ Oxytocic activity (Wichtl & Bisset, 1994)
  ○ Displays cytotoxic activity (Willuhn et al., 1994)
- Coumarins (scopoletin, umbelliferone)
- Volatile oils (thymol)
- Arnicin, a bitter compound

Nutritional Ingredients: None known

Traditional Use
- *External (creams, ointments, tinctures):* For sprains, bruises, and wound healing; anti-inflammatory; mild pain reliever; swelling due to insect bites, hemorrhoids, and venous insufficiency (Mills & Bone, 2000)
- *Internal:* For bruises and trauma injuries, dilute tea for senile heart, arteriosclerosis, angina (Weiss, 1985)

Current Use
- *External:* First aid cream used as an anti-inflammatory; mild analgesic and vulnerary for arthritis (Kneusel & Weber, 2002); swelling related to fractures; trauma injuries, especially bruises, sprains, and muscle tear (Winston, 2006)
- *Internal:* Homeopathic remedy for trauma, bruises, contusions, sprains, and strains. There are numerous clinical trials of homeopathic arnica, with mixed results. Some studies (Oberbaum et al., 2005; Seeley et al., 2006; Wolf et al., 2003) suggest benefit for reducing postoperative swelling, bleeding, and bruising, while other studies find no benefit over placebo (Ernst, 1998; Ramelet et al., 2000; Stevinson et al., 2003).

Available Forms, Dosage, and Administration Guidelines
Preparations: Dried flowers, whole or cut and sifted; creams (typically contain 15% arnica oil; salves should contain 20%–25% arnica oil); gels, ointments; tinctures; homeopathic products

Typical Dosage
* *Topical:* Apply externally, following manufacturer's instructions. Use commercial preparations rather than homemade ones because of arnica's potential toxicity.
* *Tincture* (1:10, 70% alcohol): Use internally only under the guidance of a trained practitioner; 1 to 2 gtt twice daily.

Pharmacokinetics—If Available (form or route when known): Sesquiterpene lactones are absorbed dermally after 12 hours (Tekko et al., 2006).

Toxicity: Internal use irritates mucous membranes and can cause stomach pain, diarrhea, vomiting, dyspnea, and hepatic failure. One-gram doses can damage heart and in rare cases may lead to cardiac arrest.

Contraindications: Do not use on damaged, abraded, or cracked skin.

Side Effects
* *Topical:* Contact dermatitis can occur in sensitive patients. A small skin test before general use may be helpful.
* *Internal:* GI irritation and kidney pain can occur at the normal therapeutic dosage of the tea or tincture in sensitive patients.

Long-Term Safety: Unknown

Use in Pregnancy/Lactation/Children
* Avoid during pregnancy; there is a risk of oxytocic activity and a lack of knowledge about teratogenic potential.
* Avoid during lactation or in children. No research available.
* Homeopathic preparations are safe during pregnancy and lactation and for children.

Drug/Herb Interactions and Rationale (if known): Possible reduced effectiveness of antihypertensive medications. Do not take concurrently.

Special Notes
* Best to use on a short-term basis for acute conditions.
* Avoid prolonged external use, because this increases the likelihood of contact dermatitis.

- FDA has classed arnica as an unsafe herb for internal use.
- Mexican arnica (*Heterotheca inuloides*) is a common but ineffective adulterant substituted for real arnica in some products (Mills & Bone, 2000).

BIBLIOGRAPHY

Baillargeon L, et al. (1993). The effects of *Arnica montana* on blood coagulation: A randomized, controlled trial. *Canadian Family Physician.* 39:236–267.

Brinker F. (2001). *Herb Contraindications* and *Drug Interactions* (pp. 31–32). Sandy, OR: Electic Medical Publications.

Chevallier A. (1996). *Encyclopedia of Medicinal Plants* (pp. 196–197). New York: DK Publishing.

Der Marderosian A & Beutler, J. [Eds.]. (2005). *The Review of Natural Products—Arnica Monograph.* St. Louis, MO: Facts and Comparisons.

Ernst E. (1998). Efficacy of homeopathic arnica: A systematic review of placebo-controlled clinical trials. *Archives of Surgery.* 133(11): 1187–1190.

Hart O, et al. (1997). Double-blind, placebo-controlled, randomized clinical trial of homeopathic arnica C30 for pain and infection after total abdominal hysterectomy. *Journal of the Royal Society of Medicine.* 90:73–78.

Kaziro GS. (1984). Metronidazole and *Arnica montana* in the prevention of post-surgical complications: A comparative placebo-controlled trial. *British Journal of Oral and Maxillofacial Surgery.* 22:42.

Klaas CA, et al. (2002). Studies on the anti-inflammatory activity of phytopharmaceuticals prepared from arnica flowers. *Planta Medica.* May;68(5):385–391.

Knuesel O, Weber M. (2002). *Arnica montana* gel in osteoarthritis of the knee: An open, multicenter clinical trial. *Advances in Therapy.* 19(5):209–218.

McGuffin M, et al. (1997). *American Herbal Product Association's Botanical Safety Handbook* (pp. 14–15). Boca Raton, FL: CRC Press.

Mills S, Bone K. (2000). *Principles and Practice of Phytotherapy* (pp. 269–272). Edinburgh: Churchill Livingstone.

Oberbaum M, et al. (2005). The effectiveness of the homeopathic remedies *Arnica montana* and *Bellis perennis* on mild postpartum bleeding—A randomized, double-blind, placebo-controlled study—preliminary results. Jun;12(2):87–90.

Ramelet AA, et al. (2000). Homeopathic arnica in postoperative haematomas: A double-blind study. *Dermatology.* 201(4):347–348.

Schaffner W. (1997). Granny's remedy explained at the molecular level: Helenalin inhibits NF-kappa B. *Biological Chemistry.* 378:935.

Seeley BM, et al. (2006). Effect of homeopathic *Arnica montana* on bruising in face-lifts: Results of a randomized, double-blind, placebo-controlled clinical trial. *Archives of Facial Plastic Surgery*. Jan-Feb;8(1):54–59.

Stevinson C, et al. (2003). Homeopathic arnica for prevention of pain and bruising: Randomized placebo-controlled trial in hand surgery. *Journal of the Royal Society of Medicine*. Feb;96(2):60–65.

Tekko IA, et al. (2006). Permeation of bioactive constituents from *Arnica montana* preparations through human skin in-vitro. Sep;58(9):1167–1176.

Weiss R. (1985). *Herbal Medicine* (pp. 169–170, 269–270). Gothenburg, Sweden: Ab Arcanum.

Wichtl M, Bisset N. (1994). *Herbal Drugs and Phytopharmaceuticals* (pp. 83–87). Stuttgart: CRC Press.

Willuhn G, et al. (1994). Cytotoxicity of flavonoids and sesquiterpenelactones from Arnica species against GLC4 and the COLO 320 cell lines. *Planta Medica*. 60:434–437.

Winston D. (2006). *Winston's Botanic Materia Medica*. Washington, NJ: DWCHS.

Wolf M, et al. (2003). Efficacy of arnica in varicose vein surgery: Results of a randomized, double-blind placebo-controlled pilot study. *Forsch Komplementarmed Klass Naturheilkd*. Oct;10(5):242–247.

 NAME: Artichoke (*Cynara scolymus*)

Common Names: Globe artichoke

Family: *Asteraceae*

Description of Plant

- Warm-climate perennial native to Mediterranean; 80% of the yearly crop grown in Italy, Spain, and France
- Grows about 150 cm tall
- Large, thistle-like leaves
- Large edible flower heads made up of leaf-like scales that enclose the bud

Medicinal Part: Fresh or dried leaf

Constituents and Action (if known)

- Caffeic acid derivatives (polyphenols)
  ○ Cynaroside, cynarin, cynarine are the bitter principles responsible for liver protective properties (Chevallier,

1996; Kraft, 1997). They increase bile flow (Kirchhoff et al., 1994) and assist with liver regeneration (rat livers) (Maros et al., 1968; Mills & Bone, 2000), antibacterial (Zhu et al., 2004).
   ○ 3,5 Dicaffeoylquinic acid and 4,5 dicaffeoylquinic acid have demonstrated anti-inflammatory activity in vivo (Mills & Bone, 2000), antibacterial (Zhu et al., 2004).
- Flavonoids (luteolin, apigenin, cosmoside, quercetin, rutin, hesperitin, hesperidoside) may reduce cholesterol by inhibiting cholesterol synthesis (Gebhardt, 2001; Leiss, 1998; Wegener & Fintelmann, 1999).
- Sesquiterpene lactones (cynaropicrin), antispasmodic (Emendorfer et al., 2005)
- Volatile oils (beta selinene, eugenol, deconal)

Other Actions: Antifungal (Zhu et al., 2005)

Traditional Use
- Antiemetic, bitter tonic, choleretic, diuretic, hepatoprotective
- Commonly used in Europe as a medicine since the Middle Ages. Primarily used as a digestion, liver, and urinary tract remedy and for treating dyspepsia, constipation, skin conditions, jaundice, hepatic insufficiency, urinary calculi, and nephrosclerosis.

Current Use
- Choleretic action useful to treat dyspepsia, loss of appetite, poor fat digestion, constipation, flatulence, nausea, and GERD (Holtmann et al., 2003)
- Reduces LDL cholesterol levels (Gebhardt, 2001; Saenz Rodriguez et al., 2002)
- Relieves alternating diarrhea/constipation symptoms due to IBS (Bundy et al., 2004)

Available Forms, Dosage, and Administration Guidelines
- *Leaf:* 2 g three times daily
- *Dry extract* (12:1): 0.5 g in a single daily dose
- *Fluid extract* (1:1): 2 mL three times daily
- *Tincture* (1:5, 30% alcohol): 60 to 100 gtt (3–5 mL) three times daily

Pharmacokinetics—If Available (form or route when known): Peak plasma concentrations of artichoke active constituents (caffeoylquinic acids and flavonoids) were reached in 1 hour and declined over 24 hours. Constituents dihydrocaffeic acid and dihydroferulic acids are needed for 6 to 7 hours to achieve maximum concentrations, indicating that two different metabolic pathways are used for breaking down these compounds (Wittemer et al., 2005).

Toxicity: None

Contraindications: Obstructions in biliary tract; use cautiously with gallstones

Side Effects: Handling the plant may cause allergic dermatitis in sensitive people.

Long-Term Safety: Long-term use as a food; no adverse effects expected

Use in Pregnancy/Lactation/Children: No restrictions known

Drug/Herb Interactions and Rationale (if known): None known

BIBLIOGRAPHY

Bundy R, et al. (2004). Artichoke leaf extract reduces symptoms of irritable bowel syndrome and improves quality of life in otherwise healthy volunteers suffering from concomitant dyspepsia: A subset analysis. *Journal of Alternative and Complementary Medicine.* Aug;10(4):667–669.

Chevallier A. (1996). *Encyclopedia of Medicinal Plants* (pp. 196–197). New York: DK Publishing.

Der Marderosian A, Beutler, J. [Eds.]. (2005). *The Review of Natural Products—Artichoke Monograph.* St. Louis, MO: Facts and Comparisons.

Emendorfer F, et al. (2005). Antispasmodic activity of fractions and cynaropicrin from *Cynara scolymus* on guinea-pig ileum. *Biological and Pharmaceutical Bulletin.* May;28(5):902–904.

Ensiminger A, et al. (1994). *Foods and Nutrition Encyclopedia* (2nd ed.). Boca Raton, FL: CRC Press.

Gebhardt R. (2001). Anticholestatic activity of flavonoids from artichoke (*Cynara scolymus L.*) and of their metabolites. *Medical Science Monitor.* May;7[Suppl 1]:316–320.

Holtmann G, et al. (2003). Efficacy of artichoke leaf extract in the treatment of patients with functional dyspepsia: A six-week placebo-controlled, double-blind, multicentre trial. *Alimentary Pharmacology and Therapeutics.* Dec;18(11–12):1099–1105.

Kirchhoff R, et al. (1994). Increase in choleresis by means of artichoke extract. *Phytomedicine.* 1:107–115.

Kraft K. (1997). Artichoke leaf extract: Recent findings reflecting effects on lipid metabolism, liver, and gastrointestinal tracts. *Phytomedicine.* 1:369–378.

Leiss O. (1998). Hypercholesterolemia during medication with artichoke extracts. *Deutsche Medizinische Wochenschrift.* 123(25–26):818–819.

Maros T, et al. (1968). Effects of *Cynara scolymus* extracts on the regenerations of rat liver. *Arzneimittelforschung.* 18(7):884–886.

Mills S, Bone K. (2000). *Principles and Practice of Phytotherapy* (pp. 433–438). Edinburgh: Churchill Livingstone.

Renewed proof: Inhibition of cholesterol biosynthesis by dried extract of artichoke leaves. (1999). *Fortschritte der Komplementarmedizin.* 6(3):168–169.

Saenz Rodriguez T, et al. (2002). Choleretic activity and biliary elimination of lipids and bile acids induced by an artichoke leaf extract in rats. *Phytomedicine.* Dec;9(8):687–693.

Wegener T, Fintelmann V. (1999). Pharmacological properties and therapeutic profile of artichoke. *Wien Medizinische Wochenschrift.* 149(8–10):241–247.

Wittemer SM, et al. (2005). Bioavailability and pharmacokinetics of caffeoylquinic acids and flavonoids after oral administration of artichoke leaf extracts in humans. *Phytomedicine.* Jan;12(1–2):28–38.

Zhu X, et al. (2004). Phenolic compounds from the leaf extract of artichoke (*Cynara scolymus L.*) and their antimicrobial activities. *Journal of Agriculture and Food Chemistry.* Dec 1;52(24):7272–7278.

Zhu XF, et al. (2005). Antifungal activity of *Cynara scolymus L.* extracts. *Fitoterapia.* Jan;76(1):108–111.

NAME: Ashwagandha (*Withania somnifera*)

Common Names: Winter cherry, Ashgand

Family: *Solanaceae*

Description of Plant: A native of India, this member of the nightshade family is a semihardy evergreen shrub. The small green-yellow flowers are followed by bright orange-red berries.

Medicinal Part: Root

Constituents and Action (if known)

- Alkaloids (0.4%): isopelietierine, withasamine, somniferin, anaferine; sedative, withasomnine. *Withania* alkaloids have antispasmodic activity in intestinal, bronchial, uterine, and arterial smooth muscle. The activity is similar in action to that of papaverine (Mills & Bone, 2000).
- Steroidal lactones (2.8245%): withanolides. Anti-inflammatory and inhibit synthesis of 2-macroglobin, which stimulates inflammatory cascade (Standeven, 1998). Glucocorticoid-like effect (Mills & Bone, 2000), withaferin A, immunosuppressive, hepatoprotective, sitoindosides–adaptogenic anabolic antidepressant, immunostimulant, memory aid, gastroprotective (Standeven, 1998), protects against stress-induced gastric ulcers (Bone, 1996).

Other Actions

- Ashwagandha has cardioprotective effects (Dhuley, 2000).
- Alcoholic root extract interacts with the GABA-A receptor, and it enhances benzodiazepine binding and has anticonvulsant activity.
- Root extracts have an immunomodulatory activity (Bone, 1996). Root extracts have shown the ability to work synergistically with radiation in the treatment of mouse tumors.
- A comparison of *Withania* and *Panax ginseng* showed that ashwagandha had similar potency to ginseng in its adaptogenic, tonic, and anabolic effects (Bone, 1996).

Nutritional Ingredients

- Iron

Traditional Use

- Anti-inflammatory, adaptogen, astringent, nervine, hypotensive, diuretic, antispasmodic, sedative
- Root is used in Ayurvedic and Unani medicine as an aphrodisiac, a calming tonic for exhaustion, neurasthenia, anxiety, depression, impaired memory, poor muscle tone, and as an aid in recovery from debilitating diseases. It is given in milk to children and the elderly for emaciation, debility, and anemia.

- A male reproductive tonic mixed with ghee or honey for impotence

Current Use

- Calming adaptogen, for CFS, anxiety with hypertension, insomnia, stress-induced ulcers, and impotence associated with anxiety or exhaustion (Winston & Maimes, 2007).
- Used for fibromyalgia along with black cohosh (*Cimicifuga racemosa*) and kava (*Piper methysticum*) (Winston & Maimes, 2007).
- For osteoarthritis and rheumatoid arthritis, as well as other inflammatory chronic diseases (ankylosing spondylitis, multiple sclerosis, asthma, systemic lupus erythematosus). A 32-week randomized, placebo-controlled trial found that a formula consisting of ashwagandha, boswellia, ginger, and turmeric provided substantial reduction of pain and stiffness in patients with osteoarthritis of the knees (Chopra et al., 2004).
- Supportive treatment for cancer and associated cachexia. Animal studies have demonstrated that ashwagandha can inhibit cyclophosphamide-induced damage to the bone marrow, preventing leukopenia in mice (Davis & Kuttan, 1998).
- For depleted, exhausted, underweight patients, especially the elderly with impaired memory. In a double-blind clinical trial, the effects of *Withania* (3 g/day for 1 year) on the aging process were assessed in 101 healthy men (50–59 years old). Significant improvements in hemoglobin, red blood cell count, hair melanin, and seated stature were observed. Serum cholesterol levels decreased and nail calcium was preserved. Erythrocyte sedimentation rate decreased significantly, and 71.4% of those treated with the herb reported improved sexual performance (Bone, 1996).
- Root extracts have an immunomodulatory activity (Bone, 1996). Root extracts have shown the ability to work synergistically with radiation in the treatment of mouse tumors. Another animal study indicates that *Withania* can enhance stress-depleted T-lymphocytes and Th-I cytokines (Khan et al., 2006).

Available Forms, Dosage, and Administration Guidelines

- *Dried root:* 2 to 6 g/day
- *Capsules:* Two 500-mg capsules three or four times a day
- *Tea:* 1 tsp dried root in 8 oz hot water; decoct 10 minutes and steep 20 minutes. Take 4 oz two or three times a day.
- *Tincture* (1:5, 45% alcohol): 40 to 80 gtt (2–4 mL) three times a day

Pharmacokinetics—If Available (form or route when known): Not known

Toxicity: Low potential for toxicity

Contraindications: None known

Side Effects: Rarely, nausea, dermatitis, abdominal pain, diarrhea. Animal studies indicate ashwagandha can increase serum levels of thyroid hormones. There is one recent case report suggesting that this herb caused thyrotoxicosis in a 32-year-old woman (van der Hooft et al., 2005).

Long-Term Safety: Safe; long-term history of regular use and animal and human trials show no cumulative toxicity.

Use in Pregnancy/Lactation/Children: Commonly used in India as a pregnancy tonic, as a stimulant for milk production, and for children. Use only in small amounts; large amounts (more than 3 g/day) are contraindicated during pregnancy.

Drug/Herb Interactions and Rationale (if known): May potentiate action of barbiturates and benzodiazepines. *Withania* given with paclitaxel for lung cancer enhanced its effects and reduced ROS (Senthilnathan et al., 2006).

Special Notes: Ashwagandha is considered one of the great tonic remedies in Ayurvedic medicine. Research has confirmed most, if not all, traditional uses and its very low potential for toxicity.

BIBLIOGRAPHY

Agarwal R, et al. (1999). Studies on immunomodulatory activity of *Withania somnifera* (ashwagandha) extracts in experimental immune inflammation. *Journal of Ethnopharmacology.* 67(1):27–35.

Archana R, Namasivayam A. (1999). Antistressor effect of *Withania somnifera*. *Journal of Ethnopharmacology*. 64(1):91–93.

Bhattacharya SK, Muruganandam AV. (2003). Adaptogenic activity of *Withania somnifera*: An experimental study using a rat model of chronic stress. *Pharmacology, Biochemistry and Behavior*. Jun;75(3):547–555.

Bone K. (1996). *Clinical Applications of Ayurvedic and Chinese Herbs* (pp. 137–141). Queensland, Australia: Phytotherapy Press.

Chopra A, et al. (2004). A 32-week randomized placebo-controlled clinical evaluation of RA-11, an Ayurvedic drug, on osteoarthritis of the knees. *Journal of Clinical Rheumatology*. Oct;10(5):236–245.

Davis L, Kuttan G. (1998). Suppressive effect of cyclophosphamide-induced toxicity by *Withania somnifera* extract in mice. *Journal of Ethnopharmacology*. 62(3):209–214.

Dhuley JN. (2000). Adaptogenic and cardioprotective action of ashwagandha in rats and frogs. *Journal of Ethnopharmacology*. 70(1):57–64.

Kapoor LD. (1990). *CRC Handbook of Ayurvedic Medicinal Plants* (pp. 337–338). Boca Raton, FL: CRC Press.

Khan B, et al. (2006). Augmentation and proliferation of T lymphocytes and Th-1 cytokines by *Withania somnifera* in stressed mice. *International Immunopharmacology*. Sep;6(9): 1394–1403.

Mills S, Bone K. (2000). *Principles and Practice of Phytotherapy* (pp. 595–602). London: Churchill Livingstone.

Senthilnathan P, et al. (2006). Chemotherapeutic efficacy of paclitaxel in combination with *Withania somnifera* on benzo(a)pyreneinduced experimental lung cancer. *Cancer Science*. Jul;97(7):658–664.

Standeven R. (1998). *Withania somnifera*. *European Journal of Herbal Medicine*. 4(2):17–22.

Upton, R. [Ed.]. (2000). *American Herbal Pharmacopoeia and Therapeutic Compendium—Ashwagandha Root*. Santa Cruz, CA: AHP.

van der Hooft CS, et al. (2005). Thyrotoxicosis following the use of ashwagandha. *Nederlands Tijdschrift voor Geneeskunde*. Nov 19;149(47):2637–2638.

Visavadiya NP, Narasimhacharya AV. (2007). Hypocholesteremic and antioxidant effects of Withania somnifera (Dunal) in hypercholesteremic rats. *Phytomedicine*. Feb;14(2–3):136–142. Epub 2006 May 16.

Williamson E. (2002). *Major Herbs of Ayurveda* (pp. 321–325). Edinburgh: Churchill Livingstone.

Winston D, Maimes S. (2007). *Adaptogens, Herbs for Strength, Stamina, and Stress Relief* (pp. 138–141). Rochester, VT: Inner Traditions.

NAME: Asian Ginseng (*Panax ginseng*)

Common Names: Chinese ginseng, Korean ginseng, ren shen (Chinese)

Family: *Araliaceae*

Description of Plant
- Small herbaceous plant with divided palmate leaves and clusters of red berries in the autumn. It grows in Asia above the 38th latitude (Chinese or Korean ginseng).
- The wild-harvested root is believed to be the most effective, even though the constituents are generally similar. Wild Asian *Panax* is virtually extinct and should not be used.

Medicinal Part: The root is most widely used. It is gathered in the fall just before defoliation.

Constituents and Action (if known)
- Ginsenosides (13 have been identified)
  ○ Support the adrenals by supporting the hypothalamus–pituitary–adrenal axis (Kim et al., 1999)
  ○ May reduce side effects (elevated lipid levels) in patients receiving corticosteroids
  ○ Improve cognitive function, attention span, psychomotor performance, concentration
  ○ May reduce cancer development by increasing CD4 and NK cells, increasing apoptosis and upregulating P53 (Scaglione, 1996; Yun et al., 1993; Ming et al., 2007)
  ○ Block acetylcholine and gamma-aminobutyric receptors and is an antagonist of muscarinic and histamine receptors (Tachikawa et al., 1999)
- Ginsenoside Re has significant antioxidant and hypolipidemic effects in diabetic rats (Cho et al., 2006). It also protects against diabetic retinopathy and nephropathy.
- Panaxosides A through F exert a hypoglycemic effect by increasing insulin release from the pancreas and a higher number of insulin receptors and lower glycosylated hemoglobin levels (Loi, 1996; Sotaniemi et al., 1995).
- Polysaccharides support immune function (Scaglione et al., 1996), act as antioxidants and free radical scavengers, and may reduce the development of cancer.

- Many other constituents: volatile oils, sterols, flavonoids, peptides, vitamins (B1, B2, nicotinic acid, biotin)

Nutritional Ingredients: Vitamins B1, B2, niacin, biotin

Traditional Use

- The Chinese have used ginseng for 4,000 years, and it has a reputation among the lay public as a panacea, aphrodisiac, longevity herb, and energy tonic.
- In TCM, Asian ginseng is used to tonify the original *qi* and is given for shock, syncope, shortness of breath, and weak pulse.
- Ginseng is also used to tonify the lungs, Chinese spleen, stomach, and heart. It is given in complex formulas for fatigue, impotence, asthma, lack of appetite, organ prolapse, diabetes, insomnia, poor memory, and palpitations.

Current Use

- Ginseng is an adaptogen: rather than being used to treat specific diseases, it is used to help the organism adapt to physical and mental stress.
  - Improves stamina (Kim et al., 2005)
  - Increases concentration and cognitive function (Reay, 2006b; Wesnes et al., 1997)
  - Combats mental and physical fatigue (Winston & Maimes, 2007)
  - May help to support body during and after radiation and chemotherapy
  - Aids in disease resistance (cancer, diabetes, infection) (Tachikawa et al., 1999)
  - May decrease vaginal atrophy and increase vaginal moisture during menopause
  - Enhances immune function and may protect from flu and the common cold (Scaglione et al., 1990, 1996)
  - Improves symptoms of CFIDS (Winston & Maimes, 2007)
- Ginseng has an ancient reputation for enhancing male sexual performance. Up until recently, this was thought to be a secondary action due to its adaptogenic (anabolic) function. Several recent studies (de Andrade et al., 2007; Hong et al., 2002) suggest that it has a direct ability to improve erectile dysfunction.

- Human studies also show that this root can lower blood sugar levels and enhance glycemic control (Reay et al., 2006a; Vuksan et al., 2006). In animal studies, ginseng extracts protected against diabetic-induced renal damage (Kang et al., 2006).

Available Forms, Dosage, and Administration Guidelines

Preparations: Dried root ("white"), steamed root ("red"), capsules, extracts, tablets, tinctures, teas. Fresh harvested root typically contains 2% to 3% ginsenosides, and the extracts range from 5% to 17%.

Typical Dosage

- *Capsules:* Up to four 500- to 600-mg capsules a day. For standardized products (4%–7% ginsenosides), 100 mg one or two times a day is generally recommended, or follow manufacturer or practitioner recommendations.
- *Dried roots:* 2 to 4 g/day
- *Tincture* (1:5, 35% alcohol): 60 to 100 gtt (3–5 mL) three times a day
- *Fluid extract* (1:1): 2 to 4 mL/day (34%–45% alcohol)

Pharmacokinetics—If Available (form or route when known): Ginsenosides inhibit the P450 system at the CYP 3A4 enzyme; signifigance yet unknown (Etheridge et al. 2007).

Toxicity: Nontoxic

Contraindications

- Avoid during acute infections and in patients with hypertension, schizophrenia, mania, brittle diabetes (may reduce blood sugar levels), cardiovascular disease (may elevate blood pressure), estrogen-positive cancers (may stimulate tumor growth; this is theoretical, however, and no data support this).
- Most often used in elderly, deficient, and depleted patients; less appropriate in younger, healthier persons

Side Effects: In type A people, may cause or exacerbate insomnia, anxiety, tachycardia, palpitations, high blood pressure, chest pain, and hypertension. Infrequent side effects include diarrhea, skin rash, and breast tenderness in men.

Long-Term Safety: Safe when taken as directed.

Use in Pregnancy/Lactation/Children: Do not use. Not appropriate except in rare cases of older children with chronic disease.

Drug/Herb Interactions and Rationale (if known)

- Concurrent use with caffeinated beverages increases the likelihood of overstimulation. Do not use concurrently.
- May potentiate the actions of centrally acting drugs. Do not use concurrently.
- Ginseng has a mild effect on platelets and may increase bleeding if taken concurrently with warfarin. Use cautiously.
- May potentiate the action of steroids. Use cautiously.
- Use caution with antidiabetic medications as a result of hypoglycemic activity.
- Increases side effects of monoamine oxidase inhibitors, such as headache, tremor, and mania. Avoid concurrent use.

Special Notes

- Top quality roots are extremely expensive: the best grades of Korean red may sell for $50/oz. Studies have been done on many ginseng products, and as many as 25% had no ginseng and 60% did not have enough to produce activity (Cui et al., 1994).
- Ginseng is a corruption of the Chinese name *ren shen*, which means "man root" because of the root's supposed resemblance to the human form.
- Asian ginseng, also referred to as Chinese, Korean, or *Panax ginseng*, grows in the Orient. American ginseng is of the same botanical family but grows in North America. Siberian ginseng is a distant relative of a different genus (*Eleutherococcus senticosus*). All ginsengs have known adaptogenic activity. Adaptogens show a nonspecific effect and raise the powers of resistance to toxins of a physical, chemical, or biologic nature. They bring about a normalizing or balancing action independent of the type of pathologic condition. They are relatively harmless and do

not influence normal body functions. They work through the HPA axis and SAS (sympathoadrenal system).

• Ginseng is often recommended to increase exercise performance, but several well-done studies cast doubt on this belief (Allen et al., 1998; Engels et al., 1996; Hermann et al., 1997). A recent study (Kim et al., 2005) found that ginseng extract prolonged exercise duration.

BIBLIOGRAPHY

Allen JD, et al. (1998). Ginseng supplementation does not enhance healthy young adults' peak aerobic exercise performance. *Journal of the American College of Nutritionists.* 17(5):462–466.

Bensky D, et al. (2004). *Chinese Herbal Medicine—Materia Medica* (3rd ed.; pp. 710–714). Seattle: Eastland Press.

Cho WC, et al. (2006). Ginsenoside Re of *Panax ginseng* possesses significant antioxidant and antihyperlipidemic efficacies in streptozotocin-induced diabetic rats. *European Journal of Pharmacology.* Nov 21;550(1–3):173–179.

Cui J, et al. (1994). What do commercial ginseng preparations contain? *Lancet.* 344:134.

de Andrade E, et al. (2007). Study of the efficacy of Korean Red ginseng in the treatment of erectile dysfunction. *Asian Journal of Andrology.* Mar;9(2):241–244. Epub 2006 Jul 11.

Engels HJ, et al. (1996). Failure of chronic ginseng supplementation to affect work performance and energy metabolism in healthy adult females. *Nutrition Research.* 16:1295–1305.

Etheridge AS et al. (2007). Evaluation of CYP450 Inhibition. *Planta medica.* 7(5):250–255.

Hermann J, et al. (1997). No ergogenic effects of ginseng (*Panax ginseng*) during graded maximal aerobic exercise. *Journal of the American Dietetic Association.* 97(10):1110–1115.

Hong B, et al. (2002). A double-blind crossover study evaluating the efficacy of Korean Red ginseng in patients with erectile dysfunction: A preliminary report. *Journal of Urology.* Nov;168(5): 2070–2073.

Janetsky K, Morreale AP. (1997). Probable interaction between warfarin and ginseng. *American Journal of Health-System Pharmacy.* 54(6):692–693.

Kang KS, et al. (2006). Protective effect of sun ginseng against diabetic renal damage. *Biological and Pharmaceutical Bulletin.* Aug;29(8):1678–1684.

Kim HS, et al. (1990). Antinarcotic effects of the standardized ginseng extract G115 on morphine. *Planta Medica.* 56:158–163.

Kim SH, et al. (2005). Effects of *Panax ginseng* extract on exercise-induced oxidative stress. *Journal of Sports Medicine and Physical Fitness*. Jun;45(2):178–182.

Kim YR, et al. (1999). *Panax ginseng* blocks morphine-induced thymic apoptosis by lowering plasma corticosterone level. *General Pharmacology*. 32(6):647–652.

Loi S. (1996). Ginseng. *Australian Journal of Emergency Care*. 3(3):28–29.

Ming YL et al. (2007). Anti-proliferation and apoptosis in human hepato-cellular carcinoma cells. *Cell Biol Int*.

Reay JL, et al. (2006a). The glycaemic effects of single doses of *Panax ginseng* in young, healthy volunteers. *British Journal of Nutrition*. Oct;96(4):639–642.

Reay JL, et al. (2006b). Effects of *Panax ginseng*, consumed with and without glucose, on blood glucose levels and cognitive performance during sustained 'mentally demanding' tasks. *Journal of Psychopharmacology*. Nov;20(6):771–781.

Scaglione F, et al. (1996). Efficacy and safety of the standardized ginseng extract G 115 for potentiating vaccination against common cold and/or influenza syndrome. *Drugs Under Experimental and Clinical Research*. 22(2):65–72.

Sotaniemi EA, et al. (1995). Ginseng therapy in non-insulin-dependent diabetic patients. *Diabetes Care*. 18(10):1373–1375.

Tachikawa E, et al. (1999). Effects of ginseng saponins on responses induced by various receptor stimuli. *European Journal of Pharmacology*. 369(1):23–32.

Vuksan V, et al. (2006). Korean Red ginseng (*Panax ginseng*) improves glucose and insulin regulation in well-controlled, type 2 diabetes: Results of a randomized, double-blind, placebo-controlled study of efficacy and safety. *Nutrition, Metabolism and Cardiovascular Diabetes*. Apr 20;(9):1–11. Epub 2006 Jul 21.

Wesnes KA, et al. (1997). The cognitive, subjective and physical effects of a gingko biloba/*Panax ginseng* combination in healthy volunteers with neurasthenic complaints. *Psychopharmacology Bulletin*. 33(4):677–683.

Winston D, Maimes S. (2007). *Adaptogens, Herbs for Strength, Stamina, and Stress Relief* (pp. 142–146). Rochester, VT: Inner Traditions.

Yan, Shu-Su, et al. (1998). Modulation of American ginseng on brainstem GABAergic effects on rats. *Journal of Ethnopharmacology*. 62:215–222.

Yun YS, et al. (1993). Inhibition of autochthonous tumor by ethanol insoluble fraction from *Panax ginseng* as an immunomodulator. *Planta Medica*. 59:521–524.

NAME: Astragalus (*Astragalus membranaceus,*
Astragalus membranaceus var. mongholicus)

Common Names: Milk vetch, huang chi, huang qi

Family: *Fabaceae*

Description of Plant
- Grows along forest margins in most of China, Korea, and Japan; mostly cultivated in China
- There are more than 1,750 astragalus species. Some are ornamental, some are medicinal, and others are poisonous, especially to grazing animals.
- Member of the pea family

Medicinal Part: Plants are 4 to 5 years old before the root is harvested. In most cases, astragalus is repeatedly moistened in honey water and flattened to create the typical "tongue depressor"-shaped root that is available commercially. This process is believed to make the root more tonifying.

Constituents and Action (if known)
- Polysaccharides (astragaloglucans)
  - Enhance immunologic response, stimulate white blood cell activity, increase production of antibodies and interferon (particularly effective in patients undergoing chemotherapy and radiation) (Liu et al., 1994)
  - Increase phagocytic activity Tomoda et al., 1991)
- Saponins (cycloartanes)
  - Diuretic activity, probably from local irritation of the kidney (Hostettmann et al., 1995); anti-inflammatory (Tang & Eisenbrand, 1992); hypotensive effects (Tang & Eisenbrand, 1992)
  - Stimulate growth of isolated lymphocytes (Calis et al., 1997)
- Biphenyl: antihepatoxic activity (similar to vitamin E)
- Isoflavonoid glycosides: antioxidant activity (similar to vitamin E), mucronulatol, formononetin, demethoxyisoflavin (Shirataki et al., 1997; Upton et al., 1999)
- Flavonoids (afromosin, ordoratin, calycosin, quercetin)

- Triterpenoid saponins (astragalosides I–VII): astragaloside IV inhibits diabetic peripheral neuropathy in animal studies (Yu J, et al., 2006) and is cardioprotective (Zhang, WD, 2006); antioxidants prevent shock-wave induced renal injury (Li et al., 2006)

Nutritional Ingredients: None known

Traditional Use
- The Chinese name for this herb is huang qi. *Huang* means "yellow," referring to the color of the root, and *qi* means "leader, or vital force," as it is one of the superior tonics in Chinese medicine.
- Astragalus is thought to add years of health to the aged and to increase overall vitality and health.
- It is used in TCM to tonify the Chinese spleen, for organ prolapse, as a diuretic, to strengthen the lungs, and to protect against colds and other contagious diseases.

Current Use
- To treat diabetic complications such as microalbuminuria (Lu et al., 2005) and peripheral neuropathy (Wang & Chen, 2004)
- To enhance immune function in persons with HIV infection. Several Chinese reports suggest that astragalus can induce seronegative conversion, but these reports need to be verified (Burack et al., 1996; Lu, 1995; Lu et al., 1995). A human study found that astralagus stimulated CD4 and CD8 T cells within 24 hours of ingestion, and the effect continued for 7 days (Brush et al., 2006).
- In China, it is a part of *fu-zheng* therapy, where the goal is to restore immune system function in patients with cancer and to protect them from the side effects of chemotherapy (Bensky et al., 2004).
- To treat recurrent colds, tonsillitis, and other upper respiratory tract infections (Upton et al., 1999; Yang et al., 2006)
- Chinese studies have shown increased cardiac output in 20 patients with angina after 2 weeks of treatment. The herb strengthened the function of the left ventricle and reduced oxygen free radical activity. Astragalus also increased survival

rates in in vivo studies with acute Coxsackie B-3 viral myocarditis infections (Upton et al., 1999).

Available Forms, Dosage, and Administration Guidelines

Preparations: Dried root, sliced (looks like a tongue depressor) or powdered; capsules, extracts, tablets, tinctures, combination products

Typical Dosage

- *Capsules:* Six to eight 400- to 500-mg capsules daily
- *Tincture* (1:5, 30% alcohol): 60 to 90 gtt (3–5 mL) four times a day
- *Tea:* 9 to 15 g dried sliced root, simmered for several hours in 1 qt water (the decoction is ready when the water is reduced to 1 pt)
- Or follow manufacturer or practitioner recommendations

Pharmacokinetics—If Available (form or route when known): None known

Toxicity: None known (Yu SY, et al., 2006)

Contraindications: Not recommended in acute infections

Side Effects: None known

Long-Term Safety: Used in China as a medicinal food, cooked in soups and stews. No safety issues expected.

Use in Pregnancy/Lactation/Children: No research available, but no adverse effects expected

Drug/Herb Interactions and Rationale (if known):
Astragalus given to mice with gastric carcinoma concurrently with 5-fluorouracil enhanced the antitumor effect of the medication (Zhang ZX, et al., 2006).

BIBLIOGRAPHY

Bensky D, et al. (2004). *Chinese Herbal Medicine—Materia Medica* (3rd ed.; pp. 718–723). Seattle: Eastland Press.

Burack J, et al. (1996). Pilot randomized controlled trial of Chinese herbal treatment for HIV-associated symptoms. *Journal of Acquired Immune Deficiency Syndrome and Human Retrovirology.* 12:386.

Brush J, et al. (2006). The effect of *Echinacea purpurea*, *Astragalus membranaceus* and *Glycyrrhiza glabra* on CD69 expression and immune cell activation in humans. *Phytotherapy Research*. Aug;20(8):687–695.

Calis I, et al. (1997). Cycloartane triterpene glycosides from the roots of *Astragalus melanophrurius*. *Planta Medica*. 63:183.

Dong J, et al. (2005). Effects of large dose of *Astragalus membranaceus* on the dendritic cell induction of peripheral mononuclear cell and antigen presenting ability of dendritic cells in children with acute leukemia. Oct;25(10):872–875.

He Z, et al. (1991). Isolation and identification of chemical constituents of Astragalus root. *Chemical Abstracts*. 114:58918u.

Hostettmann K, et al. (1995). *Saponins* (p. 267). Cambridge, England: Cambridge University Press.

Li X, et al. (2006). A novel antioxidant agent, astragalosides, prevents shock wave-induced renal oxidative injury in rabbits. *Urological Research*. Aug;34(4):277–282.

Liu X, et al. (1994). Isolation of astragalan and its immunological activities. *Tianran Chanwu Yaniju Yu Kaifa*. 6:23.

Lu W. (1995). Prospect for study on treatment of AIDS with traditional Chinese medicine. *Journal of Traditional Chinese Medicine*. 15:3.

Lu W, et al. (1995). A report on 8 seronegative converted HIV/AIDS patients with traditional Chinese medicine. *Chinese Medical Journal*. 108:634.

Lu ZM, et al. (2005). The protective effects of *Radix astragali* and *Rhizoma ligustici chuanxiong* on endothelial dysfunction in type 2 diabetic patients with microalbuminuria. *Sichuan Da Xue Xue Bao. Yi Xue Ban*. Jul;36(4):529–532.

Mills S, Bone K. (2000). *Principles and Practice of Phytotherapy* (pp. 273–279). Edinburgh: Churchill Livingstone.

Shirataki Y, et al. (1997). Antioxidative components isolated from the roots of *Astragalus membranaceus Bunge* (*Astragali radix*). *Phytotherapy Research*. 11:603.

Tang W, Eisenbrand G. (1992). *Chinese Drugs of Plant Origin* (pp. 191–197). Berlin: Springer-Verlag.

Upton R, et al. (1999). *American Herbal Pharmacopoeia and Therapeutic Compendium: Astragalus Root*. Santa Cruz, CA: American Pharmacopoeia.

Wang HY, Chen YP. (2004). Clinical observation on treatment of diabetic nephropathy with compound fructus arctii mixture. *Zhongguo Zhong Xi Yi Jie He Za Zhi*. Jul;24(7):589–592.

Yang Y, et al. (2006). Effects of *Astragalus membranaceus* on TH cell subset function in children with recurrent tonsillitis. *Zhongguo Dang Dai Er Ke Za Zhi*. Oct;8(5):376–387.

Yu J, et al. (2006). Inhibitory effects of astragaloside IV on diabetic peripheral neuropathy in rats. *Canadian Journal of Physiology and Pharmacology*. Jun;84(6):579–587.

Yu SY, et al. (2006). Subchronic toxicity studies of *Radix astragali* extract in rats and dogs. *Journal of Ethnopharmacology*. Mar 21;110(2):352–355. Epub 2006 Sept 27.

Zhang WD, et al. (2006). Astragaloside IV from *Astragalus membranaceus* shows cardioprotection during myocardial ischemia in vivo and in vitro. *Planta Medica*. Jan;72(1):4–8.

Zhang ZX, et al. (2006). Effect of 5-fluorouracil in combination with *Astragalus membranaceus* on amino acid metabolism in mice model of gastric carcinoma. *Zhonghua Wei Chang Wai Ke Za Zhi*. Sep;9(5):445–447.

B

NAME: Bacopa Herb (*Bacopa monniera*).
The genus is also spelled *monnieri* in some of the literature.

Common Names: Brahmi, water hyssop

Family: *Scrophulariaceae*

Description of Plant

- It is a small, succulent creeping plant native to southeast Asia. It grows in wet areas or shallow ponds.
- It is commonly sold as an aquarium plant.
- There are several bacopa cultivars sold as ornamentals that are not medicinal.

Medicinal Part: Dried herb

Constituents and Action (if known)

- Alkaloids
  - Brahmine: hypotensive (Duke, 2006)
  - Herpestine
- Glycosides: bacopaside I, II, III

- Saponins: bacoside A—neuroprotective, antioxidant; enhances SOD, catalase, and glutathione peroxidase activity, gastroprotective (Anbarasi et al., 2005). Other bacosides B and C are also present.
- Bacopasaponins: antileishmanial (Sinha et al., 2002). Other bacopasaponins D,E, and F are also present.

Nutritional Ingredients: This herb is rich in potassium.

Traditional Use

- Anticonvulsant, anti-inflammatory, antifungal, antioxidant, antispasmodic, aperient, astringent, diuretic, nervine, nootropic, mild sedative, and vulnerary
- Bacopa has a long history of use in India for nervous disorders, including anxiety, insanity, seizures, and for enhancing memory and intellect.
- It has also been used as a folk remedy in southeast Asia for asthma, bronchitis, urinary problems. scurvy, bedsores, and rheumatism.

Current Use

- Several human and animal studies confirm the traditional use of this herb for improving memory, focus, and mental acuity (Roodenrys et al., 2002). It can be used with other nootropic herbs such as ginkgo, rosemary, white peony, or holy basil to retard the progression of neurodegenerative disease and to stimulate recovery from head trauma injuries. It is also of benefit for ADD/ADHD, anxiety (with blue vervain and motherwort), nervous breakdowns, and depression (Winston & Maimes, 2007).
- In animal studies (Kar et al., 2002), bacopa increased thyroid function, suggesting that it may have benefit for mild hypothyroid conditions used along with other thyroid-stimulating herbs such as ashwagandha, bladderwrack and red ginseng.
- In another animal study, researchers suggest that bacopa is not just a nervine and nootropic but is actually an adaptogen. More research is needed to confirm this, but this herb is appropriate for use with adaptogens for chronic stress, stress-induced mental fog, nervous exhaustion, and CFIDS (Winston & Maimes, 2007).

- Topical applications of this herb are used to enhance hair growth and heal burns and sores (Williamson, 2002).

Available Forms, Dosage, and Administration Guidelines

Preparations: Tea, capsule, tincture

Typical Dosage

- *Tea:* 1 to 2 tsp dried herb to 8 oz hot water, steep 30 to 40 minutes. Take 4 oz three times a day.
- *Capsules:* Standardized extract—1 to 2 capsules twice a day
- *Tincture* (1:5, 30% alcohol): 30 to 50 gtt (1.5–2.5 mL) three or four times a day

Pharmacokinetics—If Available (form or route when known): Not known

Toxicity: None known

Contraindications: This herb is high in potassium. Avoid use in dialysis patients.

Side Effects: None known

Long-Term Safety: Safe

Use In Pregnancy/Lactation/Children: There is a lack of data to prove safety, so avoid use during pregnancy and lactation.

Drug/Herb Interactions and Rationale (if known): In animal studies, bacopa reduced liver damage and neurotoxicity caused by morphine. It also reduced cognitive dysfunction caused by the antiseizure medication phenytoin.

Special Notes: Bacopa grows in ponds, stagnant water, and sewage ditches. Be sure that any bacopa product is certified organically grown and tested to be free of heavy metals and pathogenic bacteria.

BIBLIOGRAPHY
Anbarasi K, et al. (2005). Protective effect of bacoside A on cigarette smoking-induced brain mitochondrial dysfunction in rats. *Journal of Environmental Pathology, Toxicology and Oncology*. 24(3):225–234.

Duke J. Dr. Duke's phytochemical and ethnobotanical databases. Retrieved September 25, 2006, from www.ars-grin.gov/cgi-bin/duke/chemactivities.

Jvoti A, Sharma D. (2006). Neuroprotective role of *Bacopa monniera* extract against aluminium-induced oxidative stress in the hippocampus of rat brain. *Neurotoxicology.* Jul;27(4):451–457.

Kar A, et al. (2002). Relative efficacy of three medicinal plant extracts in the alteration of thyroid hormone concentrations in male mice. *Journal of Ethnopharmacology.* Jul;81(2):281–285.

Perry LM. (1980). *Medicinal Plants of East and Southeast Asia* (p. 382). Cambridge, MA: MIT Press.

Rai D, et al. (2003). Adaptogenic effect of *Bacopa monniera* (Brahmi). *Pharmacology, Biochemistry and Behavior.* Jul;75(4):823–830.

Roodenrys S, et al. (2002). Chronic effects of Brahmi (*Bacopa monnieri*) on human memory. *Neuropsychopharmacology.* Aug;27(2):279–281.

Russo A, et al. (2003). Free radical scavenging capacity and protective effect of *Bacopa monniera L.* on DNA damage. *Phytotherapy Research.* Sep;17(8):870–875.

Sinha J, et al. (2002). Bacopasaponin C: Critical evaluation of anti-leishmanial properties in various delivery modes. *Drug Delivery.* 9(1):55–62.

Vohora D, et al. (2000). Protection from phenytoin-induced cognitive deficit by *Bacopa monniera,* a reputed Indian nootropic plant. *Journal of Ethnopharmacology.* Aug;71(3):383–390.

Williamson E. (2002). *Major Herbs of Ayurveda* (pp. 64–68). Edinburgh: Churchill Livingstone.

Winston D. (2006). *Winston's Botanic Materia Medica.* Washington, NJ: DWCHS.

Winston D, Maimes S. (2007). *Adaptogens, Herbs for Strength, Stamina, and Stress Relief* (pp. 223–224). Rochester, VT: Inner Traditions.

 NAME: Barberry (*Berberis vulgaris, B. aristata,* and other *Berberis* species)

Common Names: Berberis, jaundice berry, sourberry, Pepperidge bush, European barberry, Oregon graperoot (a related species, *B. aquifolium*)

Family: *Berberidaceae*

Description of Plant

- *Berberis vulgaris* grows wild throughout Europe and is naturalized in the eastern United States.
- Shrub grows up to 10' tall, with ovate leaves and sharp thorns.
- Flowers bloom from May to June and develop into red oblong berries.

Medicinal Part: Root bark, stem bark (less active), fruit

Constituents and Action (if known)

- Isoquinoline alkaloids: berberine (up to 6%), palmatine, berbermine, oxyacanthine, magnoflorine, jatrorrhizine, columbamine (Ivanovska & Philipov, 1996; Leung & Foster, 1996)
- Berberine (berberine chloride): antibacterial activity against *Staphylococcus epidermidis, Escherichia coli, Neisseria meningitidis,* and others (Leung & Foster, 1996), antiamoebic antithelminthic (Soffar et al., 2001).
  - Inhibits endotoxins
  - Improves watery diarrhea associated with cholera (Maung et al., 1985)
  - Anti-inflammatory (Kupeli et al., 2002)
  - Cytotoxic, antimitotic, antitumor; increases activity of other antitumor agents; inhibits carcinogens (Mills & Bone, 2000)
  - Uterine stimulant
  - Antihistaminic and anticholinergic activity (in guinea pig ileum) (Shamsa et al., 1999)
  - Antifungal (Mills & Bone, 2000)
  - Cholagogue and choleretic, increases bilirubin excretion (Mills & Bone, 2000)
  - Reduces oxygen free radicals (Ryzhikova et al., 1999)
- Berbamine: antiarrhythmic (Guo & Fu, 2005), antileukemic (Xu et al., 2006).
- Tannins

Nutritional Ingredients: The berries are rich in vitamin C, sugars, and pectin and can be made into jellies or jam.

Traditional Use
- Gastrointestinal ailments, including diarrhea and dysentery
- Bitter tonic and cholagogue; used to stimulate bile secretion, for poor fat digestion, biliousness, and constipation with clay-colored stools
- Used in alterative formulas as a blood purifier for cancers, arthritis, and skin conditions

Current Use
- Eye drops (saline solution) for trachoma and simple conjunctivitis (Mills & Bone, 2000)
- Oral use for UTIs, cystitis, urethritis, and prostatitis. In in vitro studies, berberine has been found to be as effective as metronidazole for treating *Trichomonas vaginalis* (Soffar et al., 2001)
- Oral use for amoebic infections (*Giardia, Blastocystis hominis, Dientamoeba fragilis*) and bacterial diarrhea (Winston, 2006).
- Topical use in creams for psoriasis, sores, and fungal infections
- Compounds found in berberis leaves, 5-methoxyhydnocarpin-D and pheophorbide, had strong bacterial effux pump inhibition activity against multiple-drug–resistant *Staphylococcus aureus* (Stermitz et al., 2001). The leaves of barberry may have some benefit if combined with antibiotics for MRSA and PRSA.

Available Forms, Dosage, and Administration Guidelines
Preparations: Tablets, tincture, tea
Typical Dosage
- *Berberine sulfate:* 100 mg four times a day. The oral LD50 is 329 mg/kg.
- *Tea:* 1 to 2 tsp dried root bark to 8 oz boiling water, decoct 10 minutes, steep 45 minutes; take 4 oz three times a day
- *Tincture* (1:5, 45% alcohol): 40 to 60 gtt (2–4 mL) four times a day

Pharmacokinetics—If Available (form or route when known): Rabbits given pure berberine reached a maximum blood level in 8 hours, and traces of this chemical were still

present after 72 hours. It was excreted via the stool and urine (Mills & Bone, 2000).

Toxicity: Very little

Contraindications: None known

Side Effects
- Nausea and vomiting in overdose
- Higher doses of berberine sulfate (more than 0.5 g) may cause dizziness, epistaxis, dyspnea, skin and eye irritation, GI irritation, diarrhea, and nephritis (Mills & Bone, 2000).

Long-Term Safety: No adverse effects are expected from ingestion of normal therapeutic doses of this herb.

Use in Pregnancy/Lactation/Children: Do not use in pregnancy, because it is a possible uterine stimulant.

Drug/Herb Interactions and Rationale (if known): Animal studies suggest that berberine inhibits CYP3A4 and prevents acetaminophen-induced liver damage (Janbaz & Gilani, 2000). In a human study, berberine increased the absorption and bioavailability of cyclosporine-A in renal transplant recipients, possibly due to inhibiting CYP3A4 (Wu et al., 2005; Xin et al., 2006).

Special Notes: Little scientific evidence exists as to the efficacy of the whole herb, but the major alkaloid berberine is well studied and therapeutically active. Barberry fruit is used in Middle Eastern herbal medicine for its antiarrhythmic, sedative, and neuroprotective effects (Fatehi et al., 2005).

BIBLIOGRAPHY

Der Marderosian A, Beutler J. [Eds.]. (2004). *The Review of Natural Products*. St. Louis, MO: Facts and Comparisons.

Fatehi M, et al. (2005). A pharmacological study on *Berberis vulgaris* fruit extract. *Journal of Ethnopharmacology*. Oct 31;102(1):46–52.

Guo ZB, Fu JG. (2005). Progress of cardiovascular pharmacology study on berbamine. *Zhongguo Zhong Xi Yi Jie He Za Zhi*. Aug;25(8):765–768.

Ivanovska N, Philipov S. (1996). Study on the anti-inflammatory action of *Berberis vulgaris* root extract, alkaloid fractions, and pure alkaloids. *International Journal of Immunopharmacology*. 10:553–561.

Janbaz KH, Gilani AH. (2000). Studies on preventive and curative effects of berberine on chemical-induced hepatotoxicity in rodents. *Fitoterapia.* Feb;71(1):25–33.

Kupeli E, et al. (2002). A comparative study on the anti-inflammatory, antinociceptive and antipyretic effects of isoquinoline alkaloids from the roots of Turkish Berberis species. *Life Sciences.* Dec 27;72(6):645–657.

Leung AY, Foster S. (1996). *Encyclopedia of Common Natural Ingredients Used in Food, Drugs and Cosmetics* (2nd ed.; pp. 66–67). New York: John Wiley & Sons.

Maung KU, et al. (1985). Clinical trial of berberine in acute watery diarrhea. *British Medical Journal.* 291:1601.

Mills S, Bone K. (2000). *Principles and Practice of Phytotherapy* (pp. 286–296). Edinburgh: Churchill Livingstone.

Ryzhikova MA, et al. (1999). The effect of aqueous extracts of hepatotropic medicinal plants on free-radial oxidation processes. *Eksperimentalnaia Klinicheskaia Farmakologia.* 62(2):36–38.

Shamsa F, et al. (1999). Antihistaminic and anticholinergic activity of barberry fruit (*Berberis vulgaris*) in the guinea-pig ileum. *Journal of Ethnopharmacology.* 64(2):161–166.

Soffar SA, et al. (2001). Evaluation of the effect of a plant alkaloid (berberine derived from *Berberis astrata*) on *Trichomonas vaginalis* in vitro. *Journal of the Egyptian Society of Parasitology.* Dec;31(3):893–904.

Stermitz FR, et al. (2001). *Staphylococcus aureus* MDR efflux pump inhibitors from a Berberis and a Mahonia (*Sensu strictu*) species. *Biochemical Systematics and Ecology.* Aug;29(8):793–798.

Winston D. (2006) *Winston's Botanic Materia Medica.* Washington, NJ: DWCHS

Wu X, et al. (2005). Effects of berberine on the blood concentration of cyclosporin A in renal transplanted recipients: Clinical and pharmacokinetic study. *European Journal of Clinical Pharmacology.* Sep;61(8):567–572.

Xin HW, et al. (2006). The effects of berberine on the pharmacokinetics of cyclosporin A in healthy volunteers. *Methods and Findings in Experimental and Clinical Pharmacology.* Jan-Feb;28(1):25–29.

Xu R, et al. (2006). Berbamine: A novel inhibitor of BCR/ABI fusion gene with potent anti-leukemia activity. *Leukemia Research.* Jan;30(1):17–23.

NAME: Bilberry Fruit (*Vaccinium myrtillus*) and Blueberry (*Vaccinium corymbosum, V. angustifolium*)

Common Names: Bilberries, European blueberry, whortleberries

Family: *Ericaceae* (heath family)

Description of Plant
- Known as European blueberry
- Native to northern and central Europe
- Shrubby perennial, grows in meadows and woods
- Produces shiny black berries containing many small, shiny brownish-red seeds
- Berries have a sweet taste with a slightly acrid aftertaste.
- The *Vaccinium* genus contains nearly 200 species of berries, including cranberry and American blueberry (which has similar chemistry and uses).

Medicinal Part: Ripe fruit

Constituents and Action (if known)
- Anthocyanosides (or anthocyanins)
  - Decrease vascular permeability (Colantuoni et al., 1991; Wichtl & Bissett, 1994)
  - Protect blood vessels (Grismond, 1981), particularly varicose veins, hemorrhoids, and delicate blood vessels in the elderly (Colantuoni et al., 1991; Lietti et al., 1976; Mian et al., 1977)
  - Long-term use may improve vision in persons with myopia (Gandolfo, 1990; Sala et al., 1979).
  - Antiedema (Detre et al., 1986)
  - Act as antioxidant and free radical scavenger (Lietti et al., 1976)
  - Reduce platelet stickiness; stimulate growth and reproduction of collagen (Detre et al., 1986; Monbiosse et al., 1983; Rao et al., 1981)
  - Neuroprotective and enhances mitochondrial integrity and memory (Andres-Lacueva et al., 2005; Yao & Vieira, 2007)
  - Increase prostaglandin E_2 release in stomach mucosa (Mertz-Nielsen et al., 1990)
  - Protect liver cells (Mitcheva et al., 1993)
  - Slow macular degeneration and diabetic retinopathy, speed up regeneration of rhodopsin (visual purple) (Alfieri & Sole, 1964; Gandolfo, 1990)
  - May have anticarcinogenic activity (Bomser et al., 1996), inhibit colon cancer

○ Potential anticancer activity, at least in vitro studies
  (Bomser et al., 1996)
- Polyphenols, tannins, flavonoids (hyperoside, chlorogenic
  acid, quercetin) (Fraisse et al., 1996)
- Oligomeric procyanidins (OPCs)
- Pectin

Nutritional Ingredients: Rich in vitamin C, flavonoids;
commonly eaten as a fresh fruit, in jellies and jams and in desserts.

Traditional Use
- Used to treat scurvy, urinary infections, and kidney stones
- The fruit was used to treat diarrhea, dysentery, and GI
  inflammation.
- British World War II pilots were said to have improved night
  vision with its use.
- Oral rinse for inflammation of the mouth and pharynx

Current Use
- Powerful antioxidant: reduces oxidative stress and has shown
  the ability to improve cognitive function and reduce
  inflammation (it may inhibit atherosclerosis and other
  oxidative diseases) (Andres-Lacueva et al., 2005)
- Nonspecific, acute diarrhea
- Vascular disorders: varicose veins and hemorrhoids (prevents
  and treats, particularly during pregnancy), spider veins, and
  peripheral vascular disease (improves paresthesia, pain, skin
  dystrophy, edema), nosebleeds (Colantuoni et al., 1991;
  Liette et al., 1976).
- Eye conditions: myopia, diabetic retinopathy, hypertensive
  retinopathy, macular degeneration, hemeralopia; improves
  night vision (Gandolfo, 1990; Mills & Bone, 2000).
- Gastric ulcer: protects gastric mucosa and helps to prevent
  Helicobacter pylori adhesion to the stomach lining
  (Chatterjee et al., 2004)
- Allergies: reduces production of proinflammatory substances
  such as histamine and bradykinin and stabilizes mast cells

Available Forms, Dosage, and Administration Guidelines
Preparations: Dried fruit, capsules, tablets, liquid tinctures,
fluid extracts. Standardized products contain 25%

anthocyanins. Fresh fruit contains only 0.1% to 0.25% anthocyanins.

Typical Dosage

- *Solid (native) extracts:* 0.25 to 0.5 tsp twice a day
- *Capsules and tablets:* Two or three standardized capsules or tablets a day, or follow manufacturer or practitioner recommendations.
- *Orally:* 600 to 1,800 mg/day standardized product to treat condition. Once improvement is seen, reduce dose to 200 to 300 mg/day; 200 to 300 mg/day for prevention; 60 to 120 mg/day to improve night vision.

Pharmacokinetics—If Available (form or route when known): Absorption of anthocyanins reached maximal level 15 minutes after ingestion and then decreased over time. Excretion was primarily via the liver and kidney (Ichiyanagi et al., 2006).

Toxicity: None known for fruit; long-term use of leaves can cause gastric irritation and kidney damage

Contraindications: None known

Side Effects: None known

Long-Term Safety: Very safe

Use in Pregnancy/Lactation/Children: Safe (Grismond, 1981)

Drug/Herb Interactions and Rationale (if known): Potential for increased bleeding if taken with anticoagulants and other antiplatelet drugs; use cautiously if taking medicinal quantities. Normal food quantities are safe.

Special Notes: Most studies have been performed on animals. More human research is needed.

BIBLIOGRAPHY

Alfieri R, Sole P. (1964). Influence des anthocyanosides administres par voie parenterale sur l'adaptoelectroretinogramme du lapin. *Comptes Rendu Societe de Biologie.* 158:23–38.

Andres-Lacueva C, et al. (2005). Anthocyanins I aged blueberry-fed rats are found centrally and may enhance memory. *Nutritional Neuroscience.* Apr;8(2):111–120.

Bomser J, et al. (June 1996). In vitro anticancer activity of fruit extracts from *Vaccinium* species. *Planta Medica.* 62(3):212–216.

Chatterjee A, et al. (2004). Inhibition of *Helicobacter pylori* in vitro by various berry extracts, with enhanced susceptibility to clarithromycin. *Molecular and Cellular Biochemistry.* Oct;265(1–2):19–26.

Colantuoni A, et al. (1991). Effects of *Vaccinium myrtillus* anthocyanosides on arterial vasomotion. *Arzneimittelforschung.* 41(9):905–909.

Der Marderosian A, Beutler J. [Eds.]. (2004). *The Review of Natural Products.* St. Louis, MO: Facts and Comparisons.

Detre Z, et al. (1986). Studies on vascular permeability in hypertension: Action of anthocyanosides. *Clinical Physiology and Biochemistry.* 4(2):143.

Fraisse D, et al. (1996). Polyphenolic composition of the leaf of bilberry. *Annales Pharmacie Française.* 54(6):280–283.

Gandolfo E. (1990). Perimetric follow-up of myopic patients treated with anthocyanosides and beta-carotene. *Bulletin Oculisme.* 69:57–71.

Grismond GL. (1981). Treatment of pregnancy-induced phlebopathies. *Minerva Gynecology.* 33:221–230.

Ichiyanagi T, et al. (2006). Bioavailability and tissue distribution of anthocyanins in bilberry (*Vaccinium myrtillus L.*) extract in rats. *Journal of Agricultural and Food Chemistry.* Sep 6;54(18): 6578–6587.

Lala G, et al. (2006). Anthocyanin-rich extracts inhibit multiple biomarkers of colon cancer in rats. *Nutrition and Cancer.* 54(1):84–93.

Lietti A, et al. (1976). Studies on *Vaccinium myrtillus* anthocyanosides. I. Vasoprotective and anti-inflammatory activity. *Arzneimittelforschung.* 26:829–832.

Mertz-Nielsen A, et al. (1990). A natural flavonoid, IdB 1027, increases gastric luminal release of prostaglandin E2 in healthy subjects. *Italian Journal of Gastroenterology.* 22(5):288.

Mian E, et al. (1977). Anthocyanosides and the walls of microvessels: Further aspects of the mechanism of action of their protective effect in syndromes due to abnormal capillary fragility. *Minerva Medicine.* 68:3565–3581.

Mills S, Bone K. (2000). *Principles and Practice of Phytotherapy* (pp. 297–302). Edinburgh: Churchill Livingstone.

Mitcheva M, et al. (1993). Biochemical and morphological studies on the effects of anthocyans and vitamin E on carbon tetrachloride induced liver injury. *Cellular Microbiology.* 39(4):443.

Monbiosse JC, et al. (1983). Nonenzymatic degradation of acid-soluble calf skin collagen by superoxide ion: Protective effect of flavonoids. *Biochemistry and Pharmacology.* 32:53–58.

Rao CN, et al. (1981). Influence of bioflavonoids on collagen metabolism in rats with adjuvant induced arthritis. *Italian Journal of Biochemistry.* 30:54–62.

Sala D, et al. (1979). Effect of anthocyanosides on visual performance at low illumination. *Minerva Oftalmologie.* 21:283–285.

Schmidt BM, et al. (2004). Effective separation of potent antiproliferation and antiadhesion components from wild blueberry (*Vaccinium angustifolium Ait.*) fruits. *Journal of Agricultural and Food Chemistry.* Oct 20;52(21):6433–6442.

Wichtl M, Bissett NG. (1994). *Herbal Drugs and Phytopharmaceuticals* (pp. 351–352). Stuttgart: Medpharm Scientific Publishers.

Yao Y, Vieira A. (2007). Protective activities of *Vaccinium* antioxidants with potential relevance to mitochondrial dysfunction and neurotoxicity. *Neurotoxicology.* Jan;28(1):93–100. Epub 2006 Jul 31.

 NAME: Bitter Melon (*Momordica charantia*)

Common Names: Balsam pear, cerasee, balsam apple, carilla, bitter cucumber, karela

Family: *Cucurbitaceae*

Description of Plant
- Climbing annual vine, grows up to 6' tall
- A tropical fruit used as a vegetable; it is orange-yellow when ripe and edible but very bitter
- Unripened fruit is green, cucumber-shaped with bumps on surface.
- Cultivated in Asia, Africa, Central and South America, and India

Medicinal Part: Unripe fruit, leaves, seeds, and seed oil

Constituents and Action (if known)
- Steroidal glycosides
  - Charantin and mormordin: hypoglycemic and antihyperglycemic effect (Handa et al., 1990; Raman et al., 1996)
  - Momordicosides G, F_1, F_2, I: hypoglycemic (Harinantenaina et al., 2006)
  - Momordicines I and II

- ○ Vicine: inhibits glucose absorption so blood sugar is in better control
- Insulinomimetic lectins (P-insulin): an insulin-like, hypoglycemic peptide; reduces blood sugar (Raman et al., 1996)
- Alkaloid fraction: slow-acting hypoglycemic effect (Raman et al., 1996)
- Glycoproteins (alpha and beta monorcharin): may have abortifacient activity (Cunnick et al., 1993)
- Other actions: antibiotic, antimicrobial activity (Cunnick et al., 1993), antitumor activity (Bruneton, 1999; Grover & Yaday, 2004), antilymphoma, antileukemic activity (Raman et al., 1996; Grover & Yaday, 2004), inhibits replication of viruses (polio, herpes simplex I, HIV) (Cunnick et al., 1993; Raman et al., 1996), has antifertility activity in animals (no human research available)

Nutritional Ingredients: Edible fruit contains vitamins (riboflavin, niacin, ascorbic acid) and fatty acids.

Traditional Use
- Bitter melon is used in Asia, Fiji, India, Jamaica, Mexico, Thailand, and the Caribbean for treating diabetes (Ross, 1999)
- It is used as an emmenagogue and abortifacient in the Bahamas, Australia, Brazil, Congo, Costa Rica, India, and East Africa.
- It is widely used as an anthelmintic for worms, to treat fevers (especially malaria) and gastric ulcers, and is used topically for decubitus ulcers, to relieve itching, and for snake bites (Ross, 1999).

Current Use
- Reduces blood sugar, improves glucose tolerance, reduces glycosylated hemoglobin, increases glucose utilization; does not promote insulin secretion (Ahmad et al., 1999; Platel et al., 1997; Sarkar et al., 1996; Tongia et al., 2004)
- Antiviral for HIV (experimental studies are being conducted) and herpes simplex I. It also exhibits antibacterial and antiprotozoal effects (Grover & Yaday, 2004).

- Inhibits *H. pylori*, which gives credence to its traditional use for gastric ulcers (Grover & Yadav, 2004)
- Momordica leaf extract has been shown (in vitro) to inhibit p-glycoprotein and reverse cancer cell multidrug resistance (MDR) (Limtrakul et al., 2004). It has also shown (in one human case) the ability to increase hemoglobin and reduce white blood cells in a patient with lymphacytic leukemia (Ross, 1999). Many in vitro and several in vivo (mouse and human) studies suggest that the herb has antitumor activity (Ross, 1999).

Available Forms, Dosage, and Administration Guidelines
- *Juice:* 1 to 2 oz daily
- *Powder:* 100 mg, up to three times a day, in capsules

Pharmacokinetics—If Available (form or route when known): None known

Toxicity: None known but may reduce blood sugar in susceptible patients

Contraindications: Patients with diabetes should take this herb under a practitioner's guidance. Contraindicated in hypoglycemia.

Side Effects: GI effects (nausea and vomiting), hypoglycemia

Long-Term Safety: Safe for short-term use (4–8 weeks); no long-term studies available

Use in Pregnancy/Lactation/Children
- Use in pregnancy is not recommended; may increase uterine contractions. More studies are needed.
- Use in children is not recommended. Two children, ages 3 and 4, were given the tea of the leaves and vine in the morning on an empty stomach. One to 2 hours later, they both experienced convulsions followed by a coma. Blood glucose was 1 mM (normal range 3.8–5.5 mM). Both children recovered after emergency treatment (Raman et al., 1996).

Drug/Herb Interactions and Rationale (if known):
Momordica extract was given concurrently with metformin and glibenclamide and strongly potentiated their hypoglycemic

effects (Tongia et al., 2004). This can be useful as long as the practitioner is aware of this and reduces the dosage of the prescription medication. It can be a problem if the patient adds this herb to an established drug regimen without notifying the practitioner. Severe hypoglycemia could result.

BIBLIOGRAPHY

Ahmad N, et al. (1999). Effect of *Momordica charantia* (Karolla) extracts on fasting and postprandial serum glucose levels in NIDDM patients. *Bangladesh Medical Research Council Bulletin.* Apr;25(1):11–13.

Bruneton J. (1999). *Pharmacognosy, Phytochemistry, Medicinal Plants* (2nd ed.; p. 220). Paris: Lavoisier.

Chaturvedi P, et al. (2004). Effect of *Momordica charantia* on lipid profile and oral glucose tolerance in diabetic rats. *Phytotherapy Research.* Nov;18(11):954–955.

Chevallier A. (1996). *Encyclopedia of Medicinal Plants* (p. 234). New York: DK Publishing.

Cunnick J, et al. (1993). Bitter melon (*Momordica charantia*). *Journal of Natural Medicine.* 4(1):16–21.

Der Marderosian A, Beutler J. [Eds.]. (2004). *The Review of Natural Products.* St. Louis, MO: Facts and Comparisons.

Grover JK, Yaday SP. (2004). Pharmacological actions and potential uses of *Momordica charantia*: A review. *Journal of Ethnopharmacology.* Jul;93(1):123–132.

Handa G, et al. (1990). Hypoglycemic principle of *Momordica charantia* seeds. *Indian Journal of Natural Products.* 6(1):16–19.

Harinantenaina L, et al. (2006). *Momordica charantia* constituents and antidiabetic screening of the isolated major compounds. *Chemical and Pharmaceutical Bulletin.* Jul;54(7):1017–1021.

Leatherdale B, et al. (June 6, 1981). Improvement in glucose tolerance due to *Momordica charantia*. *British Medical Journal.* 282(6279):1823–1824.

Limtrakul P, et al. (2004). Inhibition of p-glycoprotein activity and reversal of cancer multidrug resistance by *Mormordica charantia* extract. *Cancer Chemotherapy and Pharmacology.* Dec;54(6):525–530.

Platel K, et al. (1997). Plant foods in the management of diabetes mellitus: Vegetables as potential hypoglycaemic agents. *Nahrung.* 41(2):68–74.

Raman A, et al. (1996). Anti-diabetic properties and phytochemistry of *Momordica charantia* L. (Cucurbitaceae). *Phytomedicine.* 2(4):349–362.

Ross, I. (1999). *Medicinal Plants of the World*, Vol. I (pp. 213–229). Totowa, NJ: Humana Press.

Sarkar S, et al. (January 1996). Demonstration of the hypogycemic action of *Momordica charantia* in a validated animal model of diabetes. *Pharmacology Research*. 33(1):1–4.

Tongia A, et al. (2004). Phytochemical determination and extraction of *Momordica charantia* fruit and its hypoglycemic potentiation of oral hypoglycemic drugs in diabetes mellitus (NIDDM). *Indian Journal of Physiology and Pharmacology*. Apr;48(2):241–244.

NAME: Black Cohosh (*Actaea racemosa*, syn. *Cimicifuga racemosa*)

Common Names: Black snakeroot, bugbane, rattleroot, rattle weed

Family: *Ranunculaceae*

Description of Plant

- A striking plant, 3′ to 9′ tall, with deeply divided trilobate leaflets, it grows in hardwood forests in both the United States and Canada.
- Grows at edges of woods, from southern Ontario to Arkansas and northern Georgia.
- Member of the buttercup family
- Has long spikes of small white flowers; blooms from July to September

Medicinal Part: Rhizome (dug in the autumn)

Constituents and Action (if known)

- Triterpene glycosides decrease vascular spasm and reduce blood pressure; actein, racemoside, cimicifugoside, 27-deoxyacetin
- Polyphenolic compounds: acteaolactone, cimicifugic acid G, caffeic acid, ferulic acid, fukinolic acid, cimicifugic acids (A, D, D–F); antioxidants (Nuntanakorn et al., 2006)
- Salicylic acid
- Other actions
  - Luteinizing hormone and follicle-stimulating hormone levels remain normal; possible mechanism of action may be at level of neurotransmitters in the brain (Foster, 1999; Freudenstein & Bodinet, 1999).

- Does not stimulate estrogen-positive tumor growth. It actually inhibits proliferation of human breast cell lines by inducing apoptosis (Hostanska et al., 2004).
- Methanol extracts: bind to estrogen receptors (Liske & Wustenberg, 1998).
- The estrogen-like activity was believed to be due to the presence of an isoflavone-formononetin. Very careful and sensitive chemical analysis reveals that there is no formononetin in black cohosh (Jiang et al., 2006).

Nutritional Ingredients: None known

Traditional Use

- Antispasmodic, anti-inflammatory, analgesic, emmenagogue, antirheumatic, sedative
- Native Americans used it to treat arthritic joints/inflammation, fevers, and reproductive conditions, including menstrual and menopausal symptoms, as well as for stimulating childbirth. It has been used to treat menopausal women in the United States, Canada, Great Britain, and Australia since the early to mid 19th century.
- Used for bronchial spasms and coughs associated with bronchitis, pertussis, and pneumonia
- Eclectic physicians used it for uterine neuralgia, migraines associated with menses, muscle spasms, optic neuralgia, muscle pain associated with influenza, lumbago, and chronic, deep-seated muscle pain.

Current Use

- Helps to control signs and changes of menopause and those related to surgical removal of ovaries. Lengthens cycles. Fifty percent to 60% of women have reduction in symptoms in 6 to 8 weeks (Lieberman, 1998). Has worked best for women with moderate to severe symptoms (Frei-Kleiner et al., 2005), and it has been effective as low-dose transdermal estradiol (Nappi et al., 2005).
  - Reduces number and severity of hot flashes (Nappi et al., 2005)
  - Increases strength of pelvic floor muscles
  - Reduces depression, irritability, fatigue (Nappi et al., 2005)

- ○ Reduces vaginal dryness; has weak estrogen-like effects on the vaginal mucosa (Wuttke et al., 2006).
- ○ Reduces formication (skin crawling) (Nappi et al., 2005)
- ○ Alleviates insomnia and promotes sleep; has a calming effect, may be useful for menopausal insomnia (waking during the night and having difficulty falling back asleep)
- ○ A combination of black cohosh and St. John's wort reduced menopausal hot flashes by 50% and menopausal depression by 41.8% (Uebelhack et al., 2006).
- Anti-inflammatory for arthritis, especially of the muscles (fibromyalgia, bursitis), sciatica, and trigeminal neuralgia (Winston, 2006)
- Helpful during labor when a woman is irritated or very tired. Small doses under the tongue are used.
- Painful menses (dysmenorrhea) and ovulatory pain (mittelschmerz). Works well in women with low back pain.
- Lessens symptoms of endometriosis; stops spasm of uterus, reduces uterine pain, lengthens cycles
- Inhibits bone loss resulting from hormonal changes (Hunter, 2000). It stimulates osteoblast activity (Wuttke et al., 2006).
- Research has demonstrated that black cohosh can block estrogen's ability to promote tumor growth (Hostanska et al., 2004). This effect is increased with concurrent use of tamoxifen (Foster, 1999; Freudenstein & Bodinet, 1999).
- This herb has traditionally been used for prostatic and testicular pain. Recent animal studies show that *Cimicifuga* can inhibit alpha-reductase, alpha-dihydrotestosterone, and insulin-like growth factor. This data suggests that this herb may also be useful for preventing BPH and treating prostate cancer (Seidlova-Wuttke et al., 2006b).

Available Forms, Dosage, and Administration Guidelines
Preparations: Dried root, capsules, tablets, tinctures. Standardized products are available.
Typical Dosage
- *Dried root:* 1 to 2 g
- *Capsules:* Three 500-mg capsules a day of the dried root. Remifemin, a brand-name standardized extract (standardized

to 27-deoxyacetin), has been used in Germany since the 1950s for menopause symptoms (40–80 mg a day).
- *Tincture* (1:2, 60% alcohol): 10 to 20 gtt (0.5–1 mL) two to four times a day
- *Tea:* 1 tsp dried root to 8 oz boiling water, decoct 10 minutes, steep 45 minutes; take 4 oz twice a day
- *Powdered root or as tea:* 1 to 2 g

Pharmacokinetics—If Available (form or route when known): None

Toxicity: Relatively safe in normal therapeutic doses (see Long-Term Safety)

Contraindications: None known

Side Effects
- Dizziness, headaches (frontal), and visual disturbance, usually with doses of more than 8 mL/day or with higher doses of the standardized extracts
- Nausea, vomiting in overdose
- Hypotension, usually from overdose
- Can increase or start bleeding again during menopause by stimulating ovarian function. Perimenopausal bleeding should be assessed to rule out possible disease.

Long-Term Safety: There are a number of case reports, especially from Europe, linking use of black cohosh to hepatotoxicity. Many European countries now require a warning label on this product. Considering the number of women using *Cimicifuga*, the incidence of liver damage seems quite rare. When experts have analyzed the existing data, they have found that it is weak and a causal link cannot be established based on the current data (Blumenthal, 2006). A year-long study of a black cohosh extract found that it had no negative effects on endometrial tissue (Raus et al., 2006).

Use in Pregnancy/Lactation/Children
- Do not use if pregnant: increases risk of spontaneous abortion. Used in the last 2 weeks of pregnancy as a partus preparator by many midwives, herbalists, and naturopathic physicians.
- Use in children is not advised.

Drug/Herb Interactions and Rationale (if known)

- May have an additive effect with antihypertensives. Use carefully.
- Human studies found that black cohosh did not affect CYP3A4 (Gurley et al., 2006a) nor did it affect digoxin pharmacokinetics (Gurley et al., 2006b).

Special Notes: Previously, it was thought that black cohosh suppressed luteinizing hormone, had estrogenic effects, contained compounds similar to estrogen, and should not be used in women with estrogen-positive tumors. Scientific proof has negated each of these concepts.

BIBLIOGRAPHY

Blumenthal M. (2006). European health agencies recommend liver warnings on black cohosh products—ABC, herb experts and NIH workshop find no direct causal relationship between popular menopause remedy and rare reports of liver problems. *HerbalGram*. 72:56–58.

Duker E, et al. (1991). Effects of extracts from *Cimicifuga racemosa* on gonadotropin release in menopausal women and ovariectomized rats. *Planta Medica*. 57(5):420–424.

Foster S. (1999). Black cohosh: A literature review. *HerbalGram*. Winter, 45:35–49.

Frei-Kleiner S, et al. (2005). *Cimicifuga racemosa* dried ethanolic extract in menopausal disorders: A double-blind, placebo-controlled clinical trial. *Maturitas*. Aug 16;51(4):397–404.

Freudenstein J, Bodinet C. (1999). Influence of an isopropanolic aqueous extract of *Cimicifuga racemosa* rhizoma on the proliferation of MCF-7 cells. Abstracts of 23rd International LOF-Symposium on Phytoestrogens, Jan. 15, 1999, University of Ghent, Belgium.

Gurley B, et al. (2006a). Assessing the clinical significance of botanical supplementation on human cytochrome P450 3A activity: Comparison of a milk thistle and black cohosh to rafampin and clarithromycin. *Journal of Clinical Pharmacology*. Feb;46(2):201–213.

Gurley B, et al. (2006b). Effect of milk thistle (*Silybum marianum*) and black cohosh (*Cimicifuga racemosa*) supplementation on digoxin pharmacokinetics in humans. *Drug Metabolism and Disposition*. Jan;34(1):69–74.

Hostanska K, et al. (2004). *Cimicifuga racemosa* Extract inhibits proliferation of estrogen receptor-positive and negative human breast carcinoma cell lines by induction of apoptosis. *Breast Cancer Research and Treatment*. Mar;84(2):151–160.

Hunter A. (2000). *Cimicifuga racemosa*; pharmacology, clinical trials and clinical use. *European Journal of Herbal Medicine*. 5(1):19–25.

Jiang B, et al. (2006). Analysis of formononetin from black cohosh (*Actaea racemosa*). *Phytomedicine*. Jul;13(7):477–486.

Lieberman S. (1998). A review of the effectiveness of *Cimicifuga racemosa* (black cohosh) for the symptoms of menopause. *Journal of Women's Health*. Jun;7(5):525–529.

Liske E. (1998). Therapeutic efficacy and safety of *Cimicifuga racemosa* for gynecologic disorders. *Advances in Therapy*. 15(1):45–53.

Liske E, Wustenberg P. (1998). Therapy of climacteric complaints with *Cimicifuga racemosa:* Herbal medicine with clinically proven evidence. *Menopause*. 5(4):250.

Liske E, Wustenberg P. (1999). Efficacy and safety for phytomedicines for gynecological disorders with particular reference to *Cimicifuga racemosa* and *Hypericum perforatum*. First Asian-European Congress on the Menopause, Bangkok, 1998.

Mahady GB. (2005). Black cohosh (*Actaea/Cimicifuga racemosa*): Review of the clinical data for safety and efficacy in menopausal symptoms. *Treatments in Endocrinology*. 4(3):177–184.

Mills S, Bone K. (2000). *Principles and Practice of Phytotherapy* (pp. 303–309). Edinburgh: Churchill Livingstone.

Nappi RE, et al. (2005). Efficacy of *Cimicifuga racemosa* on climacteric complaints: A randomized study versus low-dose transdermal estradiol. *Gynecological Endocrinology*. Jan;20(1):30–35.

Nuntanakorn P, et al. (2006). Polyphenolic constituents of *Actaea racemosa*. *Journal of Natural Products*. Mar;69(3):314–318.

Raus K, et al. (2006). First-time proof of endometrial safety of the special black cohosh extract (*Actaea* or *Cimicifuga reacemosa* extract) CR BNO 1055. *Menopause*. Jul-Aug;13(4):678–691.

Seidlova-Wuttke D, et al. (2006a). Inhibition of 5 alpha-reductase in the rat prostate by *Cimicifuga racemosa*. *Maturitas*. 55[Suppl. 1]:S75–S82.

Seidlova-Wuttke D, et al (2006b). Inhibitory effects of a black cohosh (*Cimicifuga racemosa*) extract on prostate cancer. *Planta Medica*. May;72(6):521–526.

Struck D, et al. (1997). Flavones in extracts of *Cimicifuga racemosa*. *Planta Medica*. 63(31):289.

Uebelhack R, et al. (2006). Black cohosh and St. John's wort for climacteric complaints: A randomized trial. *Obstetrics and Gynecology*. Feb;107[2 Pt. 1]:247–255.

Winston D. (2006) *Winston's Botanic Materia Medica*. Washington, NJ: DWCHS

Wuttke W, et al. (2006). Effects of black cohosh (*Cimicifuga racemosa*) on bone turnover, vaginal mucosa, and various blood parameters in postmenopausal women: A double-blind, placebo-controlled, and conjugated estrogens-controlled study. *Menopause*. Mar-Apr;13(2):185–196.

NAME: Black Haw Bark (*Viburnum prunifolium*)

Common Names: Nannybush, wild raisin

Family: *Caprifoliaceae*

Description of Plant

- A small, shrubby, deciduous tree native to eastern North America
- Blooms in the spring with a flat cluster of white flowers, followed by purplish-black fruits

Medicinal Part: Root and stem bark

Constituents and Action (if known)

- Biflavone (amentoflavone): mildly spasmolytic
- Iridoid glycosides (2^1-0-acetyl-dihydropenstemide, patrinoside, 2^1-0-p-coumaroyl-dihydropenstemide, 2^1-0-acetylpatrinoside): uterine and intestinal antispasmodics (Upton, 2000)
- Coumarins scopoletin: spasmolytic, may effect a blockade of autonomic neurotransmitters, causing relaxation of smooth muscle (Upton, 2000); scopolin, aesculetin: spasmolytic
- Triterpenes: oleanolic acid, ursolic acid
- Tannins

Nutritional Ingredients: Edible berries

Traditional Use

- Antispasmodic, anodyne, astringent, mild hypotensive, bitter tonic, uterine tonic, uterine sedative, nervine
- Medicinal uses were learned from Native Americans, who used the bark for gastric upsets, female reproductive problems, childbirth, and muscle spasms.
- Used by eclectic physicians as a partus preparator, to alleviate postpartum pain and bleeding, to treat dysmenorrhea, and to prevent miscarriage. They also used it for diarrhea, intestinal spasms, and cardiac palpitations (Ellingwood, 1919).
- Herbalists used black haw for premenstrual irritability, spasms of the bladder and diaphragm, spasmodic coughing, asthma, hiccoughs, and spasmodic testicular pain.

Current Use
- A uterine antispasmodic useful for dysmenorrhea, pelvic congestion syndrome, low back pain associated with menses, and vaginismus. Works well with Roman chamomile, Jamaica dogwood, and black cohosh (Winston, 2006).
- Commonly used by midwives, herbalists, and naturopathic physicians to prevent miscarriage during the first and second trimester (Hoffmann, 2003).
- Can be used to control postpartum bleeding and pain, combined with yarrow, cinnamon, or shepherd's purse.
- Bark is effective for abdominal spasms, especially chronic hiccoughs, hiatus hernia, and gastric or intestinal cramps.
- Can be useful for venospasm and as an adjunctive treatment for mild to moderate hypertension (Hoffmann, 2003). Use with motherwort, hawthorn, garlic, olive leaf, dandelion leaf, or linden flower.

Available Forms, Dosage, and Administration Guidelines
- *Dried bark:* 2 to 6 g
- *Tea:* 1 to 2 tsp dried bark, 8 oz water, decoct 15 to 20 minutes, steep 30 minutes; take two or three cups a day
- *Capsules:* Two or three 500-mg capsules three times a day
- *Fresh tincture* (1:2, 40% alcohol): 80 to 160 gtt (4–8 mL) three times a day; smaller doses can be taken more frequently
- *Tincture* (1:5, 40% alcohol): 80 to 160 gtt (4–8 mL) three times a day; smaller doses can be taken more frequently

Pharmacokinetics—If Available (form or route when known): Not known

Toxicity: Safe

Contraindications: Because of the presence of oxalate acid, avoid using in patients who have kidney stones or a history of them (McGuffin et al., 1997).

Side Effects: Nausea and vomiting with large amounts

Long-Term Safety: Safe in normal therapeutic doses

Use in Pregnancy/Lactation/Children: Black haw has long been used to prevent miscarriage, and no adverse effects have been reported. No adverse effects are expected in lactating women or children.

Drug/Herb Interactions and Rationale (if known): None known

Special Notes: Has a long history of empirical use as an antispasmodic, and animal studies have confirmed this activity

BIBLIOGRAPHY

Cometa MF, et al. (1998). Preliminary studies on cardiovascular activity of *Viburnum prunifolium L.* and its iridoid glucosides. *Fitoterapia.* 69(5):23.

Ellingwood F. (1919). *American Materia Medica, Therapeutics, and Pharmacognosy* (pp. 474–476). Evanston, IL: Ellingwood's Therapeutist.

Hoffmann D. (2003). *Medical Herbalism* (pp. 593–594). Rochester, VT: Healing Arts Press.

Leung A, Foster S. (1996). *Encyclopedia of Common Natural Products* (2nd ed.; pp. 89–90). New York: John Wiley & Sons.

McGuffin M, et al. (1997). *Botanical Safety Handbook* (p. 122). Boca Raton, FL: CRC Press.

Moermann DE. (1998). *Native American Ethnobotany* (p. 595). Portland, OR: Timber Press.

Tomassini L, et al. (1998). Iridoid glucosides from *Viburnum prunifolium* and preliminary pharmacological studies. Proceedings of the Societa Italiana di Fitochimica 9th National Congress, Florence, Italy.

Upton R. [Ed.]. (2000). *American Herbal Pharmacopoeia and Therapeutic Compendium: Black Haw Bark.* Santa Cruz, CA: AHP.

Wichtl M, Bissett NG. [Eds.]. (1994). *Herbal Drugs and Phytopharmaceuticals* (pp. 525–526). Stuttgart: Medpharm Science.

Winston D. (2006). *Winston's Botanica Materia Medica.* Washington, NJ: DWCHS.

 NAME: Blessed Thistle (*Cnicus benedictus*)

Common Names: Cardo Santo thistle, holy thistle, Chardon, St. Benedict thistle

Family: *Asteraceae*

Description of Plant
- Small, annual thistle found primarily in Europe
- Has small yellow flowers, and the leaves have weak, innocuous spines, unlike many of the more prickly thistles

Medicinal Part: Leaves and flowers

Constituents and Action (if known)

- Sesquiterpene lactones
  - Cnicin (bitter compound) has antibacterial activity (Barrero et al., 1997; Skenderi, 2003), stimulates taste buds, increases secretion of saliva and gastric juice and appetite (Bradley, 1992)
  - Salonitenolide (Gruenwald et al., 1998)
- Lignan lactones (lignanalides): trachelogenin, arctigenin, nortracheloside
- Tannins (8%)
- High mineral content (K^+, Mg^{++}, Ca^{++}, manganese)
- Flavonoids
- Volatile oils

Nutritional Ingredients: Ca^{++}, Mg^{++}, K^+, manganese

History: Originally cultivated in monastery gardens and was considered a panacea, thus the epithet *benedictus*

Traditional Use

- Bitter tonic and cholagogue, antipyretic, antibacterial, aperient, galactagogue
- It is used to enhance digestion and absorption, for poor fat digestion, anorexia, and biliousness
- It was used in England to help pubescent girls who had delayed puberty and a lack of breast development

Current Use

- Cholagogue: for inadequate bile secretion, clay-colored stools, and poor fat digestion with elevated blood lipids
- It is used to treat dyspepsia and biliousness with nausea, flatulence, bloating, and constipation.
- Loss of appetite: stimulates secretion of saliva and gastric juices, useful for achlorhydria, along with orange peel, angelica, and dandelion root (Winston, 2006)

Available Forms, Dosage, and Administration Guidelines

Preparations: Dried herb, capsules, tablets, tonics, tinctures
Typical Dosage
- *Capsules:* Three 500- to 600-mg capsules a day

- *Tea:* Steep 1 to 2 tsp dried herb in 8 oz of hot water for 10 to 15 minutes; take 2 to 4 oz up to three times a day 15 minutes before meals; or follow practitioner's recommendations.
- *Tincture* (1:5, 30% alcohol): 30 to 80 gtt (1.5–4 mL) three times a day
- *Fluid extract:* (1:1 g/mL), 2 mL three times a day

Pharmacokinetics—If Available (form or route when known): None known

Toxicity: None known

Contraindications: None known

Side Effects
- Nausea, vomiting with excess dosage
- Contact dermatitis
- Allergic reaction: possible cross sensitivity to other members of the *Asteraceae* family (feverfew, mugwort, chamomile)
- Avoid use in women who have PMS-induced breast tenderness, as it may exacerbate symptoms (Winston, 2006).

Long-Term Safety: Long history of use in European herbal medicine and in liquors. No safety issues expected at usual therapeutic doses.

Use in Pregnancy/Lactation/Children: Not recommended (Blumenthal et al., 2000; McGuffin, 1997). Blessed thistle has a long history of use as a galactogogue to stimulate milk flow, so safe during lactation.

Drug/Herb Interactions and Rationale (if known): None known

Special Notes: Little scientific research is available on this herb.

BIBLIOGRAPHY

Barrero AF, et al. (1997). Biomimetic cyclization of cnicin to malacitanolide, a bytotoxic eudesmanolide from *Centaurea malacitana. Journal of Natural Products.* 60:1034–1035.

Blumenthal M, et al. (2000). *Herbal Medicine: Expanded Commission E Monographs* (pp. 27–29). Austin: American Botanical Council.

Bradley PR. [Ed.]. (1992). *British Herbal Compendium*, Vol. 1 (pp. 126–127). Bournemouth: British Herbal Medicine Association.

Gruenwald J, et al. (2004). *PDR for Herbal Medicines* (pp. 111–112). Montvale, NJ: Medical Economics Co.

McGuffin T. (1997). *Botanical Safety Handbook* (p. 33). Boca Raton, FL: CRC Press.

Reynolds JEF, et al. [Eds.]. (1996). *Martindale, The Extra Pharmacopoeia* (31st ed.). London: Royal Pharmaceutical Society of Great Britain.

Skenderi G. (2003). *Herbal Vade Mecum* (pp. 53–54). Rutherford, NJ: Herbacy Press.

Winston D. (2006). *Winston's Botanic Materia Medica*. Washington, NJ: DWCHS.

 NAME: Blue Cohosh (*Caulophyllum thalictroides*)

Common Names: Blue ginseng, papoose root

Family: *Berberidaceae*

Description of Plant
- Perennial herb that grows to 2′ to 3′; has small pale yellow-green flowers
- Forest plant that grows from Georgia to Canada

Medicinal Part: Dried rhizome

Constituents and Action (if known)
- Triterpene saponins: caulosaponin and caulophyllosaponin are uterine stimulants; can constrict coronary blood vessels; in rats, can inhibit ovulation (Baillie & Rasmussen, 1997; Gunn & Wright, 1996)
- Quinolizidine alkaloids
  - *N*-methylcytisine: a quinolizidine alkaloid, pharmacologically similar to nicotine (10%–40% less active), which can raise blood pressure and stimulate small intestine and may cause hyperglycemia. Teratogenic in in vitro rat embryo culture (Kennelly et al., 1999). Also contains anagyrine and baptifoline, which are teratogenic.
  - Taspine: embryo toxicity in in vitro rat embryo culture (Kennelly et al., 1999), stimulates topical wound healing (Dong et al., 2005)

- Magnoflorine (aporphine alkaloid): hypotensive, uterine stimulant (Der Marderosian & Beutler, 2004).

Nutritional Ingredients: None known

Traditional Use
- Native Americans used small amounts of a decoction for several weeks before birth to ease delivery.
- The eclectic physicians used it to treat spasmodic pain, arthritis of the small joints (fingers, toes, wrists), uterine pain with fullness, amenorrhea, dysmenorrhea, ovarian pain, pain due to uterine prolapse, and to stimulate labor (Ellingwood, 1919).
- Used to induce sweating and lower fevers

Current Use
- Menstrual disorders (amenorrhea, dysmenorrhea), premenstrual symptoms, mastalgia, ovarian pain, mittelschmerz, functional ovarian cysts, pain of endometriosis (Winston, 2006)
- Used by skilled midwives to stimulate labor and to help pass the placenta after delivery (usually mixed with other herbs); the safety of this practice is questionable.

Available Forms, Dosage, and Administration Guidelines
Preparations: Dried root, cut and sifted; capsules, tablets, tinctures, combination products, teas
Typical Dosage
- *Dried root:* 0.3 to 1 g three times a day
- *Capsule:* 1 (00) capsule two times a day
- *Tincture* (1:5, 60% alcohol): 5 to 20 gtt (0.25–1 mL) up to three times a day

Pharmacokinetics—If Available (form or route when known): None known

Toxicity
- May cause congestive heart failure in newborns when used prepartum
- Overdose causes symptoms similar to nicotine overdose. In a 2002 case report, a woman who used blue cohosh to attempt to induce abortion developed tachycardia, sweating,

abdominal pain, vomiting, and muscle weakness (Rao & Hoffmann, 2002).

- Poisoning has been reported in children after ingestion of blue fruits.
- Ingestion of the fresh plant or root can cause gastritis.

Contraindications

- Avoid in pregnancy or when trying to get pregnant; may act as an abortifacient.
- Taken as a partus preparator, it has been associated with congestive heart failure in newborns (Jones & Lawson, 1998).
- Avoid in heart disease

Side Effects

- May inhibit luteinizing hormone release and ovulation (may have some benefit as a contraceptive, but more research is needed)
- GI irritation, diarrhea, cramping
- Hypertension

Long-Term Safety: Unknown. Not recommended for long-term daily use. Recent concerns about congestive heart failure in newborns create serious doubts as to the safety of using blue cohosh as a partus preparatory or to stimulate labor. There are indications that at least in some of the cases reported, patients were taking this herb in double the normal dose.

Use in Pregnancy/Lactation/Children

- Do not use during pregnancy; appropriate only after labor has begun
- Contraindicated during lactation and in children

Drug/Herb Interactions and Rationale (if known)

- May increase side effects and toxicity of nicotine products. If used concurrently, observe for possible potentiation.
- Theoretical possibility of interaction with antihypertensives and antiangina agents exists. Use cautiously.

Special Notes: When used in small, appropriate doses by clinicians for short periods of time in healthy adults (men and nonpregnant women), blue cohosh may be a relatively safe and useful herb. More research is needed.

BIBLIOGRAPHY

Baillie N, Rasmussen P. (1997). Black and blue cohosh in labor. *New Zealand Medical Journal*. 110:20–21.

Bone K. (2000). Adverse reaction reports. *Modern Phytotherapist*. 5(3):11–16.

Der Marderosian A, Beutler J. [Eds.]. (2004). *The Review of Natural Products*. St. Louis, MO: Facts and Comparisons.

Dong Y, et al. (2005). Enhancement of wound healing by taspine and its effect on fibroblast. *Zhong Yao Cai*. Jul;28(7):579–582.

Elder NC, et al. (March/April 1997). Use of alternative health care by family practice patients. *Archives of Family Medicine*. 6:181–184.

Ellingwood F. (1919). *American Materia Medica, Therapeutics, and Pharmacognosy* (pp. 480–481). Evanston, IL: Ellingwood's Therapeutist.

Gunn TR, Wright IMR. (1996). The use of blue and black cohosh in labour. *New Zealand Medical Journal*. 109:410–411.

Jones TK, Lawson BM. (1998). Profound neonatal congestive heart failure caused by maternal consumption of blue cohosh herbal medication. *Journal of Pediatrics*. 132[3 Pt. 1]:550–552.

Kennelly EJ, et al. (1999). Detecting potential teratogenic alkaloids from blue cohosh rhizomes using an in vitro rat embryo culture. *Journal of Natural Products*. 62(10):1385–1389.

Rao RB, Hoffmann RS. (2002). Nicotinic toxicity from tincture of blue cohosh (*Caulophyllum thalictroides*) used as an abortifacient. *Veterinary and Human Toxicology*. Aug;44(4):221–222.

Winston D. (2006). *Winston's Botanic Materia Medica*. Washington, NJ: DWCHS.

Wright IM. (1999). Neonatal effects of maternal consumption of blue cohosh. *Journal of Pediatrics*. 134(3):384–385.

 NAME: Borage (*Borago officinalis*)

Common Names: Common borage, beebread, starflower, ox's tongue

Family: *Boraginaceae*

Description of Plant
- Hardy annual that grows 2′ tall and is covered with coarse hairs
- Has oval leaves and star-shaped bright-blue flowers with black anthers

- Flowers bloom from May to September.
- Grows throughout Europe and is cultivated in North America
- Has cucumber-like odor and taste

Medicinal Part: Borage seed oil, herb

Constituents and Action (if known)
Herb

- Mucilage: may cause expectorant effect
- Malic acid and potassium nitrate: cause mild diuretic effect (Awang, 1990)
- Rosmarinic acid: antioxidant (Bandoniene et al., 2005)
- Tannins
- Pyrrolizidine alkaloids: potentially hepatotoxic

Seed Oil: Fatty acids are a source of gamma-linolenic acid (GLA), which may reduce prostaglandins (E_1), inhibit platelet aggregation, and have anti-inflammatory properties (Engler et al., 1992; Fan & Chapkin, 1998; Karlstad et al., 1993; Leventhal et al., 1993; Pullman-Mooar et al., 1990).

Nutritional Ingredients

- Flowers can be used to garnish salads.
- Stems and leaves have been eaten raw or cooked like spinach.
- Seeds contain gamma-linolenic acid, a dietary source of essential fatty acids (Leung & Foster, 1996).

Traditional Use

- No traditional use for the seed oil
- Adrenal tonic, galactagogue, demulcent, diuretic, refrigerant
- Leaves and flowers were seeped in wine to dispel melancholy.
- The herb is used by European herbalists as a mild adaptogenic tonic to the HPA axis. It is still frequently used in the UK for mental exhaustion and adrenal depletion. The leaf was also used to treat gastric and urinary tract irritation, coughs, and sore throats.

Current Use: Borage seed oil is a source of GLA, which has been studied as an anti-inflammatory. Studies indicate that the seed oil can relieve dry skin in the elderly (Brosche & Platt, 2000), improve infantile seborrhea (Tollesson & Frithz,

1993), and reduce symptoms of rheumatoid arthritis (Kast, 2001). It may also have benefit for PMS symptoms and atopic eczema.

Available Forms, Dosage, and Administration Guidelines: Capsules contain borage seed oil, which is 20% to 26% gamma-linolenic acid. Typical dosage is three or four 300-mg capsules a day, or follow manufacturer or practitioner recommendations.

Pharmacokinetics—If Available (form or route when known): None known

Toxicity: Seed oil is not associated with toxicity. Leaf contains potentially hepatoxic pyrrolizidine alkaloids (supinin, lycopsamin).

Contraindications: None known

Side Effects: None

Long-Term Safety: Appears safe. Canadian government has approved this product as a dietary supplement.

Use in Pregnancy/Lactation/Children: The seed oil appears safe; approved as a dietary supplement with no restrictions. Avoid using the herb while pregnant, nursing, or with young children (Brinker, 2001).

Drug/Herb Interactions and Rationale (if known): One researcher has postulated that concurrent use of NSAIDs would interfere with the effects of borage seed oil (Kast, 2001). Additional research is needed to determine the accuracy of his assertions.

BIBLIOGRAPHY

Awang DVC. (1990). Herbal medicine: Borage. *Canadian Pharmacy Journal*. 123:121.

Bandoniene D, et al. (2005). Determination of rosmarinic acid in sage and borage leaves by high-performance liquid chromatography with different detection methods. *Journal of Chromatographic Science*. Aug:43(7):372–376.

Bard JM, et al. (1997). A therapeutic dosage (3 g/day) of borage oil supplementation has no effect on platelet aggregation in healthy volunteers. *Fundamentals of Clinical Pharmacology*. 11(2):143–144.

Bartram T. (1995). *Encyclopedia of Herbal Medicine* (p. 65). Dorset: Grace Publishers.

Brinker F. (2001). *Herb Contraindications and Drug Interactions* (pp. 46–47). Sandy, OR: Eclectic Medical Publications.

Brosche R, Platt D. (2000). Effect of borage oil consumption on fatty acid metabolism, transepidermal water loss and skin parameters in elderly people. *Archives of Gerontology and Geriatrics*. Mar-Apr;30(2):139–150.

Engler MM, et al. (1992). Dietary gamma-linolenic acid lowers blood pressure and alters aortic reactivity and cholesterol metabolism in hypertension. *Journal of Hypertension*. 10(10):1197–1204.

Fan YY, Chapkin RS. (1998). Importance of dietary gamma-linolenic acid in human health and nutrition. *Journal of Nutrition*. 128:1411–1414.

Henz BM, et al. (1999). Double-blind, multicentre analysis of the efficacy of borage oil in patients with atopic eczema. *British Journal of Dermatology*. 140(4):685–688.

Karlstad MD, et al. (1993). Effect of intravenous lipid emulsions enriched with gamma-linolenic acid on plasma n-6 fatty acids and prostaglandin biosynthesis after burn and endotoxin injury in rats. *Critical Care Medicine*. 21:1740–1749.

Kast RE. (2001). Borage oil reduction of rheumatoid arthritis activity may be mediated by increased cAMP that suppresses tumor necrosis factor-alpha. *International Immunopharmocology*. 2001 Nov;1(12):2197–2199.

Leung A, Foster S. (1996). *Encyclopedia of Common Natural Ingredients* (pp. 98–99) (2nd ed.). New York: John Wiley & Sons.

Leventhal LJ, et al. (1993). Treatment of rheumatoid arthritis with gamma-linolenic acid. *Annals of Internal Medicine*. 119:867–873.

Mancuso P, et al. (1997). Dietary fish oil and fish and borage oil suppress intrapulmonary proinflammatory eicosanoid biosynthesis and attenuate pulmonary neutrophil accumulation in endotoxic rats. *Critical Care Medicine*. 25:1198–1206.

Mills DE. (1989). Dietary fatty acid supplementation alters stress reactivity and performance in man. *Journal of Human Hypertension*. 3:111–116.

Pullman-Mooar S, et al. (1990). Alteration of the cellular fatty acid profile and the production of eicosanoids in human monocytes by gamma-linolenic acid. *Arthritis and Rheumatism*. 33:1526–1533.

Tollesson A, Frithz A. (1993). Borage oil, an effective new treatment for infantile seborrhoeic dermatitis. *British Journal of Dermatology*. 129(1):95.

NAME: Boswellia (*Boswellia serrata*)

Common Names: Shallaki (Sanskrit), sallai guggal (Hindi)

Family: *Burseraceae*

Description of Plant: A small- to medium-sized tree that grows on dry hills throughout most of India but is especially common in the northwestern mountainous region

Medicinal Part: The gum resin that oozes from the bark when the tree is cut

Constituents and Action (if known)
- Triterpene acids (alpha, beta, and gamma boswellic acids)
- Boswellic acids reduce leukotriene formation, which in turn slows progression of inflammatory conditions (Ammon et al., 1993; Banno et al., 2006; Gupta VN et al., 1997; Kulkarni et al., 1991; Wildfeuer et al., 1998). Antiviral: inhibits EBV and is cytotoxic against neuroblastoma cell lines (Akihisa et al., 2006).
  - Reduce morning stiffness and increase joint activity in persons with inflammatory conditions (Kulkarni et al., 1991)
  - Reduce symptoms in asthma (Gupta et al., 1998)
  - Reduce inflammation and increase remission rates in ulcerative colitis (Gupta I et al., 1997)
- Quercetin: blocks proinflammatory 5-lipoxygenase and leukotrienes (Anonymous, *Alternative Medicine Review*, 1998)
- Terpenoids
- EOs (alpha-thujene and p-cymene, alpha-pinene, alpha-phellandrine): antifungal activity (Anonymous, *Selected Medicinal Plants of India*, 1992).

Nutritional Ingredients: None

Traditional Use
- Anti-inflammatory, expectorant, astringent
- Used in Ayurvedic medicine in India to treat liver disease, cancer, diarrhea, dysentery, skin diseases, ulcers, and as a general tonic and blood purifier
- Used as an expectorant and to reduce inflammation in the respiratory tract—coughs, bronchitis, and asthma.
- Used topically to treat boils, wounds, fungal infections, and sores

Current Use

- Inflammatory conditions of the musculoskeletal system: rheumatoid arthritis, osteoarthritis, tendinitis, bursitis, and repetitive motion injuries. Improves blood flow to joints, decreases pain, and increases flexion (Kimmatkar et al., 2003; Kulkarni et al., 1991).
- A multiherb formula consisting of boswellia, turmeric, ginger, and ashwagandha showed significant benefit over placebo for osteoarthritis of the knees (Chopra et al., 2004).
- Grade II or III ulcerative colitis: studies show that this herb is as effective as sulfasalazine (Gupta I et al., 1997; Gupta I et al., 2001).
- In human studies, 40 patients with bronchial asthma were given boswellia for 6 weeks. Significant (moderate or better) improvement was seen in 70% of the participants (Gupta et al., 1998).
- Boswellia is traditionally used in Ayurvedic medicine for treating cancer. In vitro studies suggest that it has antitumor activity and can induce programmed cell death in leukemic cells and in melanoma (Winston, 2006).

Available Forms, Dosage, and Administration Guidelines

- Standardized ethanol extracts containing 60% to 65% boswellic acids: follow label directions
- *Capsule:* (300–400 mg standardized extract): two capsules two or three times a day

Pharmacokinetics—If Available (form or route when known): None known

Toxicity: None known

Contraindications: None known

Side Effects: Occasional mild gastric upset and skin rashes

Long-Term Safety: Safe

Use in Pregnancy/Lactation/Children: Use cautiously in pregnancy.

Drug/Herb Interactions and Rationale (if known): None known

Special Notes: Boswellia is closely related to the gum-resin frankincense. They share similar uses and have many constituents in common.

BIBLIOGRAPHY

Akihisa T, et al. (2006). Cancer chemopreventive effects and cytotoxic activities of the triterpene acids from the resin of *Boswellia carteri*. *Biological and Pharmaceutical Bulletin*. Sep;29(9):1976–1979.

Ammon HPT, et al. (1993). Mechanism of anti-inflammatory actions of curcumine and boswellic acids. *Journal of Ethnopharmacology*. 38:113–119.

Anonymous. (1998). Monograph: *Boswellia serrata*. *Alternative Medicine Review*. 3(4):306–307.

Anonymous. (1992). *Selected Medicinal Plants of India*. (pp. 64–66). Bombay: Chemexeil.

Banno N, et al. (2006). Anti-inflammatory activities of the triterpene acids from the resin of *Boswellia carteri*. *Journal of Ethnopharmacology*. Sep 1;107(2):249–253.

Chopra A, et al. (2004). A 32-week randomized, placebo-controlled clinical evaluation of RA-11, an Ayurvedic drug, on osteoarthritis of the knees. *Journal of Clinical Rheumatology*. Oct;10(5):236–245.

Etzel R. (1996). Special extract of *Boswellia serrata* (H15) in the treatment of rheumatoid arthritis. *Phytomedicine*. 3(1):91–94.

Gupta I, et al. (1997). Effects of *Boswellia serrata* gum resin in patients with ulcerative colitis. *European Journal of Medical Research*. 2(1):37–43.

Gupta I, et al. (1998). Effects of *Boswellia serrata* gum resin in patients with bronchial asthma: Results of a double-blind, placebo-controlled, 6-week clinical study. *European Journal of Medical Research*. 3(11):511–514.

Gupta I, et al. (2001). Effects of gum resin of *Boswellia serrata* in patients with chronic colitis. *Planta Medica*. Jul;67(5):391–395.

Gupta VN, et al. (1997). Chemistry and pharmacology of gum-resin of *Boswellia serrata*. *Indian Drugs*. 24:221–231.

Kimmatkar N, et al. (2003). Efficacy and tolerability of *Boswellia serrata* extract in treatment of osteoarthritis of knee—A randomized double blind placebo controlled trial. *Phytomedicine*. Jan;10(1):3–7.

Kulkarni RR, et al. (1991). Treatment of osteoarthritis with a herbomineral formula: A double-blind, placebo-controlled, cross-over study. *Journal of Ethnopharmacology*. 33 (1-2):91–95.

McCaleb R, et al. (2000). *Encyclopedia of Popular Herbs*. Roseville, CA: Prime Publishing. (pp. 84–89).

Singh BG, Atal CK. (1986). Pharmacology of an extract of sallai guggal ex-boswellia serrata, a new non-steroidal anti-inflammatory agent. *Agents and Actions*. 18(3–4):407–412.

Wildfeuer A, et al. (1998). Effects of boswellic acids extracted from an herbal medicine on the biosynthesis of leukotrienes and the course of experimental autoimmune encephalomyelitis. *Arzneimittelforschung.* 48(6):668–674.

Winston D. (2006). *Winston's Botanic Materia Medica.* Washington, NJ: DWCHS.

NAME: Burdock (*Arctium lappa, A. minus, A. pubens, A. tomentosum*)

Common Names: Beggar's buttons, greater burdock (*A. lappa*), lesser burdock (*A. minus*)

Family: *Asteraceae*

Description of Plant
- Common weed that grows throughout much of the world's temperate regions
- Biennial, with large leaves; grows 3′ to 9′ tall
- Pinkish-purple flowers that develop into a spiny burr containing the seeds

Medicinal Part: Roots (may be 5–6′ long), leaves, seeds

Constituents and Action (if known)
- Polyacetylene compounds: antibacterial activity
- Arctopicrin (bitter component): antibacterial activity
- Bitter glycoside (arctin): reduces symptoms of common cold (Sun, 1992; Wang et al., 1993)
- Lignans: antimutagenic effect (Leung & Foster, 1996), antiproliferative activity against leukemia cells (Matsumoto et al., 2006); cytotoxic (Awale et al., 2006).
- Polyphenolic acids (caffeic, chlorogenic): may decrease urinary stones (Grases et al., 1994)
- Volatile acids (acetic, butyric, isovaleric)
- Fixed oil (from seeds)
- Inulin: a nonabsorbable polysaccharide; source of fructooligosaccharides:prebiotic (Palframan et al., 2002). Also contains fructofuranan, which is an antitussive and immunomodulator (Kardosova et al., 2003).

Nutritional Ingredients

- In Japan, roots are used as a vegetable called *gobo*. The root contains 11% protein, 19% lipids, and 34% inulin (Tadeda et al., 1991).
- The central stalk, with the outer skin removed, is a tasty raw vegetable.
- Young greens can be cooked as a bitter vegetable.

Traditional Use

Internal

- Root
  - Blood purifier (alterative) to treat skin conditions (eczema, psoriasis), cancer, arthritis, and obesity. Burdock root is one of four ingredients in the "cancer formula" known as Essiac.
  - Mild diuretic and laxative
  - Used to stimulate lymphatic circulation, especially with chronically enlarged lymph nodes, mastitis, and lymphedema
- Seed tincture used by eclectic physicians to treat dry, crusty, or scaly skin conditions

Topical: Leaves were used as a poultice or wash to help heal wounds, boils, and styes.

Current Use

- Antimutagenic activity; dietary use may reduce chemically induced carcinogenesis. A number of in vitro and animal studies suggest that the traditional use of this herb for cancer may have some validity (Awale et al., 2006; Kardosova et al., 2003; Matsumoto et al., 2006).
- In animal studies, burdock root enhanced SOD and reduced levels of compounds associated with "wear and tear" and aging, MDA, and lipofuscin in the liver, brain and blood (Liu et al., 2005).
- The leaves are strongly antibacterial, especially topically for furuncles (boils).
- Seeds, called *niu bang zi* in TCM, are used for red, painful sore throats; coughs; mumps; and painful enlarged lymph nodes. The seeds show significant in vitro inhibitory effect against *Streptococcus pneumoniae* and many pathogenic fungi.

Available Forms, Dosage, and Administration Guidelines

Preparations: Dried root, tea, capsules, tablets, tinctures
Typical Dosage

- *Capsules:* Up to six 500- to 600-mg capsules a day
- *Tea:* Steep 1 to 2 tsp dried root in 8 to 10 oz of hot water, decoct 15 to 20 minutes, steep 40 minutes; take up to three times a day.
- *Tincture* (1:5, 30% alcohol): 40 to 90 gtt (2–4 mL) three times a day
- *Seeds:* In TCM, dose averages 3 to 10 g a day.

Pharmacokinetics—If Available (form or route when known): None known

Toxicity: Poisoning has been reported, but this is from contamination with deadly nightshade root. The adverse effects are consistent with atropine toxicity. This type of dangerous adulteration is inexcusable and fortunately rare.

Contraindications: None

Side Effects: Topical: contact dermatitis from handling the plant has been reported (Rodriguez et al., 1995)

Long-Term Safety: Traditional use as a food; no toxicity expected

Use in Pregnancy/Lactation/Children: Uterine-stimulating activity has been seen in in vivo animal studies.

Drug/Herb Interactions and Rationale (if known): Use cautiously with insulin or oral antidiabetic agents because of possible increased hypoglycemia.

Special Notes: Burdock burrs, and their ability to stick to pet hair and clothing, were the inspiration for Velcro.

BIBLIOGRAPHY

Awale S, et al. (2006). Identification of arctigenin as an antitumor agent having the ability to eliminate the tolerance of cancer cells to nutrient starvation. *Cancer Research.* Feb 1;66(3):1751–1757.

Bensky D, et al. (2004). *Chinese Herbal Medicine, Materia Medica* (pp. 49–52). Seattle: Eastland Press.

Der Marderosian A, Beutler J. [Eds.]. (2004). *The Review of Natural Products*. St. Louis, MO: Facts and Comparisons.

Grases F, et al. (1994). Urolithiasis and phytotherapy. *International Urology and Nephrology*. 26(5):507.

Integrative Medicine Access. (2000). *Burdock Monograph*. Newton, MA: Integrative Medicine Communications.

Kardosova A, et al. (2003). A biologically active fructan from the roots of *Arctium lappa* L., var. *Herkules*. *International Journal of Biological Macromolecules*. Nov;33(103):135–140.

Leung A, Foster, S. (1996). *Encyclopedia of Common Natural Ingredients* (2nd ed.; pp. 107–108). New York: John Wiley & Sons.

Lin SC, et al. (2002). Hepatoprotective effects of *Arctium lappa* linne in liver injuries induced by chronic ethanol consumption and potentiated by carbon tetrachloride. *Journal of Biomedical Science*. Sep-Oct;9(5):401–409.

Liu S, et al. (2005). An experimental research into the anti-aging effects of *Radix arctii* lappae. *Journal of Traditional Chinese Medicine*. Dec;25(4):296–299.

Matsumoto T, et al. (2006). Antiproliferative and apoptotic effects of butyrolactone lignans from *Arctium lappa* on leukemic cells. *Planta Medica*. Feb;72(3):276–278.

Palframan RJ, et al. (2002). Effect of pH and dose on the growth of gut bacteria on prebiotic carbohydrates in vitro. *Anaerobe*. Oct;8(5):287–292.

Rodriguez P, et al. (1995). Allergic dermatitis due to burdock (*Arcticum lappa*). *Contact Dermatitis*. 33(3):134.

Sun W. (1992). Determination of arctin and arctigenin in *Fructus arctii* by reverse-phase HPLC. *Acta Pharmaceutica Sinica*. 27(7):549.

Tadeda H, et al. (1991). Effect of feeding amaranth (Food Red #2) on the jejunal sucrase and digestion-absorption capacity of the jejunum in rats. *Journal of Nutrition Science and Vitamins*. 37(6):611.

Wang H, et al. (1993). Studies on the chemical constituents of *Arcticum lappa* L. *Acta Pharmaceutica Sinica*. 28(12):911.

C

NAME: Calendula (*Calendula officinalis*)

Common Names: Pot marigold

Family: *Asteraceae*

Description of Plant
- Believed to have originated in Egypt, but now is cultivated worldwide
- Grows to 2' tall
- Orange or yellow ray flowers bloom from May to October.

Medicinal Part: Dried flower

Constituents and Action (if known)
- Triterpenoid esters: anti-inflammatory activity (Akihisa et al., 1996; Della Loggia et al., 1994; Hamburger et al. 2003; Zitterl-Eglseer et al., 1999)
- Faradiol monoester: equals indomethacin in activity
- EOs: antibacterial
- Sesquiterpene glycosides (DeTommasi et al., 1990)
- Sterols and fatty acids; calendic and oleanic acid
- Oleanolic acid glycosides (Szakiel & Kasprzky, 1989)
- Flavonols (Pietta et al., 1992)
- Tocopherols: antioxidant
- Carotenoid: lutein and other carotenoid pigments including flavoxanthin, lycopene, and rubixanthin; anti-inflammatory, antioxidant
- Other actions: an aqueous ethanol extract of the flowers exhibited spasmolytic and spasmogenic effects in vitro (Bashir et al., 2006). In an animal study, a unique extract of calendula showed significant cytotoxic activity, and it stimulated lymphocyte activation (Jimenez-Medina et al., 2006). Reduces HIV-1, rhinovirus, and stomatitis virus activity in vitro (DeTommasi et al., 1990; Kalvatchev et al., 1997).

Nutritional Ingredients: Dried petals have a saffron-like quality and have been used in cooking and in salads.

Traditional Use
- Topically to promote wound healing and reduce inflammation, particularly for slow-to-heal wounds
- European folk use as a diaphoretic, bitter tonic, lymphatic tonic, and as treatment for jaundice
- Eclectic physicians used calendula for conjunctivitis, gastric ulcers, and topically for burns and rashes.
- Mouthwash: heals gums after tooth extraction

Current Use
Internally
- Postmastectomy lymphedema and pain (Newell et al., 1996; Zitterl-Eglseer et al., 1999). In a phase III clinical trial, researchers compared calendula with trolamine for preventing of radiation-induced dermatis in breast cancer patients. Patients using the herb had less pain, less inflammation of the skin, and fewer interruptions of radiotherapy (Pommier et al., 2004).
- Chronic colitis (Chakurski et al., 1981)
- Reduces inflammation of oral and pharyngeal mucosa (gingivitis, apthous stomatata)
- Promotes bile production
- Treatment of gastric and duodenal ulcers (Blumenthal et al., 2000), gastritis (Der Marderosian & Beutler, 2004).

Topically: Enhances epithelization of surgical wounds; reduces varicose veins; heals cracked nipples after breast-feeding, bruises, and decubitus ulcers. Liquid preparations also show antibacterial, antiviral, and antifungal activity. In a clinical trial, a calendula ointment accelerated wound healing in patients with venous leg ulcers (Duran et al., 2005).

Available Forms, Dosage, and Administration Guidelines
Preparations: Dried flowers; salves, tinctures
Typical Dosage
- *Dried flowers:* 3 to 6 g three times a day
- *Tincture:* (1:5, 70% alcohol), 30 to 60 gtt (1.5–3 mL) three times a day
- For external use, apply tincture to affected area (dilute tincture 1:2 in water for open wounds) or follow manufacturer or practitioner recommendations.

Pharmacokinetics—If Available (form or route when known): None known

Toxicity: None known

Contraindications: None known

Side Effects: Allergy possible due to cross sensitivity to plants such as feverfew, ragweed, chamomile, dandelion flower pollen.

There are cases in the literature of contact sensitization from calendula.

Long-Term Safety: Generally recognized as safe; no adverse effects expected

Use in Pregnancy/Lactation/Children: Traditionally, calendula has been used as an emmenagogue, so avoid oral use during early pregnancy (Brinker, 2001).

Drug/Herb Interactions and Rationale (if known):
Unknown

Special Notes
- Do not confuse with the African marigold (Tagetes).
- Most studies have been performed in animals, although there is now some research done in humans.

BIBLIOGRAPHY
Akihisa T, et al. (1996). Triterpene alcohols from the flowers of compositae and their anti-inflammatory effects. *Phytochemistry.* 43(6):1255–1260.

Bashir S, et al. (2006). Studies on spasmogenic and spasmolytic activities of *Calendula officinalis* flowers. *Phytotherapy Research.* Oct;20(10):906–910.

Blumenthal M, et al. (2000). *Herbal Medicine: Expanded Commission E Monographs.* Austin, TX: American Botanical Council.

Brinker, F. (2001). *Herb Contraindications and Drug Interactions* (3rd ed., p. 52). Sandy, OR: Eclectic Medical Publications.

Chakurski I, et al. (1981). Treatment of chronic colitis with an herbal combination of *Taraxacum officinale, Hypericum perforatum, Melissa officinalis, Calendula officinalis* and *Foeniculum vulgare. Vutreshni Bolesti.* 20(6):51–54.

Della Loggia R, et al. (1994). The role of triterpenoids in the topical anti-inflammatory activity of *Calendula officinalis* flowers. *Planta Medicine.* 60(6):516–520.

Der Marderosian A, Beutler J. [Eds.]. (2004). *The Review of Natural Products.* St. Louis, MO: Facts and Comparisons.

DeTommasi N, et al. (1990). Structure and in vitro antiviral activity of sesquiterpene glycosides from *Calendula arvensis. Journal of Natural Products.* 53(4):830.

Duran V, et al. (2005). Results of the clinical examination of an ointment with marigold (*Calendula officinalis*) extract in the treatment of venous leg ulcers. *International Journal of Tissue Reactions.,* 2005;27(3):101–106.

Hamburger M, et al. (2003). Preparative purification of the major anti-inflammatory triterpenoid esters from marigold (*Calendula officinalis*). *Fitoterapia*. Jun;74(4):328–338.

Jiminez-Medina E, et al. (2006). A new extract of the plant *Calendula officinalis* produces a dual in vitro effect: Cytotoxic anti-tumor activity and lymphocyte activation. *BMC Cancer*. May 5;6:119.

Kalvatchev Z, et al. (1997). Anti-HIV activity of extracts from *Calendula officinalis* flowers. *Biomedical Pharmacotherapy*. 51(4): 176–180.

Kishimoto S, et al. (2005). Analysis of carotenoid composition in petals of calendula (*Calendula officinalis* L.). *Bioscience, Biotechnology, and Biochemistry*. Nov;69(11):2122–2128.

Newell C, et al. (1996). *Herbal Medicines* (pp. 58–59). London: Pharmaceutical Press.

Pietta P, et al. (1992). Separation of flavonol-2-O-glycosides from *Calendula officinalis* and *Sambucus nigra* by high-performance liquid and micellar electrokinetic capillary chromatography. *Journal of Chromatography*. 593(1–2):165.

Pommier P, et al. (2004). Phase III randomized trial of *Calendula officinalis* compared with trolamine for the prevention of acute dermatitis during irradiation for breast cancer. *Journal of Clinical Oncology*. Apr 15;22(8):1447–1453.

Szakiel A, Kasprzky Z. (1989). Distribution of oleanolic acid glycosides in vacuoles and cell walls isolated from protoplasts and cells of *Calendula officinalis* leaves. *Steroids*. 53(3–5):501.

Zitterl-Eglseer K, et al. (1999). Anti-oedematous activities of the main triterpenoid esters of marigold (*Calendula officinalis* L.) *Ethnopharmacology*. 57(2):139–144.

 NAME: Catnip (*Nepeta cataria*)

Common Names: Catmint

Family: *Lamiaciae*

Description of Plant

- Catnip is a small- to medium-sized aromatic herbaceous perennial with fuzzy, grey-green leaves.
- It is easily grown as a garden plant and is commonly found growing wild in open fields and waste places.
- The volatile oil content is highest in plants grown in poor soil.

Medicinal Part: The dried herb

Constituents and Action (If Known)
- Volatile oils: antispasmodic, sedative (Skenderi, 2003)
  - β-caryophyllene: analgesic, anti-inflammatory, gastroprotective, sedative (Duke), antioxidant, antibacterial, antifungal (Jutea et al., 2002)
  - Citronellal: insect repellant, sedative (Duke)
  - Geranial: antibacterial (Moleyar & Narasimham, 1992), antispasmodic, sedative (Duke, 2006)
  - Thymol: antibacterial, anti-inflammatory (Braga et al., 2006a), antioxidant (Braga et al., 2006b), carminative (Duke)
- Nepetalactone (Iridoid): bitter tonic (Skenderi, 2003), insect repellant, sedative (Duke, 2006)

Nutritional Ingredients: In England before the introduction of Chinese tea (black tea), catnip was used as a beverage tea. In France the young leaves of this herb have been used as a seasoning.

Traditional Use
- It is a mild analgesic, antispasmodic, carminative, diaphoretic, insect repellent, and sedative.
- Catnip has a long history of use as a remedy for infants and children. The tea is taken by nursing women to prevent or treat colic in babies. The tea was (and still is) given to children for stomachaches, colds, fevers (as a tea and as an enema), teething pain, nausea, flatulence, and irritability.

Current Use
- Catnip is a safe, time-tested children's remedy for fevers (use it with elder flower and/or peppermint), intestinal viruses (use it with chamomile and ginger), digestive upset, intestinal colic, painful flatulence with abdominal distention, and vomiting (use it with ginger).
- Adults who internalize stress in the GI tract respond well to the use of catnip along with chamomile and hops. It is effective for treating stress-induced nausea, flatulence, diarrhea, IBS, and esophageal spasms (Winston, 2006). It can also be used for other GI disturbances, including belching, hiccoughs, and hyperchlorhydria (use it with

meadowsweet, marshmallow, and licorice) as well as simple
dysmenorrhea with nausea.
* Studies on catnip show that it has antifungal and
antibacterial activity (Nostro et al., 2001), and the essential
oil helps to repel mosquitoes.

Available Forms, Dosage, and Administration Guidelines

Preparations: Tea, tincture, glycerite

Typical Dosage
* *Tea:* 1 to 2 tsp dried herb, 8 oz hot water, steep 15 to 20
minutes, take up to three cups a day
* *Tincture:* (1:2 or 1:5; 35% alcohol), 80 to 100 gtt (4–5 mL)
three or four times a day
* *Glycerite:* (1:4), 1 tsp four times a day

Pharmacokinetics–If Available (form or route when known): Not known

Toxicity: There is some mention in the scientific and popular
literature of catnip altering human consciousness, as it does
with felines. There is little evidence to promote this idea, but
there is a case report of a toddler exhibiting central nervous
system depression after consuming a large quantity of catnip
(Osterhoudt et al., 1997).

Contraindications: None known

Side Effects: None known

Long-Term Safety: Safe

Use in Pregnancy/Lactation/Children: Avoid large quantities
during pregnancy (Brinker, 2001) although small amounts are
probably safe. This herb has a long history of safe use in lactating
women, infants (via breast milk), and with children.

Drug/Herb Interactions and Rationale (if known): None
known in humans. In mice, the essential oil and nepetalic acid
given IP increased the sedative effects of hexobarbitol (Brinker,
2001).

Special Notes: Catnip is known for its mind-altering effects
on felines (cats, tigers, lions, etc.)

BIBLIOGRAPHY

Amer A, Mehlhorn H. (2006). Repellency effect of forty-one essential oils against aedes, anopheles, and culex mosquitoes. *Parasitology Research.* Sep;99(4):478–490.

Braga PC, et al. (2006a). Antiinflammatory activity of thymol: Inhibitory effect on the release of human neutrophil elastase. *Pharmacology.* 77(3):130–136.

Braga PC, et al. (2006b). Antioxidant potential of thymol determined by chemiluminescence inhibition in human neutrophils and cell-free systems. *Pharmacology.* 76(2):61–68.

Brinker F. (2001). *Herb Contraindications and Drug Interactions* (3rd ed.; pp. 56–57). Sandy, OR: Eclectic Medical Publications.

Duke J. Dr. Duke's phytochemical and ethnobotanical databases. Retrieved September 30, 2006, from www.ars-grin.gov/cgi-bin/duke/chemactivities.

Jutea F, et al. (2002). Antibacterial and antioxidant activities of *Artemisia annua* essential oil. *Fitoterapia.* Oct;73(6):532–535.

Moleyar V, Narasimham P. (1992). Antibacterial activity of essential oil components. *International Journal of Food Microbiology.* Aug;16(4):337–342.

Nostro A, et al. (2001). The effect of *Nepeta cataria* extract on adherence and enzyme productin of *Staphylococcus aureus*. *International Journal of Antimicrobial Agents.* Dec;18(6):583–585.

Osterhoudt KC, et al. (1997). Catnip and alteration of human consciousness. *Veterinary and Human Toxicology.* Dec;39(6):373–375.

Skenderi G. (2003). *Herbal Vade Mecum* (pp. 85–86). Rutherford, NJ: Herbacy Press.

Winston D. (2006). *Winston's Botanic Materia Medica.* Washington, NJ: DWCHS.

 NAME: Cat's Claw (*Uncaria tomentosa, U. guianensis*)

Common Names: Una de gato, saventaro, samento

Family: *Rubiaceae*

Description of Plant

- Large woody vine (liana) found in the highlands of the Peruvian rain forest
- Vine can grow 100′ long and climbs on trees.
- Has somewhat large, curved thorns that resemble a cat's claw

Medicinal Part: Inner bark of plant (root is undisturbed), whole stem, root bark

Constituents and Action (if known)

- Oxinadole alkaloids, isomitraphylline, uncarine F., speciophylline; anti-inflammatory activity (Sandoval-Chacon et al., 1998); immune-enhancing activity (Hemingway & Phillipson, 1974; Rizzi et al., 1993); antileukemic activity (Bacher et al., 2006; Stuppner et al., 1993); antimutagenic (Rizzi et al., 1993)
  - Mitrophylline: diuretic activity (Jones, 1994)
  - Rynchophylline: inhibits platelet activity and thrombosis (Chen et al., 1992; Jones, 1994), decreases peripheral vascular resistance, has antihypertensive activity, decreases cholesterol (Jones, 1994)
  - Pteropodine, isopteropodine: modulates neurotransmitter 5-HT(2), possible antidepressant effect (Roth et al., 2001); antileukemic (Bacher et al., 2006)
  - Hirstutine: local anesthetic properties on bladder (Jones, 1994); may have an effect on Ca^{++} movement, reduces blood pressure and dilates blood vessels (Taylor, 2005)
- Indole alkaloid glucosides (cadambine, 3-dihydrocadambine, 3-isohydrocadambine)
- Six quinovic acid glycosides have antiviral activity in vitro (Aquino et al., 1989), anti-inflammatory activity (Aquino et al., 1991)
- Proanthocyanidins and phenolic esters (caffeic acid): antioxidant, antitumor, and immune boosting (Goncalves et al., 2005)
- Triterpinoid saponins
- Catechins (D-catechol)
- Carboxyl alkyl esters: strongly anti-inflammatory (Taylor, 2005)
- Other actions: cytotoxic, antiviral, antibacterial, immunomodulatory (Heitzman et al., 2005)

Nutritional Ingredients: None known

Traditional Use: Long history of traditional ethnomedical use by the native peoples of the Amazonian rain forest. It has been used for a large number of conditions, including:

- As an anti-inflammatory for arthritis, asthma, gastritis, gastric ulcers
- For genitourinary pain, hematuria, profuse menstrual bleeding
- Topically for wounds, mouth sores, fungal infections

Current Use

- Heals the mucosal membranes in persons with Crohn's disease, inflammatory bowel disease, gastritis, irritable bowel disorder, and leaky gut syndrome (Winston, 2006)
- Reduces side effects of cancer chemotherapy and AZT therapy for HIV (Taylor, 2005). A human study found that *Uncaria tomentosa* prevented oxidation-induced DNA damage and enhanced DNA repair (Sheng et al., 2001).
- Used in clinical practice in Europe for cancer, HIV
- Forty patients with rheumatoid arthritis took cat's claw or a placebo for 52 weeks. Patients receiving the herb had 53.2% less joint pain (24.1% for placebo) and a reduction in the number of swollen joints (Mur et al., 2002). In a study of patients with osteoarthritis of the knees, patients taking cat's claw had significant reductions in pain (Piscoya et al., 2001).

Available Forms, Dosage, and Administration Guidelines

Preparations: Dried root and stem, capsules, extracts, tablets, tinctures; powdered extracts standardized for total alkaloid content are available

Typical Dosage

- *Capsules:* Six to nine 500- to 600-mg capsules a day
- *Decoction:* Simmer 1 tbsp powdered root in 16 oz water for 45 minutes; take 1/2 to 1 cup daily for minor problems. A therapeutic dose can be up to 3 cups a day.
- *Tincture* (1:5, 60% alcohol): 20 to 40 gtt (1–2 mL) up to five times a day. The tincture has higher antioxidant activity than did the decoction (Pilarski et al., 2006).

Pharmacokinetics—If Available (form or route when known): None known

Toxicity: None known

Contraindications: Avoid using in patients receiving immunosuppressive therapies or women attempting to get pregnant.

Side Effects: Mild constipation, mild diarrhea, or digestive upset; rarely, mild lymphocytosis. Monitor for signs of bleeding.

Long-Term Safety: Unknown

Use in Pregnancy/Lactation/Children: Contraindicated during pregnancy because of its traditional use as a contraceptive

Drug/Herb Interactions and Rationale (if known)
- Avoid concurrent use with blood thinners.
- May potentiate activity of antihypertensives; use cautiously together.
- Although there is no research to confirm these beliefs, European physicians recommend against using this herb with insulin, hormone therapies, vaccines, or immunosuppressive medications.

Special Notes
- Little human research exists. Well-designed human studies are needed to verify or disprove folk and current clinical use.
- A company marketing a specific "cat's claw" product has claimed that there are two chemotypes of *Uncaria tomentosa*, one with tetracyclic oxindole alkaloids (TOAs) and another with pentacyclic oxindole alkaloids (POAs). Supposedly, the POAs are the "good alkaloids," and the TOAs counteract the beneficial effects of the former compound. There is no independent confirmation of this theory, and it contradicts 30 years of study and research (Taylor, 2005).

BIBLIOGRAPHY
Aquino R, et al. (1989). Plant metabolites, structure and in vitro antiviral activity of quinovic acid glycosides from *Uncaria tomentosa* and *Guettarda platypoda*. *Journal of Natural Products*. 52(4):679–685.

Aquino R, et al. (1991). Plant metabolites: New compounds and antiinflammatory activity of *Uncaria tomentosa*. *Journal of Natural Products*. 54(2):453–459.

Bacher N, et al. (2006). Oxindole alkaloids from *Uncaria tomentosa* induce apoptosis in proliferating G0/G1-arrested and BCl-2-expressing acute lymphobiastic leukaemia cells. *British Journal of Haematology.* Mar;132(5):615–622.

Chen CX, et al. (1992). Inhibitory effect of rhynchophylline on platelet aggregation and thrombosis. *Acta Pharmacologica Sinica.* 13:126–130.

Der Marderosian A, Beutler J. [Eds.]. (2004). *The Review of Natural Products.* St. Louis, MO: Facts and Comparisons.

Goncalves C, et al. (2005). Antioxidant properties of proanthocyandins of *Uncaria tomentosa* bark decoctin: A mechanism for anti-inflammatory activity. *Phytochemistry.* Jan;66(1):89–98.

Heitzman ME, et al. (2005). Ethnobotany, phytochemistry, and pharmacology of *Uncaria* (Rubiaceae). *Phytochemistry.* Jan;66(1):5–19.

Jones K. (1994). The herb report: Una de gato, life-giving vine of Peru. *American Herb Association.* 10(3):4.

Keplinger K, et al. (1999). Ethnomedicinal use and new pharmacological, toxicological, and botanical results. *Journal of Ethnopharmacology.* 64(1):23–34.

McCaleb R, et al. (2000). *Encyclopedia of Popular Herbs* (p. 95). Roseville, CA: Prima Publishers.

Mur E, et al. (2002). Randomized double-blind trial of an extract from the pentacyclic alkaloid-chemotype of *Uncaria tomentosa* for the treatment of rheumatoid arthritis. *Journal of Rheumatology.* Apr;29(4):678–681.

Pilarski R, et al. (2006). Antioxidant activity of ethanolic and aqueous extracts of *Uncaria tomentosa* (Willd.) DC. *Journal of Ethnopharmacology.* Mar 8;104(1–2):18–23.

Piscova J, et al. (2001). Efficacy and safety of freeze-dried cat's claw in osteoarthritis of the knee: Mechanisms of action of the species *Uncaria guianensis. Inflammation Research.* Sep;50(9): 442–448.

Reinhard KH. (1999). *Uncaria tomentosa. Journal of Alternative and Complementary Medicine.* 5(2):143–151.

Rizzi R, et al. (1993). Mutagenic and antimutagenic activities of *Uncaria tomentosa* and its extracts. *Journal of Ethnopharmacology.* 38(1):63.

Roth BL, et al. (2001). Insights into the structure and function of 5-HT(2) family serotonin receptors reveal novel strategies for therapeutic target development. *Expert Opinion on Therapeutic Targets.* Dec 5;(6):685–695.

Sandoval-Chacon M, et al. (1998). Antiinflammatory actions of cat's claw: The role of NF-kappaB. *Alimentary Pharmacologic Therapy.* 12(12):1279–1289.

Sheng Y, et al. (2001). DNA repair enhancement of aqueous extracts of *Uncaria tomentosa* in a human volunteer study. *Phytomedicine*. Jul;8(4):275–282.

Stuppner H, et al. (1993). A differential sensitivity of oxindole alkaloids to normal and leukemic cell lines. *Planta Medica*. 59[Suppl.]:A583.

Taylor L. (2005). *The Healing Power of Rainforest Herbs* (pp. 217–224). Garden City Park, NY: Squire One Publishers.

Winston D. (2006). *Winston's Botanic Materia Medica*. Washington, NJ: DWCHS.

 NAME: Cayenne (*Capsicum frutescens, C. annuum*)

Common Names: Chili pepper, cayenne pepper, red pepper, Mexican chili, hot pepper, jalapeno

Family: *Solanaceae*

Description of Plant

- An oblong pungent fruit; a member of the *Capsicum* genus (nightshades). This same genus also includes paprika, bell, and sweet peppers.
- Originally grew in tropical America, but now is grown worldwide

Medicinal Part: Fruit (pepper)

Constituents and Action (if known)

- Capsaicinoids (up to 1.5%)
  - Oleoresin capsaicin (1.5%): powerful irritant that causes a reflex vasodilatation, probably mediated by substance P. After initial topical application, substance P is released, causing the sensation of pain. After repeated applications, substance P is depleted and a lack of pain impulses ensues. This effect usually occurs within 3 days of regular application.
  - Capsaicin combined with the green tea catechin, epigallocatechin gallate EGCG, had a synergistic effect (10 to 100 times more active than either compound alone) for inhibiting the cancer-specific cell surface protein tNOX and inducing apoptosis (Morre et al., 2006).

- ○ 6,7 dihydrocapsaicin, nordihydrocapsaicin, homodihydrocapsaicin, homocapsaicin
- Steroid glycosides: capsicosides, A to D

Nutritional Ingredients
- Carotenoids (capsanthin, capsorubin, alpha and beta carotene, lutein)
- Vitamins C, E, A, B_1, B_2, B_3
- Capsaicin is responsible for the pungency of the pepper
- Flavonoids

Traditional Use
- To treat mouth sores (ancient Mayans)
- To stimulate digestive power; GI stimulant and carminative
- To strengthen the blood vessels and normalize blood pressure
- A local counterirritant for sore muscles
- To stop local capillary bleeding (nose bleeds, bleeding ulcers, cuts)
- A catalyst to increase absorption in herbal formulas, commonly used in neo-Thomsonian, traditional Mexican, and southeast Asian medicine for this purpose

Current Use
- Topical application to control pain in osteoarthritis and rheumatoid arthritis; herpes zoster, shingles (Zostrix cream contains either 0.025% or 0.075% capsaicin), and back pain (Frerick et al., 2003); diabetic, postsurgical, and trigeminal neuralgias (Robbins et al., 1998); psoriasis (Ellis et al., 1993)
- Korean research has found that capsicum plasters placed on acupuncture points for pain control (stomach 36) can significantly reduce pain from postsurgical hernia repair (Kim et al., 2006a) and abdominal hysterectomy (Kim et al., 2006b) as well as reduce postsurgical nausea and vomiting (Misra et al., 2005).
- Nasal spray used once weekly for 5 weeks reduces chronic, nonallergic rhinitis, runny nose, and sneezing. Nasal spray may also be helpful in decreasing the pain and number of cluster headaches.
- Used internally to stimulate digestion, reduce dyspepsia (Bortolotti et al., 2002), reduce blood lipids (Ahuja & Ball,

2006), improve peripheral circulation (this use has not been proven scientifically)
- Cayenne has shown inhibitory activity against *Helicobacter pylori,* and studies show that people who regularly consume hot peppers have a lower incidence of duodenal and peptic ulcers than those who do not.

Available Forms, Dosage, and Administration Guidelines
Preparations: Fresh or dried powdered fruit; capsules, tablets, tinctures
Typical Dosage
- *Spice:* Use freely in flavoring food.
- *Capsules:* Up to three 400- to 500-mg capsules a day
- *Tea:* Steep 0.25 to 0.5 tsp powdered spice in a cup of hot water for 10 to 15 minutes. If patient can tolerate the tea, small sips should be taken throughout the day.
- *Tincture* (1:10, 90% alcohol): 5 to 10 gtt (0.25–0.5 mL) diluted in water
- Or follow manufacturer or practitioner recommendations

Pharmacokinetics—If Available (form or route when known): None known

Toxicity
- *Topically:* Intolerable sensation of heat and burning; milk may blunt effect
- *Internal:* Intense GI pain and burning

Contraindications
Internal
- Acid indigestion, gastroesophageal reflux (GERD): a recent study indicated that hot peppers can induce or exacerbate esophageal reflux (Milke P et al., 2006)
- Popular wisdom has stated that cayenne peppers should be avoided if a patient has hemorrhoids. In a recent study, researchers found no basis for this belief (Altomare et al., 2006).
Topical
- Do not use on open, broken skin and in or near eyes or vaginal mucosa.
- Do not apply additional heat.

Side Effects

- External: contact dermatitis; does not cause blistering or redness because it does not act on capillary beds; transient stinging
- Internal: GI distress

Long-Term Safety: Safe; long-term food use

Use in Pregnancy/Lactation/Children

- Pregnancy: safe as a food. Internally, large quantities should be used cautiously because this herb may cause uterine contractions.
- Lactation: safe as a food
- Do not use in young children.

Drug/Herb Interactions and Rationale (if known): None known

Special Notes

- Hot peppers cause skin burning and irritation. Use rubber gloves when preparing fresh peppers. Wash hands thoroughly after preparing peppers or using the creams.
- Capsaicin is not water soluble, so it is difficult to wash off after handling peppers.
- Avoid contact with eyes.

BIBLIOGRAPHY

Ahuja KD, Ball MJ. (2006). Effects of daily ingestion of chilli on serum lipoprotein oxidation in adult men and women. *British Journal of Nutrition.* Aug;96(2):239–242.

Altomare DF, et al. (2006). Red hot chili pepper and hemorrhoids: The explosion of a myth—Results of a prospective, randomized, placebo-controlled, crossover trial. *Diseases of the Colon and Rectum.* Jul;49(7):1018–1023.

Blumenthal M, et al. (2000). *Herbal Medicine: Expanded Commission E Monographs* (pp. 52–56). Austin, TX: American Botanical Council.

Bortolotti M, et al. (2002). The treatment of functional dyspepsia with red pepper. *Alimentary Pharmacology and Therapeutics.* Jun;16(6):1075–1082.

Ellis CN, et al. (1993). A double-blind evaluation of topical capsaicin in pruritic psoriasis. *Journal of the American Academy of Dermatology.* 29:438–442.

Frerick H, et al. (2003). Topical treatment of chronic low back pain with a capsicum plaster. *Pain.* Nov;106(1–2):59–64.

Kim KS, et al. (2006a). The analgesic effects of capsicum plaster at the Zusanli point after abdominal hysterectomy. *Anesthesia and Analgesia*. Sep;103(3):709–713.

Kim KS, et al. (2006b). The effect of capsicum plaster in pain after inguinal hernia repair in children. *Paediatric Anesthesia*. Oct;16(10):1036–1041.

McCaleb R, et al. (2000). *Encyclopedia of Popular Herbs* (pp. 96–104). Roseville, CA: Prima Publishers.

Milke P, et al. (2006). Gastroesophageal reflux in healthy subjects induced by two different species of chilli (*Capsicum annum*). *Digestive Diseases*. 24(1–2):184–188.

Misra MN, et al. (2005). Prevention of PONV 6y acustimulation with capsicum plaster is comparable to ondansetron after middle ear surgery. *Can J. Anaesth*. May:52(5):485–489.

Morre DM, et al. (2006). Catechin-vanilloid synergies with potential clinical applications in cancer. *Rejuvenation Research*. Spring;9(1):45–55.

Robbins WR, et al. (1998). Treatment of intractable pain with topical large-dose capsaicin: Preliminary report. *Anesthesia and Analgesia*. 86:579–583.

NAME: German or Hungarian Chamomile (*Matricaria recutita*), Roman or English Chamomile (*Chamaemelum nobile*)

Common Names: Common chamomile, true chamomile, wild chamomile, sweet false chamomile (*C. nobile*)

Family: *Asteraceae*

Description of Plant: *M. recutita* is an erect annual, growing 1' to 2.5' tall; has small daisy-like flowers in clusters. *C. nobile* is a hardy, low-growing perennial with daisy-like flowers.

Medicinal Part: Flower head; gather just before blooming and then dry

Constituents and Action (if known)

- Volatile oils: carminative activity, anti-inflammatory, antidiuretic, antispasmodic, sedative, muscle relaxing, antibacterial (Aggag & Yousef, 1972)
  - Alpha-bisabolol (50% of EO): anti-inflammatory, antipyretic (Habersang et al., 1979; Isaac, 1979), antiulcer effect (Fidler et al., 1996)

- ° Alpha-bisabolol oxides A and B: papaverine-like antispasmodic activity (Achterath-Tuckerman et al., 1980)
- ° Matricine: anti-inflammatory (Della Loggia et al., 1996)
- ° Chamazulene: formed during steam distillation, makes up 5% of EO; anti-inflammatory
- Flavonoids (0.5%–3%): contain significant anti-inflammatory activity (Della Loggia et al., 1996)
  - ° Apigenin-7-glucoside and luteolin: bind to benzodiazepine receptors and have anxiolytic and mild relaxing effects with no sedation; anti-inflammatory activity may be greater than that of indomethacin (Hamon, 1989; Paladini et al., 1999)
  - ° Quercetin: equal to apigenin in strength; antispasmodic effects (Achterath-Tuckerman et al., 1980)
- Sesquiterpene lactones: matricin, matricarin

Nutritional Ingredients: German chamomile is commonly used in Europe as a calming beverage tea.

Traditional Use
Internal
- As a remedy for teething babies
- To relieve upset stomachs, intestinal colic, and menstrual cramps
- To reduce tension and induce sleep. It is often used with lemon balm, passion flower, or linden flower.

Topical: For hemorrhoids, mastitis, eczema, and leg ulcers; reduces inflammation; soothes aches; heals cuts, sores, and bruises

Current Use
Internal—German Chamomile
- Inflammation, irritation, or spasm of the GI tract; indigestion, IBS, IBD, gastritis, peptic and gastric ulcers, GERD, diarrhea with bowel spasms, flatulence, and for colic in infants (give the tea to the mother and the oils pass through the breast milk to the infant) (Winston, 2006). A chamomile/apple pectin product was used in a study of acute diarrhea in 255 children aged 6 months to 6 years. It was effective for reducing stool frequency and the duration of the condition (Becker et al., 2006).

- Chamomile is a nervine used for mild anxiety, stress-induced insomnia, and bruxism.
- The flower tea and tincture have long been used for mild to moderate dysmenorrhea, PMS anxiety, and a combination product containing German chamomile and *Angelica sinensis* was very effective in relieving menopausal hot flashes, fatigue, and sleep disturbances (Kupfersztain et al., 2003).

Topical–German Chamomile

- Anogenital irritation: hemorrhoids, vulval irritation (use as a sitz bath)
- Wound healing (Glowania et al., 1987): chamomile tea used as a mouthwash reduces pain and helps to heal apthous stomatata, gingivitis, or 5-FU- and methotrexate-induced oral mucositis (Fidler et al., 1996; Mazokopakis et al., 2005)
- Eczema: ointment is as effective as hydrocortisone and superior to nonsteroidal anti-inflammatories (Aertgeerts et al., 1985)

Internal–Roman Chamomile

- Is less useful than German chamomile for digestive upsets but is a stronger antispasmodic for dysmenorrhea and intestinal spasms.

Available Forms, Dosage, and Administration Guidelines

Preparations: Dried flowers; capsules, cream salve, tea, tincture, bath products

Typical Dosage

- *Bath:* For hemorrhoids or irritated skin, soak 1 lb dried flowers in a tub of hot water.
- *Capsules:* Up to six 300- to 400-mg capsules a day
- *Tea:* Steep 1 to 2 tbsp dried flowers in a cup of hot water for 5 to 10 minutes; take three or four times a day.
- *Tincture* (1:5, 40% alcohol): 60 to 120 gtt (3–6 mL) three times a day
- Or follow manufacturer or practitioner recommendations
- *Topical:* For insect bites, mix 1 tsp aloe vera gel with 2 gtt chamomile EO and apply to bite.

Pharmacokinetics—If Available (form or route when known): None known

Toxicity: None known

Contraindications: None known

Side Effects: Topical—allergic skin reactions. Internal— bronchial constriction. Persons with severe allergies to plants in the *Asteraceae* family (ragweed, asters, chrysanthemums) should avoid chamomile. Allergic reactions are rare (Mann & Staba, 1986).

Long-Term Safety: Safe

Use in Pregnancy/Lactation/Children: German chamomile has a long history of use during pregnancy and breast-feeding and as a children's remedy. It is a common beverage tea throughout Europe and South America. Roman chamomile has been found to be an abortifacient in animals. Avoid use during pregnancy.

Drug/Herb Interactions and Rationale (if known): Anticoagulants may potentiate effect. Use cautiously together.

Special Notes: German chamomile is better tasting and milder in action than Roman chamomile. It is more appropriate for pregnant women and children.

BIBLIOGRAPHY
Achterath-Tuckerman U, et al. (1980). Investigations on the spasmolytic effect of compounds of chamomile and kamillosan on the isolated guinea pig ileum. *Planta Medica.* 39:38.
Aertgeerts P, et al. (1985). [Comparative testing of Kamillosan cream and steroidal (0.25% hydrocortisone, 0.75% fluocortin butyl ester) and non-steroidal (5% bufexamac) dermatologic agents in maintenance therapy of eczematous diseases] (In German). *Zeitschrift fur Hautkrankheiten.* 60(3):270–277.
Becker B, et al. (2006). Double-blind, randomized evaluation of clinical efficacy and tolerability of an apple pectin-chamomile extract in children with unspecific diarrhea. *Arzneimittelforschung.* 56(6):387–393.
Blumenthal M, et al. (2000). *Herbal Medicine, Expanded Commission E Monographs* (pp. 57–61). Austin, TX: American Botanical Council.
Della Loggia R, et al. (1996). The role of flavonoids in the anti-inflammatory activity of Chamomilla recutita. In: Cody V, et al.

[Eds.]. *Plant Flavonoids in Biology and Medicine: Biochemical, Pharmacological and Structure-Activity Relationships*. New York: Alan R. Liss.

Der Marderosian A, Beutler J. [Eds.]. (2004). *The Review of Natural Products*. St. Louis, MO: Facts and Comparisons.

Fidler P, et al. (1996). Prospective evaluations of a chamomile mouthwash for prevention of 5-FU-induced oral mucosites. *Cancer*. 77:522–524.

Ganzera M, et al. (2006). Inhibitory effects of the essential oil of chamomile (*Matricaria recutita L*.) and its major constituents on human cytochrome P450 enzymes. *Life Sciences*. Jan 18;78(8):856–861.

Glowania HJ, et al. (1987). Effect of chamomile on wound healing: A clinical double-blind study (In German). *Zeitschrift fur Hautkrankheiten*. 62(17):1262–1271.

Habersang S, et al. (1979). Pharmacological studies with compounds of chamomile IV. *Planta Medica*. 37:115.

Hamon NW. (1989). *Herbal medicine: The chamomiles. Canadian Pharmaceutical Journal*. Nov:612.

Isaac O. (1979). Pharmacological investigations with compounds of chamomile I. *Planta Medica*. 35:118.

Kupfersztain C, et al. (2003). The immediate effect of natural plant extract *Angelica sinensis* and *Matricaria chamomilla* (Climex) for the treatment of hot flushes during menopause. A preliminary report. *Clinical and Experimental Obstetrics and Gynecology*. 30(4):203–206.

Mann C, Staba EJ. (1986). The chemistry, pharmacology, and commercial formulations of chamomile. In: Craker LE, Simons JE. [Eds.]. *Herbs, Spices, and Medicinal Plants: Recent Advances in Botany, Horticulture, and Pharmacology*, Vol. 1 (pp. 235–280). Phoenix, AZ: Oryx Press.

Mazokopakis EE, et al. (2005). Wild chamomile (*Matricaria recutita L*.) mouthwashes in methotrexate-induced oral mucositis. *Phytomedicine*. Jan;12(1–2):25–27.

McKay DL, Blumberg JB. (2006). A review of the bioactivity and potential health benefits of chamomile tea (*Matricaria recutita L*.). *Phytotherapy Research*. Jul;20(7):519–530.

Mills S, Bone K. (2000). *Principles and Practice of Phytotherapy* (pp. 319–327). Edinburgh: Churchill Livingstone.

Paladini AC, et al. (1999). Flavonoids and the central nervous system: From forgotten factors to potent anxiolytic compounds. *Journal of Pharmacy and Pharmacology*. 51(5):519–526.

Rodriguez-Serna M, et al. (1998). Allergic and systemic contact dermatitis from *Matricaria chamomilla* tea. *Contact Dermatitis*. 39(4):192–193.

Segal R, Pilote L. (2006). Warfarin interaction with *Matricaria chamomilla*. *Canadian Medical Association Journal*. Apr 25;174(9):1281–1282.

Winston D. (2006). *Winston's Botanic Materia Medica*. Washington, NJ: DWCHS.

 NAME: Chaparral (*Larrea tridentata*)

Common Names: Creosote bush, grease wood

Family: *Zygophyllaceae*

Description of Plant: A very long-lived evergreen perennial shrub that grows in the deserts of Mexico and the American Southwest. The aromatic leaves smell like creosote.

Medicinal Part: Leaves

Constituents and Action (if known)

- Lignans: nordihydroguaiaretic acid (antioxidant), selective lipoxygenase inhibitor, inhibits platelet derived growth factor and protein kinase intracellular signaling (McDonald et al., 2001), norisoguaiasin, dihydroguariaretic acid, larreatricin, many others
- Flavonoids: quercitin, kaempherol, rutin—antioxidant, anti-inflammatory
- Triterpenes: larreagenin A, larreic acid
- Other actions: methanolic extracts of this herb were found to have antiulcerogenic and anti-inflammatory effects in animal studies (Pedernera et al., 2006)

Traditional Use

- Antioxidant, expectorant, alterative, diuretic, antitumor, antifungal, anti-inflammatory, antirheumatic
- Ethnobotanical use by Native Americans and Hispanics for arthritis, bursitis, neuralgias (orally and topically), uterine fibroids, cancer, respiratory infections, and skin conditions (orally and topically)

Current Use

- Chaparral has a long history of use by peoples of the Southwest and Mexico (Native Americans and Hispanics).

It was widely used during the 1960s and 1990s as a treatment for cancer, arthralgias, uterine fibroids, and the like. In the late 1980s and early 1990s, a small number of cases of what was believed to be chaparral-induced hepatotoxicity were reported. Initially, phytochemists could not determine any hepatotoxic compounds in the plant, and the cases were believed to be idiosyncratic reactions to a powerful plant. Recent in vitro animal studies suggest that a major constituent of the plant, NDGA, has pro-oxidant effects on hepatic tissue. This may explain the underlying cause of the reported problems. These studies are not on the whole plant, nor was it studied in humans, so more research is needed. The preliminary studies indicate that the liver-damaging effect is dose dependent, and a very small clinical trial suggests that low-dose oral use and topical use of the plant is relatively safe (Heron & Yarnell, 2001).

- Topical use (baths) for arthralgias, sciatica, bursitis, psoriasis, and fungal infections. Ethanolic extracts of chaparral were found to inhibit fungal growth (Quiroga et al., 2004).
- Research is ongoing for the use of this nordihydroguaiaretic acid (NDGA) and its analogues in treating lymphoma and breast cancer. Intratumoral injection has shown the greatest activity. A new derivative of NDGA (compound 4) is 10 times more potent than NDGA for inhibiting small cell lung cancer cell proliferation (McDonald et al., 2001).

Available Forms, Dosage, and Administration Guidelines: Avoid using capsules or tablets of this herb. No toxicity observed from tea (1 tsp dried leaf to 8 oz water). The strongly unpleasant taste may limit the amount taken and thus the possibility of side effects.

Pharmacokinetics—If Available (form or route when known): The half-life of NDGA (in mice) is 135 minutes.

Toxicity: Potentially hepatotoxic (Anesini et al., 1997; Katz et al., 1990; Sheikh et al., 1997). Recent in vitro studies indicate that NDGA in large doses has pro-oxidant (hepatotoxic) effects on rat hepatocyte tissue (Sahu et al., 2006).

Contraindications: Liver disease, pregnancy, kidney disease

Side Effects
- Chaparral-induced hepatitis (has occurred in a few people taking chaparral tablets or capsules)
- Contact dermatitis

Long-Term Safety: Not recommended for long-term use

Use in Pregnancy/Lactation/Children: Do not use.

Drug/Herb Interactions and Rationale (if known): None known

Special Notes: NDGA was previously used as an antioxidant in the food industry (1940s–1970) until rat feeding studies (0.5%–1% NDGA for 74 weeks) showed lymph node and kidney lesions.

BIBLIOGRAPHY

Anesini C, et al. (1997). In vivo antitumoural activity and acute toxicity study of *Larrea divarcata C.* extract. *Phytotherapy Research.* 11(7):521–523.

Anesini C, et al. (1998). In vivo antitumor activity of *Larrea divaricata C.* extract. *Phytomedicine.* 5(1):41–46.

Heron S, Yarnell E. (2001). The safety of low-dose *Larrea tridentata* (DC) Coville (creosote bush or chaparral): A retrospective clinical study. *Journal of Alternative and Complementary Medicine.* Apr;7(2):175–185.

Katz M, et al. (1990). Herbal hepatitis: Subacute hepatic necrosis secondary to chaparral leaf. *Journal of Clinical Gastroenterology.* 12:203.

Lambert JD, et al. (2002). Nordihydroguaiaretic acid: Hepatotoxicity and detoxification in the mouse. *Toxicon.* Dec;40(12):1701–1708.

Leung A, Foster S. (1996). *Encyclopedia of Common Natural Ingredients* (2nd ed.; pp. 148–150). New York: John Wiley & Sons.

Mabry JT, et al. (1977). *Creosote Bush: Biology and Chemistry of Larrea in New World Deserts.* Stroudsburg, PA: Dowden, Hutchinson and Ross.

McDonald RW, et al. (2001). Synthesis and anticancer activity of nordihydroguaiaretic acid (NDGA) and analogues. *Anti-Cancer Drug Design.* Dec;16(6):261–270.

Quiroga EN, et al. (2004). In vitro fungitoxic activity of *Larrea divaricata* cav. extracts. *Letters in Applied Microbiology.* 39(1):7–12.

Pedernera AM, et al. (2006). Anti-ulcerogenic and anti-inflammatory activity of the methanolic extract of *Larrea divariacata* cav. in rats. *Journal of Ethnopharmacology.* May 24;105(3):415–420.

Sahu SC, et al. (2006). Prooxidant activity and toxicity of nordihydroguaiaretic acid in clone-9 rat hepatocyte cultures. *Food and Chemical Toxicology*. Oct;44(10):1751–1757.

Sheikh NM, et al. (1997). Chaparral: Associated hepatotoxicity. *Archives of Internal Medicine*. 157:913–919.

NAME: Chaste Tree (*Vitex agnus-castus*)

Common Names: Monk's pepper, chasteberry

Family: *Verbenaceae*

Description of Plant: A woody shrub that grows abundantly in southern Europe and the Mediterranean; likes moist riverbanks; has purple flowers in summer, gray fruit in autumn

Medicinal Part: Dried fruit

Constituents and Action (if known)

- Bicyclic diterpenes: rotundifuran—dopaminergic activity (Jarry et al., 2006)
- Iridoid glycosides: agnuside (0.6%), aucubin (0.3%)
- Flavonoids and flavones (glucosides): casticin, iso-orientin, isovitexin (Brown, 1994; Snow, 1996), penduletin and apigenin-estrogenic (Jarry et al., 2006)
- EOs (0.5%–1.22%)
  - Monoterpenes: cineol (25%), alpha-pinene, beta-pinene, limonene, sabinene (Kustrak et al., 1992); sedative properties
  - Sesquiterpenes: beta-caryophyllene, germacrene B; may assist with regulation of luteal phase of female cycle (Milewicz et al., 1993)
- Other actions: binds to dopamine receptors and inhibits release of prolactin (Jarry et al., 1994; Snow, 1996)

Nutritional Ingredients: None known

History: Symbol of chastity in medieval European church; where it is native (Mediterranean, Greek islands), in pre-Christian times its use was sacred to Hera, the protectress of women

Traditional Use

- Anaphrodisiac, diaphoretic, diuretic, carminative, galactagogue
- Has been used for more than 2,000 years to treat female problems, such as menstrual cramps, irregular cycles, breast pain, and abnormal bleeding and to stimulate milk production in lactating women
- Believed to be an "anaphrodisiac" for men, it was called *monk's pepper*. Was grown around monasteries, and monks used it regularly as a tea to lessen sexual desires.
- Used for digestive upsets, to promote sweating in fevers, to increase urination, and to relieve hysteria

Current Use

- Treats perimenopausal symptoms (hot flashes, vaginal dryness, formication); most effective if used with black cohosh, dong quai, and omega-3 fatty acids (Hoffmann, 2003; Winston, 2006)
- Relieves moderate to severe premenstrual anxiety and other premenstrual symptoms caused by elevated estrogen levels or deficient progesterone levels (migraines, breast tenderness, cramps, edema, constipation) (ESCOP, 2003; Prilepskaya et al., 2006)
- Relieves breast pain (mastodynia) and helps to treat fibrocystic breast disease (Gorkow et al., 2002; Wuttke et al., 2003)
- Relieves dysmenorrhea; use along with antispasmodics such as black haw, motherwort, or Roman chamomile (Winston, 2006)
- In latent hyperprolactinemia, inhibits prolactin secretion by directly binding to the dopamine receptor in the pituitary (Kilicdag et al., 2004). Used for corpus luteum insufficiency (often caused by hyperprolectinemia) and associated symptoms (hypermenorrhea, infertility, polymenorrhea, oligomenorrhea, anovulation, primary and secondary amenorrhea, menorrhagia) (ESCOP, 2003; Mills & Bone, 2000).
- May be useful for women who have stopped using birth control pills and have irregular menstrual cycles (Winston, 2006)

- Increases milk production during lactation. Studies on 100 nursing mothers found that *Vitex* increased milk flow and eased milk release (Hoffmann, 2003).
- Useful for polycystic ovarian disease, along with saw palmetto, licorice, and white peony root (Winston, 2006)
- Can reduce the size of uterine fibroids (smooth muscle or subserous) and ovarian cysts; takes 2 to 6 months to see improvement
- Teenage acne: in a controlled study of 161 patients (male and female), after 3 months of treatment with *Vitex*, 70% reported significant improvement compared with patients using a placebo (Hoffmann, 2003)
- Some herbalists use *Vitex* to reduce cravings and withdrawal symptoms from opiates (heroin, methadone, oxycodone) due to its ability to bind with the mu-opiate receptor (Webster et al., 2006).

Available Forms, Dosage, and Administration Guidelines

Preparations: Dried fruit; capsules, tinctures, tablets, and combination products. Many clinical studies in Europe used a proprietary extract and capsules called Agnolyt.

Typical Dosage

- *Capsules* (nonstandardized): Up to three 650-mg capsules a day
- *Standardized extracts* (standardized for 0.5% agnuside): 175 to 225 mg/day
- *Tea:* Steep 1 scant tsp dried, ground berries in 1 cup of hot water for 10 to 15 minutes; take two cups a day.
- *Tincture* (1:5, 45% alcohol): 20 to 40 gtt (1–2 mL) once or twice a day
- Or follow manufacturer or practitioner recommendations

Pharmacokinetics—If Available (form or route when known): Not known

Toxicity: Nontoxic

Contraindications: May aggravate spasmodic dysmenorrhea that is not associated with premenstrual symptoms (Mills & Bone, 2000)

Side Effects: Reports of mild nausea, urticaria with itching, headache, increased menstrual flow, and acne have been noted.

Long-Term Safety: Safe (Daniele et al., 2005); safe in women with estrogen-positive cancers, no effect on estrogen receptors

Use in Pregnancy/Lactation/Children: Do not use until after menarche. Use cautiously in early pregnancy for insufficient corpus luteum function. Studies on lactating women show benefits and no toxicity.

Drug/Herb Interactions and Rationale (if known):
Haloperidol may weaken or block the effects of *Vitex*.

Special Notes: This herb's ability to reduce prolactin secretions may make it useful for benign prostatic hypertrophy in men.

BIBLIOGRAPHY

Betz W. (1998). Commentary. *Forschende Komplementarmedizen.* 5:146–147.

Bone K. (1994). *Vitex agnus castus:* Scientific studies and clinical applications. *European Journal of Herbal Medicine.* 1(2):12–15.

Brown DJ. (1994). *Vitex agnus castus* clinical monograph. *Quarterly Review of Natural Medicine.* Summer:111–121.

Daniele C, et al. (2005). *Vitex agnus castus:* A systematic review of adverse events. *Drug Safety.* 2005;28(4):319–332.

European Scientific Cooperative on Phytotherapy. (2003). *ESCOP Monographs* (pp. 8–13). New York: Thieme.

Gorkow C, et al. (2002). Effectiveness of *Vitex agnus-castus* preparations, *Wiener Klinische Wochenschrift.* 152(15–16):364–372.

Halaska M, et al. (1998). Treatment of cyclical mastodynia using an extract of *Vitex agnus castus:* Results of a double-blind comparison with a placebo. *Ceska Gynekologie.* 63(5):388–392.

Hirobe C, et al. (1997). Cytotoxic flavonoids from *Vitex agnus-castus.* *Phytochemistry.* 46(3):521–524.

Hoffmann, D. (2003). *Medical Herbalism, the Science and Practice of Herbal Medicine* (pp. 595–596). Rochester, VT: Inner Traditions.

Jarry H, et al. (1994). In vitro prolactin but not LH and FSH release is inhibited by compounds in extracts of *Agnus castus:* Direct evidence for a dopaminergic principle by the dopamine receptor assay. *Experimental and Clinical Endocrinology.* 102:448–454.

Jarry H, et al. (2006). In vitro assays for bioactivity-guided isolation of endocrine active compounds in *Vitex agnus-castus.* *Maturitas.* 55:S26–S36.

Kilicdag EB, et al. (2004). *Fructus agni casti* and bromocriptine for treatment of hyperprolactinemia and mastalgia. *International Journal of Gynaecology and Obstetrics.* Jun;85(3):292–293.

Kustrak KJ, et al. (1992). The composition of the essential oil of *Vitex agnus castus. Planta Medica.* 58[Suppl. 1]:A681.

Lauritzen D, et al. (1997). Treatment of premenstrual tension syndrome with *Vitex agnus-castus.* Controlled, double-blind study versus pyridoxine. *Phytomedicine.* 4(3):183–189.

Loch EG, et al. (2000). Treatment of premenstrual syndrome with a phytopharmaceutical formulation containing *Vitex agnus-castus. Journal of Women's Health and Gender-Based Medicine.* 9(3):315–320.

Milewicz A, et al. (1993). *Vitex agnus castus* extract in the treatment of luteal phase defects due to a latent hyperprolactinemia. Results of a randomized placebo-controlled double-blind study. *Arzneimittelforschung.* 45:752–756.

Mills S, Bone K. (2000). *Principles and Practice of Phytotherapy* (pp. 328–334). Edinburgh: Churchill Livingstone.

Prilepskaya VN, et al. (2006). *Vitex agnus-castus:* Successful treatment of moderate to severe premenstrual syndrome. *Maturitas.* 55:S55–S63.

Snow J. (1996). *Vitex. Protocol Journal of Botanical Medicine.* 1(4):20–23.

Webster DE, et al. (2006). Activation of the mu-opiate receptor by *Vitex agnus-castus* methanol extracts: Implication for its use in PMS. *Journal of Ethnopharmacology.* Jun 30;106(2):216–221.

Winston D. (2006). *Winston's Botanic Materia Medica.* Washington, NJ: DWCHS.

Wuttke W, et al. (2003). Chaste tree (*Vitex Agnus-castus*)— Pharmacology and clinical indications. *Phytomedicine.* May;10(4):348–357.

NAME: Cinnamon (*Cinnamomum verum,* syn. *C. zeylanicum*)

Common Names: Ceylon cinnamon, true cinnamon; Chinese cinnamon, which has similar uses, is *C. aromaticum* (*C. cassia*)

Family: *Lauraceae*

Description of Plant: A small evergreen tree native to southern India and Sri Lanka, now cultivated in India, Sri

Lanka, Malaysia, Madagascar, Vietnam, Zanzibar, Java, and Egypt

Medicinal Part: Bark and occasionally the leaves or buds

Constituents and Action (if known)

- Volatile oils (aldehydes): halt growth of *Aspergillus* (Tantaoui-Elaraki & Beraoud, 1994) and *Escherichia coli* (De et al., 1999); antifungal, antiviral, bactericidal effects (Leung & Foster, 1996)
  - Cinnamaldehyde (60%–85%): antiulcer activity, antibacterial, antifungal (Ooi et al., 2006)
  - Terpenes (eugenol, beta phellandrene, carvacrol, and others): anesthetic and antiseptic activity, inhibits *Candida albicans* growth (Tampieri et al., 2005)
  - Cinnamyl alcohol and acetate, limonene
- Condensed tannins
- Other actions: methylene chloride extracts have inhibitory effect on *Helicobacter pylori* (Tabak et al., 1999)
- Cinnamon extract has strong antioxidant activity (Lin et al., 2003; Mancini-Filho et al., 1988).

Nutritional Ingredients: Used as a spice and flavoring

Traditional Use

- Antibacterial, antifungal, carminative, antihemorrhagic
- EO used to treat GI upset, dysmenorrhea, hemorrhages (with oil of *Erigeron*), menorrhagia, hemoptysis, hematuria, nosebleeds (Ellingwood, 1919)
- Used to treat diarrhea, dysentery, vomiting, nausea, indigestion
- Flavoring agent for unpleasant-tasting medicines

Current Use

- May be useful for treating gastric ulcers and inhibiting *H. pylori* (Tabak et al., 1999). Only one human trial has been conducted, and in that trial, cinnamon in a low dose was not effective (Nir et al., 2000). The authors of the study admit that a larger dose or combining it with other antimicrobials might be more effective. This brings up a serious point when looking at the way that herbs are studied. In herbal medicine, it is rare to use single herbs; rather, they are almost always used in formulas to enhance activity or absorption or to reduce side effects. A 2005 study found that cinnamon inhibited *H. pylori* growth but that tumeric, ginger, oregano, and licorice killed the bacterium (O'Mahony et al., 2005). In traditional herbal practice, combining cinnamon, ginger, and licorice is a common practice that would make a flavorful and most likely effective treatment for gastric ulcers.

- Relieves GI system problems: useful for flatulence, nausea, bloating, borborygmus, mild gastric upset, poor fat digestion
- Adjunct therapy for insulin resistance (metabolic syndrome) and adult-onset insulin-resistant diabetes. Cinnamon increases the utilization of endogenous insulin (Khan et al., 1990), moderately lowers blood sugar levels (Khan et al., 2003; Verspohl et al., 2005), and helps with glycemic control (Mang et al., 2006). Regular intake of cinnamon also reduced triglycerides, LDL cholesterol, and total cholesterol in type 2 diabetics (Khan et al., 2003).
- In Chinese medicine, cinnamon (*C. aromaticum*) is used in several forms. The sliced twigs (Gui Zhi) are used to stimulate sweating, for cold/damp arthralgias, amenorrhea, cold/damp coughs, and edema (Chen & Chen, 2004). The bark (Rou Gui) is used for impotence, cold/damp coughs, poor peripheral circulation, asthma, edema, GI upset, dysmenorrhea, and arthritis (bi-pain) (Chen & Chen, 2004).

Available Forms, Dosage, and Administration Guidelines

- Used in combination with other herbs; rarely used alone
- *Bark:* Unless otherwise prescribed, 2 to 4 g/day of ground bark
- *Infusion or decoction:* 0.25 to 0.5 tsp powdered bark in 8 oz hot water; steep covered 20 minutes; take 2 to 4 oz three times a day
- *Fluid extract* (1:1): 10 to 25 gtt (0.5–1 mL) three times a day
- *Tincture* (1:5, 70% alcohol): 30 to 50 gtt (1.5–2.5 mL) three times a day
- *EO:* 1 to 2 gtt three times a day

Pharmacokinetics—If Available (form or route when known): Not known

Toxicity: Large amounts increase heart rate and intestinal motility, followed by sleepiness and depression (Wichtl & Bisset, 1994).

Contraindications: None known

Side Effects: There are case reports of skin irritation from contact with cinnamon powder and oral lesions from chewing cinnamon gum.

Long-Term Safety: As a spice, long-term use is safe.

Use in Pregnancy/Lactation/Children: Use as a spice is fine; avoid large doses.

Drug/Herb Interactions and Rationale (if known): None known

Special Notes: Cinnamon has been found to kill *Escherichia coli* O157, the potentially fatal bacteria that causes serious food poisoning. Along with cloves and garlic, cinnamon added to meats and unpasteurized apple cider killed 99.5% of the bacteria (Friedman, et al., 2004).

BIBLIOGRAPHY

Blumenthal M, et al. (2000). *Herbal Medicine: Expanded Commission E Monographs*. Austin, TX: American Botanical Council.

Chen J, Chen T. (2004). *Chinese Medical Herbology and Pharmacology* (pp. 40–42, 447–449). City of Industry, CA: Art of Medicine Press.

De M, et al. (1999). Antimicrobial screening of some Indian spices. *Phytotherapy Research*. 13(7):616–618.

Ellingwood F. (1919). *American Materia Medica, Therapeutics, and Pharmacognosy* (p. 353). Evanston, IL: Ellingwood's Therapeutist.

Friedman M, et al. (2004). Antibactrial activities of plant essential oils and their components against Escherichia coli O157:H7 and Salmonella enterica in apple juice. *Journal Agricul Food Chem*. Sep. 22:52(19):6042–6048.

Khan A, et al. (1990). Insulin potentiating factor and chromium content of selected foods and spices. *Biological Trace Elements Research*. 24:183–188.

Khan A, et al. (2003). Cinnamon improves glucose and lipids of people with type 2 diabetes. *Diabetes Care*. Dec;26(12):3215–3218.

Leung AY, Foster S. (1996). *Encyclopedia of Common Natural Ingredients Used in Food, Drugs and Cosmetics* (2nd ed.; pp. 167–170). New York: John Wiley & Sons.

Lin CC, et al. (2003). Antioxidant activity of *Cinnamomum cassia*. *Phytotherapy Research*. Aug;17(7):726–730.

Mancini-Filho J, et al. (1988). Antioxidant activity of cinnamon (*Cinnamomum zeylanicum*, Brene) extracts. *Bollettino Chimico Farmaceutico*. 137(11):443–447.

Mang B, et al. (2006). Effects of a cinnamon extract on plasma glucose, HbA, and serum lipids in diabetes mellitus type 2. *European Journal of Clinical Investigation*. May;36(5):340–344.

Nir Y, et al. (2000). Controlled trial of the effect of cinnamon extract on *Helicobacter pylori*. *Helicobacter*. Jun;5(2):94–97.

O'Mahony R, et al. (2005). Bactericidal and anti-adhesive properties of culinary and medicinal plants against *Helicobacter pylori*. *World Journal of Gastroenterology*. Dec 21;11(47):7499–7507.

Ooi LS, et al. (2006). Antimicrobial activities of cinnamon oil and cinnamaldehyde from the Chinese medicinal herb *Cinnamomum cassia* Blume. *American Journal of Chinese Medicine*. 34(3):511–522.

Tabak M, et al. (1999). Cinnamon extracts' inhibitory effect on *Helicobacter pylori*. *Journal of Ethnopharmacology*. 67(3):269–277.

Tampieri MP, et al. (2005). The inhibition of *Candida albicans* by selected essential oils and their major components. *Mycopathologia*. Apr;159(3):339–345.

Tantaoui-Elaraki A, Beraoud L. (1994). Inhibition of growth and aflatoxin production in *Aspergillus parasiticus* by essential oils of selected plant materials. *Journal of Environmental Pathology, Toxicology, and Oncology*. 13(1):67.

Verspohl EJ, et al. (2005). Antidiabetic effect of *Cinnamomum cassia* and *Cinnamomum zeylanicum* in vivo and in vitro. *Phytotherapy Research*. Mar;19(3):203–206.

Wichtl N, Bisset NG. [Eds.]. (1994). *Herbal Drugs and Phytopharmaceuticals* (pp. 148–150). Stuttgart: Medpharm Scientific Publishers.

 NAME: Coltsfoot (*Tussilago farfara*)

Common Names: Bullfoot, coughwort, foalswort, Kuan Dong Hua (Chinese name for the flowers)

Family: *Asteraceae*

Description of Plant: Creeping weedy perennial that flowers before leafing out. Flowers are yellow, followed by a white dandelion-like puffball.

Medicinal Part: Leaf, flowers

Constituents and Action (if known)

- Mucilage (6%–10%)

- Tannins (5%)
- Triterpenes: beta-amyrin, arnidol, faradiol
- Pyrrolizidine alkaloids: trace amounts of tussilagine, isotussilagine, senkirkine, senecionin in some samples
- Flavonoids

History: Painted pictures of coltsfoot leaves were used as a sign of an herbalist in medieval France.

Nutritional Ingredients: The leaves, burned to ash, have been used as a salt substitute.

Traditional Use
- Expectorant, pectoral, demulcent
- Dry coughs, bronchitis, bronchial catarrh, asthma, sore throat, chest colds, tonsillitis
- Irritation of the bladder

Current Use
- Dry, irritable, ticklish coughs; chronic irritation of the mouth and throat with hoarseness
- In Chinese medicine, the flowers are often used with other respiratory tonics for coughs, wheezing, and mild asthma (Chen & Chen, 2004).

Available Forms, Dosage, and Administration Guidelines: *Tea:* 1 tsp dried herb in 8 oz water, steep 20 minutes; take 4 oz three times a day

Pharmacokinetics—If Available (form or route when known): Not known

Toxicity: Contains trace amounts of pyrrolizidine alkaloids, a cumulative liver toxin associated with veno-occlusive disease. The FDA classifies it as an herb of "undefined safety."

Contraindications: Pregnancy, breast-feeding, use in children, liver disease

Side Effects: None known

Long-Term Safety: The German Commission E warns against use for more than 28 days a year. Short-term use only. Even when used for a few days, daily intake of PAs should not exceed 10 mcg a day (Gruenwald et al., 2004).

Use in Pregnancy/Lactation/Children: Do not use

Drug/Herb Interactions and Rationale (if known): None known

Special Notes

- There are PA-free varieties of coltsfoot and PA-free extracts available from Europe.
- Source of the herb is important: two common adulterants, Western coltsfoot (Petasites) and *Adenostyles alliariae*, contain dangerous levels of PAs
- Coltsfoot flowers used in TCM have higher levels of the toxic PA senkirkine, which is potentially carcinogenic. Avoid using the flowers.

BIBLIOGRAPHY

Brinker F. (2001). *Herb Contraindications and Drug Interactions* (3rd ed.; p. 74). Sandy, OR: Eclectic Medical Publications.

Chen J, Chen T. (2004). *Chinese Medical Herbology and Pharmacology* (pp. 729–730). City of Industry, CA: Art of Medicine Press.

Der Marderosian AH, Beutler J. [Eds.]. (2005). *The Review of Natural Products*. St Louis, MO: Facts and Comparisons.

Gruenwald J, et al. (2004). *PDR for Herbal Medicines* (pp. 200–201). Montvale, NJ: Thompson-PDR.

Schultz V, et al. (1998). *Rational Phytotherapy: A Physician's Guide to Herbal Medicine* (3rd ed.; p. 34). Berlin: Springer-Verlag.

Sperl W, et al. (1995). Reversible hepatic veno-occlusive disease in an infant after consumption of pyrrolizidine-containing herbal tea. *European Journal of Pediatrics*. 154(2):112–116.

Wichtl M, Bisset NG. (1994). *Herbal Drugs and Phytopharmaceuticals* (pp. 197–199). Boca Raton, FL: CRC Press.

 NAME: Comfrey Leaf or Root (*Symphytum officinale*)

Common Names: Knitbone

Family: *Boraginaceae*

Description of Plant

- Comfrey is a large-leafed herbaceous perennial with prickly leaves and white, pink, or pale blue flowers.

- It is a very easy plant to grow, and the leaves added to a compost pile accelerate and enhance compost fermentation.

Medicinal Part: Leaf or root

Constituents and Action (if known)
- Allantoin (13,000 ppm, leaf; 6,000–8,000 ppm, root): anti-inflammatory, antioxidant (Koll et al., 2004)
- Caffeic acid (root): antioxidant, neuroprotective (Zhou et al., 2006), anti-inflammatory (Norata et al., 2006)
- Rosmarinic acid (leaf): antioxidant, anti-inflammatory, antibacterial, antiviral (Peterson et al., 2003), neuroprotective (Iuvone et al., 2006)
- Pyrrolizidine alkaloids (root and leaf)
  - Symphytine: hepatotoxic (Betz et al., 1994)
  - Intermedicine: hepatotoxic (Betz et al., 1994)
  - Echimidine: hepatotoxic (Betz et al., 1994)
  - Symlandine: hepatotoxic (Betz et al., 1994)
  - Lycopasamine: hepatotoxic (Betz et al., 1994)
- Sulphur containing amino acids (cysteine, methionone): radioprotective (Wan et al., 2006), antioxidant (Shoveller et al., 2005)
- Mucilage: demulcent, anti-inflammatory (Winston, 2006)
- Protein

Nutritional Ingredients: In the 1960s and 1970s, comfrey leaves were commonly juiced and mixed with other juices to make "green drinks." This practice is not recommended.

Traditional Use
- Demulcent, vulnerary, styptic, astringent, anti-inflammatory
- Comfrey has a long tradition of use topically to heal fractures, sprains, muscle tears, bruises, joint injuries, and abrasions
- Internally, comfrey has been used to heal inflammation and ulceration of the stomach, and small and large intestines (gastric and duodenal ulcers, ulcerative colitis, ileitis, regional enteritis).
- Due to its abundant mucilage, it has also been used for irritation of the throat and upper respiratory tract (dry coughs, sore throat, bronchitis).

Current Use

● In July, 2001, the FDA recommended that comfrey not be
used internally due to the potentially hepatotoxic PAs that it
contains. There are four relatively well-documented cases of
comfrey-induced veno-oclusive disease (VOD) in the
literature. There are still some practitioners in the herbal and
naturopathic communities who dispute that comfrey has
significant potential for harm (Denham, 1996). There are a
number of issues that need to be recognized. First, comfrey
root contains much higher levels of PAs than the leaf.
Mature leaves contain lower levels of PAs than young leaves.
An infusion (tea) of the leaf only extracts about one third of
the alkaloids found in the plant (Roitman, 1981). So, if this
herb is going to be used internally, the mature leaf tea would
be the safest preparation. It is also important to note that
Symphytum officinale contains fewer and less toxic PAs than
S. uplandicum or Russian comfrey. The lack of definite
botanical identification and hybridization between the two
species may play a role in some of the four reported VOD
cases. Determining the actual risk of using this herb orally is
problematic. During the 1960s through the 1990s, hundreds
of thousands to millions of Americans routinely (many
daily) ingested comfrey in the form of "green drinks,"
capsules, or tablets (comfrey-pepsin), teas, and tinctures.
One would suspect that if comfrey was as toxic as stated in
the literature, there would be many more reported cases of
VOD. The concern with this belief is that veno-oclusive
disease is a very slow, chronic problem that can be "invisible"
until very late in its progression. The only way to determine
if someone has VOD is a liver biopsy, and since this
procedure is not commonly performed, there is no idea as to
whether there are a significant number of subclinical cases of
VOD in the population of people who at one time used this
herb. Much of the literature about the toxicity of PAs has
studied isolated PAs, not a whole herb or comfrey, and most
of the research studied rats. This is unfortunate, because rats
and mice are very susceptible to PA toxicity, while humans
are less so (Rode, 2002). Interestingly, not only is there a
wide difference in susceptibility to PAs from species to
species, there is a substantial difference in susceptibility to

various types of PAs. Pigs are quite susceptible to poisoning from the PA-containing plant Senecio, but even when fed comfrey at levels as high as 4% of their diet, they had no liver damage (Rode, 2002). Chickens are also sensitive to PAs from other plants but suffered no liver damage from regular ingestion of comfrey.

- There are numerous human studies showing that comfrey gels or ointments can help to speed healing of ankle sprains and muscle and back pain (Kucera et al., 2005; Predel et al., 2005). Dermal absorption of PAs is limited, and comfrey products for topical use are widely available in countries that have banned or controlled the use of it internally (Brauchli et al., 1982; Koll et al., 2004).

Available Forms, Dosage, and Administration Guidelines

Preparations: Tea, PA-free tincture, ointment, poultice

Typical Dosage

- *Tea* (made from the dried, mature leaves): 1 to 2 tsp dried leaf to 8 oz hot water, steep 30 to 40 minutes, take 4 oz twice a day. If used internally, recommended for short-term use only.
- *PA-free tincture* (1:5; 65% alcohol): 10 to 20 gtt (0.5–1 mL) three times a day
- *Topical applications:* The maximum dosage of PAs in topical preparations allowed by the German government is 100 mcg a day, and the length of the treatment is limited to 4 to 6 weeks a year.

Pharmacokinetics—If Available (form or route when known): PAs are well absorbed orally, they are excreted mainly via the urine (50–80%). Dermal absorption is minimal in intact skin (EAEMP, 1999).

Toxicity: Chronic internal use of comfrey has been linked to four cases of VOD. The FDA has recommended against using comfrey topically on open wounds due to the possible dermal absorption of PAs.

Contraindications: Avoid using topically for puncture wounds, as it can quickly heal the surface, preventing drainage of wounds.

Side Effects: See Toxicity

Long-Term Safety: Problematic, due to potentially hepatotoxic PAs

Use in Pregnancy/Lactation/Children: Avoid internal use during pregnancy, lactation, and with children.

Drug/Herb Interactions and Rationale (if known): One animal study suggests taking glycyrrhizin or glycyrrhetinic acid (compounds from licorice) with PAs may decrease their hepatotoxicity (Lin et al., 1999). Avoid using comfrey with eucalyptus, which may increase the toxicity of the PAs (Brinker, 2001).

Special Notes: There is a PA-free comfrey tincture available from Germany and Switzerland. This product still contains trace amounts of PAs (less than one part per million) but is considered safe for internal use.

BIBLIOGRAPHY

Altamirano JC, et al. (2005). Investigation of pyrrolizidine alkaloids and their N-oxides in commerical comfrey-containing products and botanical materials by liquid chromatography electrospray ionization mass spectrometry. *Journal of AOAC International.* Mar-Apr;88(2):406–412.

Bartram T. (1995). *Encyclopedia of Herbal Medicine* (pp. 124–125). Dorset, UK: Grace Publishers.

Betz JM, et al. (1994). Determination of pyrrolizidine alkaloids in commercial comfrey products (*Symphytum* sp.). *Journal of Pharmacological Science.* May;83(5):649–653.

Brauchli J, et al. (1982). Pyrrolizidine alkaloids from *Symphytum officinale* L. and their percutaneous absorption in rats. *Cellular and Molecular Life Sciences.* 38(9):1085–1087.

Brinker F. (2001). *Herb Contraindications and Drug Interactions* (3rd ed.; p. 75). Sandy, OR: Eclectic Medical Publications.

Denham A. (1996). Using herbs that contain pyrrolizidine alkaloids. *European Journal of Herbal Medicine.* Autumn;2(3):27–38.

EAEMP, European Agency for the Evaluation of Medicinal Products. Symphyti Radix Summary Report, August 1999.

Iuvone T, et al. (2006). The spice sage and its active ingredient rosmarinic acid protect PC12 cells from amyloid-beta peptide-induced neurotoxicity. *Journal of Pharmacology and Experimental Therapeutics.* Jun;317(3):1143–1149.

Koll B, et al. (2004). Efficacy and tolerance of a comfrey root extract (Extr. Rad. Symphyti) in the treatment of ankle distortions: Results of a multicenter, randomized, placebo-controlled, double-blind study. *Phytomedicine.* Sep;11(6):470–477.

Kucera M, et al. (2004). Efficacy and safety of topically applied Symphytum herb extract cream in the treatment of ankle distortion: Results of a randomized controlled clinical double blind study. *Wiener Medizinische Wochenschrift.* Nov;154(21–22):498–507.

Kucera M, et al. (2005). Topical Symphytum herb concentrate cream against myalgia: A randomized controlled double-blind clinical study. *Advances in Therapy.* Nov-Dec;22(6):681–692.

Lin G, et al. (1999). The effects of pretreatment with glycyrrhizin and glycyrrhetinic acid on the retrorsine-induced hepatotoxicity in rats. *Toxicon.* Sep;37(9):1259–1270.

Norata GD, et al. (2006). Anti-inflammatory and anti-atherogenic effects of cathechin, caffeic acid and trans-resveratrol in apolipoprotein E deficient mice. *Atherosclerosis.* 191(2):265–271.

Petersen M, et al. (2003). Rosmarinic acid. *Phytochemistry.* Jan;62(2):121–125.

Predel HG, et al. (2005). Efficacy of a comfrey root extract ointment in comparison to a diclofenac gel in the treatment of ankle distortions: Results of an observer-blind, randomized, multicenter study. *Phytomedicine.* Nov;12(10):707–714.

Rode D. (2002). Comfrey toxicity revisited. *Trends in Pharmacological Sciences.* Nov;23(11):497–499.

Roitman JN. (1981). Comfrey and liver damage. *Lancet,* Apr 25;1 (8226):944.

Shoveller AK, et al. (2005). Nutritional and functional importance of intestinal sulfur amino acid metabolism. *Journal of Nutrition.* Jul;135(7):1609–1612.

Wan XS, et al. (2006). Protection against radiation-induced oxidative stress in cultured human epithelial cells by treatment with antioxidant agents. *International Journal of Radiation Oncology, Biology, Physics.* Apr 1;64(5):1475–1481.

Winston D. (2006). *Winston's Botanic Materia Medica.* Washington, NJ: DWCHS.

Zhou Y, et al. (2006). Caffeic acid ameliorates early and delayed brain injuries after focal cerebral ichemia in rats. *Acta Pharmacologica Sinica.* Sep;27(9):1103–1110.

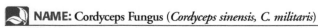

NAME: Cordyceps Fungus (*Cordyceps sinensis, C. militaris*)

Common Names: Caterpillar fungus, Dong Chong Xia Cao (Chinese)

Family: *Clavicipitaceae*

Description of Plant

- This is a small mushroom that parasitizes the caterpillar of the Thitarodes moth.
- The mushrooms are collected in the grasslands of the Himalayan plateau in Tibet, Bhutan, and Nepal.

Medicinal Part: The fungus or the mycelium, which is grown on soybeans, rice, or in fermentation tanks

Constituents and Action (if known)

- Adenosine: anti-inflammatory (Linden, 2006)
- Cordycepic acid (mannose)
- Cordycepin: antitumor (Yoshikawa et al., 2004), antibacterial (Ng & Wang, 2005)
- Ecdysterones: antioxidant, anabolic, adaptogenic, hepatoprotective (Kholodova, 2001)
- Ergosterol: antitumor, immunomodulatory (Ng & Wang, 2005)
- Polysaccharides: CSP-1—hypoglycemic, antioxidant (Li et al., 2006), immunomodulatory (Wu et al., 2006)
- Other actions: antileukemic (Stamets, 2002), hypocholesteremic (Yamaguchi et al., 2000)

Nutritional Ingredients: The fungus is prized in Chinese medicine as a nutritive tonic. The emperor was given duck stuffed with cordyceps as a longevity-enhancing food. The caterpillar fungus is still used today, cooked with chicken or duck as a strengthening food.

Traditional Use

- Adaptogen, antiasthmatic, antibacterial, antileukemic, antioxidant, hepatoprotective, hypocholesteremic, immune amphoteric, nephroprotective, sedative
- Cordyceps is used in Chinese medicine for deficient kidney *yin* and *yang* conditions causing weakness, fatigue, low back pain, poor memory, tinnitus, dizziness, and impotence.
- It is also frequently used for *yin* deficient (dry) asthma with a chronic cough. Combined with Prince Seng, licorice, and Ophiopogon, it relieves asthma, dry coughs, and hemoptysis (Winston, 2006).

Current Use

- Cordyceps is nephroprotective and improves kidney function in patients with chronic nephritis with degeneration and glomerulonephritis (Chen & Chen, 2004; Winston & Maimes, 2007).

- In a Chinese study (Lu, 2002), a combination of cordyceps and artemisinin was given to 31 patients (30 additional patients were in the control group) who were in remission from lupus nephritis. The cordyceps-artemisinin protocol prevented recurrence in 83.9% of patients, whereas 50% of the control group relapsed.

- This mushroom is an immunomodulator; it increases Kupffer cell, macrophage, and NK cell activity. It increases levels of erythroid (bone marrow) cells and platelets suppressed by medication (Nakamura et al., 1999a; Stamets, 2005). Many in vivo animal studies as well as in vitro studies show that this mushroom stimulates immune response, preventing streptococcal infections (Kuo et al., 2005), liver metastasis of Lewis lung carcinoma, and B16 melanoma cells (Nakamura et al., 1999b). It is also used for autoimmune conditions and allergies, especially allergic asthma and allergic rhinitis (Winston & Maimes, 2007).

- Cordyceps has a long history of use for impotence and lack of libido. In a Chinese study, cultivated cordyceps improved sexual performance in 64.5% of patients who took 1 gram three times a day (Chen & Chen, 2004).

- Olympic athletes from China have used this mushroom to enhance athletic performance and improve recovery time. In 2004, there were two negative studies using a standardized extract of cordyceps with endurance-trained cyclists. The limitations of both studies are they were short—2 weeks and 5 weeks—and it raises questions about the activity of the specific product (Parcell et al., 2004). It is an adaptogen helping to re-regulate the HPA axis, the immune system, and nervous system. Hot water mycelial extracts increased swimming endurance in mice. It also prevented stress-induced weight changes to the thymus, adrenals, spleen, and thyroid (Koh et al., 2003). It also has antiarrhythmic (Chen & Chen, 2004), bronchodilating (Stamets, 2005), hypocholesteremic (Koh et al., 2003), and hepatoprotective (Koh et al., 2003) effects.

- Many herbalists and naturopathic physicians use cordyceps as an immune amphoteric to help support the immune and endocrine systems for patients undergoing orthodox therapies for leukemia, cancer, hepatitis B and C, autoimmune diseases, and Lyme disease (Winston, 2006).

Available Forms, Dosage, and Administration Guidelines

Preparations: Dried mushroom, tincture, capsule

Typical Dosage

- *Dried mushroom:* 5 to 10 g a day
- *Tincture* (1:4, 25% alcohol): 20 to 40 gtt (2–4 mL) three times a day
- *Capsules* (5:1 extract): 2 capsules twice a day

Pharmacokinetics—If Available (form or route when known): Not known

Toxicity: Excessive doses of cordyceps have been reported to cause immune suppression in animals and to cause headache, edema, and anxiety in humans.

Contraindications: Avoid in people with mushroom allergies.

Side Effects: In overdose, side effects can include immune suppression, headache, anxiety, edema, and nosebleeds.

Long-Term Safety: Safe in normal therapeutics doses. Animal studies indicate that cordyceps has very little acute or chronic toxicity.

Use In Pregnancy/Lactation/Children: Safe

Drug/Herb Interactions and Rationale (if known): Some texts recommend against using this mushroom with patients who are taking immunosuppressive medication. A Chinese study found no interaction and that taking cordyceps prevented cyclosporine-induced nephrotoxicity (Xu et al., 1995). Cordyceps reduced nephrotoxicity in mice and humans caused by gentamicin, amikacin, and kanamycin (Brinker, 2001).

Special Notes: There is controversy as to whether the cultivated *Cordyceps mycelium* is as effective as the natural caterpillar fungus. Several studies show that both have activity

(Yu et al., 2006), and there is a possibility of the wild mushrooms being contaminated with other fungi and bacteria. Occasionally, unscrupulous traders will put lead wires inside the fungi to increase the weight.

BIBLIOGRAPHY

Brinker F. (2001). *Herb Contraindications and Drug Interactions* (3rd ed.; p. 76). Sandy, OR: Eclectic Medical Publications.

Chen J, Chen T. (2004). *Chinese Medical Herbology and Pharmacology* (pp. 883–885). City of Industry, CA: Art of Medicine Press.

Kholodova Y. (2001). Phytoecdysteroids: Biological effects, application in agriculture and complementary medicine (as presented at the 14th Ecdysone Workshop, July, 2000, Rapperswil, Switzerland). *Ukrainskii Biokhimicheskii Zhurnal.* May-Jun;73(3):21–29.

Koh JH, et al. (2003). Antifatigue and antistress effect of the hot-water fraction from mycelia of *Cordyceps sinensis*. *Biological and Pharmaceutical Bulletin.* May;26(5):691–694.

Kuo CF, et al. (2005). *Cordyceps sinensis* mycelium protects mice from group a streptococcal infection. *Journal of Medical Microbiology.* Aug;54[Pt. 8]:795–802.

Li SP, et al. (2006). Hypoglycemic activity of polysaccharide, with antioxidation, isolated from cultured *Cordyceps mycelia*. *Phytomedicine.* Jun;13(6):428–433. Epub 2005 Sep 19.

Linden J. (2006). New insights into the regulation of inflammation by adenosine. *Journal of Clinical Investigation.* Jul;116(7):1835–1837.

Lu L. (2002). Study on effect of *Cordyceps sinensis* and artemisinin in preventing recurrence of lupus nephritis. *Zhongguo Zhong Xi Yi Jie He Za Zhi.* Mar;22(3):169–171.

Nakamura K, et al. (1999a). Activation of in vivo Kupffer cell function by oral administration of *Cordyceps sinensis* in rats. *Japanese Journal of Pharmacology.* Apr;79(4):505–508.

Nakamura K, et al. (1999b). Inhibitory effect of *Cordyceps sinensis* on spontaneous liver metastasis of Lewis lung carcimona and B16 melanoma cells in syngeneic mice. *Japanese Journal of Pharmacology.* Mar;79(3):335–341.

Ng TB, Wang HX. (2005). Pharmacological actions of cordyceps, a prized folk medicine. *Journal of Pharmacy and Pharmacology.* Dec;57(12):1509–1519.

Parcell AC, et al. (2004). *Cordyceps sinensis* (CordyMax Cs-4) supplementation does not improve endurance exercise performance. *International Journal of Sport Nutrition and Exercise Metabolism.* Apr;14(2):236–242.

Stamets P. (2002). *Mycomedicinals* (pp. 57–62). Olympia, WA: Mycomedia Productions.

Winkler D. (2004). Yartsa gunbu—*Cordyceps sinensis*. Economy, ecology, & ethno-mycology of a fungus endemic to the Tibetan plateau. In: Bosei A, Cardi F [Eds.]. *Wildlife and Plants in Traditional and Modern Tibet: Conceptions, Exploitation and Conservation. Memorie della Societa Italiana di Scienze Naturali.* 34(1–2).

Winston D. (2006). *Winston's Botanic Materia Medica.* Washington, NJ: DWCHS.

Winston D, Maimes S. (2007). *Adaptogens, Herbs for Strength, Stamina, and Stress Relief.* (pp. 150–154). Rochester, VT: Inner Traditions.

Wu Y, et al. (2006). Effect of various extracts and a polysaccharide from the edible mycelia of *Cordyceps sinensis* on cellular and humoral immune response against ovalbumin in mice. *Phytotherapy Research.* Aug;20(8):646–652.

Xu F, et al. (1995). Amelioration of cyclosporin nephrotoxicity by *Cordyceps sinensis* in kidney-transplanted recipients. *Nephrology, Dialysis, Transplantation.* 10(1):142–143.

Yamaguchi Y, et al. (2000). Inhibitory effects of water extracts from fruiting bodies of cultured *Cordyceps sinensis* on raised serum lipid peroxide levels and aortic cholesterol deposition in atherosclerotic mice. *Phytotherapy Research.* Dec;14(8):650–652.

Yoshikawa N, et al. (2004). Antitumour activity of cordycepin in mice. *Clinical and Experimental Pharmacology and Physiology.* Dec;31[Suppl. 2]:S51–S53.

Yu HM, et al. (2006). Comparison of protective effects between cultured *Cordyceps militaris* and natural *Cordyceps sinensis* against oxidative damage. *Journal of Agricultural and Food Chemistry.* Apr 19;54(8):3132–3138.

Zhu J, et al. (1999a). The scientific rediscovery of an ancient Chinese herbal medicine—*Cordyceps sinensis*, Part I. *Journal of Alternative and Complementary Medicine.* 4(3):289–303.

Zhu J, et al. (1999b). The scientific rediscovery of an ancient Chinese herbal medicine—*Cordyceps sinensis*, Part II. *Journal of Alternative and Complementary Medicine.* 4(4):429–457.

 NAME: Cranberry (*Vaccinium macrocarpon*)

Common Names: Swamp cranberry, small cranberry, southern mountain cranberry, marsh apple

Family: *Ericaceae*

Description of Plant: Small trailing evergreen vine producing pink-purple flowers from May to August, loves water, grows well in acidic bogs but also in acidic mountain forests

Medicinal Part: Ripe fruit and juice

Constituents and Action (if known)
- Anthocyanins or proanthocyanidins: high-molecular-weight anthocyanins (flavonoids) prevent *Escherichia coli* from adhering to bladder wall (Howell et al., 1998; Ofek et al., 1991; Zafiri et al., 1989; Zopf & Roth, 1996) as well as the teeth and gums (Weiss et al., 1998)
- Organic acids (citric, malic, guinic, benzoic, glucuronic): slow biotransformation of acids, which increases excretion of hippuric acid, which acidifies the urine. Quinic and benzoic acids break down and form hippuric acid in urine (Avorn et al., 1994; Der Marderosian, 1977; Kahn et al., 1967; Walsh, 1992).
- Flavonoids: quercitin and flavonol compounds—antiproliferative and antioxidant (He & Liu, 2006).
- Triterpenoids: ursolic acid—antiproliferative (He & Liu, 2006), anti-inflammatory, antibacterial (He & Liu, 2006)
- Fructose: prevents adhesion of type 1 *E. coli* to the urinary tract (Zafiri et al., 1989)
- Carbohydrates (10%), ascorbic acid (10 mg)

Nutritional Ingredients: Can be used to make relish or sauces and juice. The bitter and sour taste of cranberries makes added sweeteners a necessity. Unsweetened cranberries are low in calories (209 calories/lb), are a good source of fiber, and are high in vitamin C and flavonoids.

Traditional Use
- Used as a refrigerant to reduce fever
- To acidify the urine, treat urinary tract infections, and prevent formation of urinary calculi
- To prevent and treat scurvy
- To soothe swollen glands and wounds (topically as a poultice)

Current Use

- Lowers incidence of and prevents urinary tract infections (Avorn et al., 1994; Gibson et al., 1991; Howell et al., 1998; Stothers, 2002)
- Decreases incidence of urinary stones (McHarg et al., 2003)
- Decreases symptoms in chronic pyelonephritis (6 oz juice twice a day)
- Reduces odor in urine in incontinent patients (Walsh, 1992)
- Unsweetened juice may prevent coaggregation of gum bacteria and reduce plaque formation (Weiss et al., 1998).
- Cranberry juice also exhibits an antiadhesion effect against *Helicobacter phylori* and can reduce infections by this organism and the gastric ulcers and gastritis that it can cause (Zhang et al., 2005).

Available Forms, Dosage, and Administration Guidelines

Preparations: Whole fruit, raw or jellied; juice, fruit concentrate, capsules

Typical Dosage

- *Capsules:* One capsule morning and night, but up to nine 300- to 500-mg capsules a day
- *Food:* 3 to 8 oz fresh fruit a day
- *Juice:* 5 to 20 oz cranberry juice cocktail a day (make sure that juice contains real cranberry; most contain 10%–33% cranberry)
- Or follow manufacturer or practitioner recommendations

Pharmacokinetics—If Available (form or route when known): Studies have found a high degree of absorption of cranberry anthocyanins, and urinary excretion reached a maximum between 3 to 6 hours after ingestion (Ohnishi et al., 2006).

Toxicity: None known

Contraindications: Do not use in urinary obstruction.

Side Effects: None with normal doses; large doses (3–4 L/day) may result in diarrhea

Long-Term Safety: Very safe

Use in Pregnancy/Lactation/Children: None known; safe

Drug/Herb Interactions and Rationale (if known):
Drinking large amounts of cranberry juice may affect warfarin levels and potential for increased bleeding (Aston et al., 2006). A human study looked at the effects of cranberry juice, grape juice, and tea on flurbiprofen clearance. While all three beverages altered CYP2C9-mediated clearance of the medication in vitro, none had this effect in humans. The authors of the study state that since warfarin is metabolized by this pathway, interactions between any of these substances and warfarin are highly unlikely (Greenblatt et al., 2006). Cranberry juice did not affect cyclospone disposition in humans (Grenier et al., 2006) but did alter nifedipine pharmacokinetics in rats and inhibited CYP3A4 (Uesawa & Mohri, 2006).

Special Notes

- Should not be used as a substitute for anti-infectives when a urinary tract infection is present
- Persons with diabetes should use sugar-free juices.
- Always drink at least six to eight glasses of water a day.

BIBLIOGRAPHY

Aston JL, et al. (2006). Interaction between warfarin and cranberry juice. *Pharmacotherapy*. Sep;26(9):1314–1319.

Avorn J, et al. (1994). Reduction of bacteriuria and pyuria after ingestion of cranberry juice. *Journal of the American Medical Association*. 271:751.

Bruyere F. (2006). Use of cranberry in chronic urinary tract infections. *Médecine et. Maladies Infectieses*. Jul;36(7):358–363.

Der Marderosian AH. (1997). Cranberry juice. *Drug Therapy*. 7:151.

Gibson L, et al. (1991). Effectiveness of cranberry juice in preventing urinary tract infections in long-term care facility patients. *Journal of Naturopathic Medicine*. 2:45–47.

Greenblatt DJ, et al. (2006). Interaction of flurbiprofen with cranberry juice, grape juice, tea, and fluconazole: In vitro and clinical studies. *Clinical Pharmacology and Therapeutics*. Jan;79(1):125–133.

Grenier J, et al. (2006). Pomelo juice, but not cranberry juice, affects the pharmacokinetics of cyclosporine in humans. *Clinical Pharmacology and Therapeutics*. Mar;79(3):255–262.

He X, Liu Rh. (2006). Cranberry phytochemicals: Isolation, structure elucidation, and their antiproliferataive and antioxidant activities. *Journal of Agricultural and Food Chemistry*. Sep 20;54(19): 7069–7074.

Howell AB, et al. (1998). Inhibition of the adherence of P-fimbriated *Escherichia coli* to uroepithelial-cell surfaces by proanthocyanidin extracts from cranberries. *New England Journal of Medicine.* 339(15):1085–1086.

Kahn DH, et al. (1967). Effect of cranberry juice on urine. *Journal of the American Dietetic Association.* 51:251.

McCaleb R, et al. (2000). *Encyclopedia of Popular Herbs* (pp. 114–119). Roseville, CA: Prima Publishers.

McHarg T, et al. (2003). Influence of cranberry juice on the urinary risk factors for calcium oxalate kidney stone formation. *BJU International.* Nov;92(7):765–768.

Ofek I, et al. (1991). Anti-*Escherichia coli* adhesion activity of cranberry and blueberry juices. *New England Journal of Medicine.* 324:1599.

Ohnishi R, et al. (2006). Urinary excretion of anthocyanins in humans after cranberry juice ingestion. *Bioscience, Biotechnology, and Biochemistry.* Jul;70(7):1681–1687.

Stothers L. (2002). A randomized trial to evaluate effectiveness and cost effectiveness of naturopathic cranberry products as prophylaxis against urinary tract infection in women. *Canadian Journal of Urology.* Jun;9(3):1558–1562.

Uesawa Y, Mohri K. (2006). Effects of cranberry juice on nifedipine pharmacokinetics in rats. *Journal of Pharmacy and Pharmacology.* Aug;58(8):1067–1072.

Walsh BA. (1992). Urostomy and urinary pH. *Journal of ET Nursing.* 19:110.

Weiss EI, et al. (1998). Inhibiting interspecies coaggregation of plaque bacteria with a cranberry juice constituent. *Journal of the American Dental Association.* 129(12):1719–1723. Retrieved October 3, 2006, from www.phytochemicals.info/phytochemi-cals/ursolic-acid.php.

Zafiri D, et al. (1989). Inhibitory activity of cranberry juice on adherence of type 1 and type P fimbriated *Escherichia coli* to eucaryotic cells. *Antimicrobial Agents and Chemotherapy.* 33:92–98.

Zhang L, et al. (2005). Efficacy of cranberry juice on *Helicobacter pylori* infection: A double-blind, randomized placebo-controlled trial. *Helicobacter.* Apr;10(2):139–142.

Zopf D, Roth S. (1996). Oligosaccharide anti-infective agents. *Lancet.* 347:1017–1021.

D

 NAME: Dandelion (*Taraxacum officinale*)

Common Names: Lion's tooth, priest's crown, *pissenlit* (French), *diente de leon* (Spanish)

Family: *Asteraceae*

Description of Plant
- Member of the aster family, closely related to chicory
- Perennial; grows 12″ high
- Spatula-like leaves are deeply toothed, shiny, and hairless.
- Yellow flowers bloom much of the year and are light-sensitive, opening in the morning and closing in the evening and in wet weather.

Medicinal Part: Root and leaf, dried or fresh. Fresh root preparations are more potent than dried root.

Constituents and Action (if known)
Leaf
- Sesquiterpene lactones (eudesmanolides): increase bile secretions (Duke, 1992; Newall et al., 1996); may contribute to mild anti-inflammatory activity (Leung & Foster, 1996; Newall et al., 1996); contribute to the allergenic component of dandelion; may cause mild gastrointestinal discomfort (Wichtl & Bisset, 1994); diuretic effect, may reduce blood pressure (Wichtl & Bisset, 1994)
- Triterpenes
  - Taxarerol: antiulcer and dyspepsia effects (Duke, 1992)
  - Taraxol, beta-amyrin and cycloartenol
- Carotenoids (lutein, violaxanthin)
- Flavonoids (apigenin, luteolin)
- Phenolic acids (caffeic and chlorogenic acids)
- Minerals (Calcium, potassium)
Root
- Sesquiterpene lactones
- Triterpenes: taraxasterol, taraxol
- Chicoric acid
- Lactopictine (taraxacin)
- Inulin (2% in spring, 40% in autumn): a source of fruto-oligo-saccharides—ketose, nystose, fructofuranosylnystose
Flowers
- Flavonoids
- Coumaric acid
- Carotenoids

- An extract of dandelion flower inhibited reactive oxygen species (ROS) and nitric oxide (NO) and prevents lipid peroxidation (Hu & Kitts, 2005)

Nutritional Ingredients

- Rich source of vitamins A, D, B complex, C (the cooked leaves contain more vitamin A than an equal serving of carrots, up to 15,000 IU per 100 g)
- Rich source of minerals: iron, silicon, magnesium, sodium, potassium, zinc, manganese, calcium, copper, and phosphorus
- Substantial amounts of choline, a nutrient for the liver
- Rich source of fiber and fructo-oligo-saccharides

Traditional Use

- Both leaf and root have been used for centuries to treat liver and gallbladder conditions as well as digestive problems. The root and, to a lesser degree, the leaves, are used as cholagogues, bitter tonics, aperients, and liver tonics.
- The leaf is a nonirritating, potassium-sparing diuretic and has been used for dysuria, edema, obesity, and hypertension.
- Topical application of milky latex to warts

Current Use

Herb

- As a nonirritating, potassium-sparing diuretic, dandelion leaf contains high levels of K^+ (Blumenthal et al., 2000; ESCOP, 2003). It can be used for hypertension in the elderly, PMS water weight gain, and edema (Winston, 2006).
- For the prevention of urinary calculi (Grases et al., 1994)
- The leaf is a bitter tonic, enhancing bile secretion and digestion (Bradley, 1992).

Root

- As a mild laxative (aperient), especially with clay-colored stools
- Stimulates digestion and appetite (root and leaf); used for anorexia, inadequate bile secretion, dysbiosis, impaired hepatic and biliary function, gallstones (ESCOP, 2003), and digestive torpor (flatulence, bloating, constipation). In an animal study, dandelion protected against cholecystokinin-induced pancreatitis (Seo et al., 2005).

- Anti-inflammatory properties: indicated for rheumatic conditions (Bradley, 1992)
- Dandelion root infusion stimulated growth of 14 strains of bifidobacteria. This herbal medicine has a long history of use for enhancing digestive health and may be effective for stimulating normal bowel flora after antibiotic use (Troianova et al., 2004).
- The root and leaf also have been used to lower blood sugar levels, and animal studies seem to confirm hypoglycemic activity (Der Marderosian & Beutler, 2004).

Nutritional Use: Tender leaves can be used in salads or lightly cooked as a nutritious vegetable, flowers can be used to make wine, root can be roasted and used to make a coffee-like beverage.

Available Forms, Dosage, and Administration Guidelines

- *Food:* Eat young leaves raw or lightly cooked in the spring.
- *Tea* (leaf): Steep 1 to 2 tsp of the dried leaf in 8 oz of hot water, steep 20 to 30 minutes; take 1 cup 2 to 3 times a day.
- *Tea* (root): Steep 1 to 2 tsp cut and sifted dried root in 8 oz of hot water for 40 minutes; take 4 oz three times a day.
- *Tinctures*: Leaf (1:5, 30% alcohol): 60 to 80 gtt (3–4 mL) three times a day; fresh root (1:2, 30% alcohol): 80 to 100 gtt (4–5 mL) three times a day
- *Powdered extract* (4:1): 250 to 500 mg a day

Pharmacokinetics—If Available (form or route when known): None known

Toxicity: None reported

Contraindications: Do not use with obstruction of the bile ducts, gallbladder, empyema and ileus; may exacerbate these conditions (Newall et al., 1996).

Side Effects: Milky latex in leaves may cause contact dermatitis; bitterness may exacerbate hyperacidity.

Long-Term Safety: Safe

Use in Pregnancy/Lactation/Children: Long-time use as food; no adverse reactions expected

Drug/Herb Interactions and Rationale (if known)

- Use cautiously with antihypertensives because the leaf is a diuretic. Treat it as you would a prescription diuretic.
- Avoid concurrent use of diuretics because there is a strong possibility of potentiating effects (but not K^+ loss, because dandelion contains K^+).

BIBLIOGRAPHY

Bartram T. (1995). *Encyclopedia of Herbal Medicine* (pp. 140–141). Dorset, UK: Grace Publishers.

Blumenthal M, et al. (2000). *Herbal Medicine: Expanded Commission E Monographs* (pp. 78–83). Austin, TX: American Botanical Council.

Bradley P. [Ed.]. (1992). *British Herbal Compendium*, Vol. I (pp. 73–77). Dorset, UK: British Herbal Medicine Association.

Der Marderosian A, Beutler J. [Eds.]. (2004). *The Review of Natural Products*. St. Louis, MO: Facts and Comparisons.

Duke JA. (1992). *Handbook of Biologically Active Phytochemicals and Their Activities*. Boca Raton, FL: CRC Press.

European Scientific Cooperative on Phytotherapy. (2003). *ESCOP Monographs* (pp. 499–504). New York: Thieme.

Foster S. (1998). *101 Medicinal Herbs*. Loveland, CO: Interweave Press.

Grases F, et al. (1994). Urolithiasis and phytotherapy. *International Urology and Nephrology.* 26(5):507–511.

Hobbs C. (1989). *Taraxacum officinale:* A monograph and literature review. In: *Eclectic Dispensatory of Botanical Therapeutics*. Alstat, E [Ed.] Portland, OR: Eclectic Medical Publications.

Hu C, Kitts DD. (2005). Dandelion (*Taraxecum officianale*) flower extract suppresses both reactive oxygen species and nitric oxide and prevents lipid oxidation in vitro. *Phytomedicine.* Aug;12(8):588–597.

Leung A, Foster S. (1996). *Encyclopedia of Common Natural Ingredients* (2nd ed.; pp. 205–207). New York: John Wiley & Sons.

Newall C, et al. (1996). *Herbal Medicines* (pp. 96–97). London: Pharmaceutical Press.

Seo SW, et al. (2005). *Taraxacum officinale* protects against cholecystokinin-induced acute pancreatitis in rats. *World Journal of Gastroenterology.* Jan 28;11(4):597–599.

Swanston-Flatt SK, et al. (1989). Glycaemic effects of traditional European plant treatments for diabetes. Studies in normal and streptozotocin diabetic mice. *Diabetes Research.* 10(2):69–73.

Troianova I, et al. (2004). The bifidogenic effect of *Taraxacum officinale* root. *Fitoterapia.* Dec;75(7–8):760–763.

Wichtl M, Bisset NG. [Ed.]. (1994). *Herbal Drugs and Phytopharmaceuticals* (pp. 486–489). Boca Raton, FL: CRC Press.

Winston D. (2006). *Winston's Botanic Materia Medica*. Washington, NJ: DWCHS.

 NAME: Dan Shen (*Salvia miltiorrhiza*)

Common Names: Red root sage, tan sheng (Wade-Giles)

Family: *Lamiaceae*

Description of Plant: A small perennial in the mint family with reddish-purple flowers. The best roots are cultivated and are a rich purple-black color inside with a red outer bark.

Medicinal Part: Root

Constituents and Action (if known)

- Diterpene quinones: tanshiones, 1, IIA (0.5%): reduce calcium uptake by myocardium; IIB is an anti-inflammatory anticoagulant with cytotoxic activity against human carcinoma lines in vitro. Antibacterial, antioxidant, antineoplastic (Wang et al., 2007).
- Cryptotanshinone (inhibits metalloproteinases, NF-kappa B and AP-1, which promote atherosclerosis [Suh et al., 2006]), isotanshinones 1, IIA, IIB
- Salvianolic acids A, B, C: inhibited peroxidation of rat liver microsomes (Bone, 1996), calcium channel inhibitor (Lam et al., 2006)
- Flavonoids: baicalin—antipyretic, antitumor (Franek et al., 2005)
- Phenolic acids: caffeic acid, rosmarinic acid, ferulic acid, protocatechuic aldehyde—antioxidant, anti-ischemia, antithrombotic, hypotensive, antiviral, and antitumor activities (Jiang et al., 2005)

Nutritional Ingredients: None

Traditional Use

- Antibacterial, antioxidant, renal protective, hepatoprotective, emmenagogue, anti-inflammatory, mild sedative

- In TCM, used to "move blood" (enhance circulation and relieve stagnation), promoting menstrual flow, removing blood stasis and the resultant pain (dysmenorrhea, abdominal pain, hepatomegaly, angina). It is also used for insomnia and palpitations and topically for bruises (Chen & Chen, 2004).

Current Use

- Cardiovascular disease: studies have shown the benefits of this herb for angina pectoris, hypertension, and angiitis. It is not cardiotonic but potentiates other cardiotonic herbs such as astragalus and *Angelica sinensis*. In a controlled study, dan shen reduced lipid peroxidation, and in 20 patients with hyperviscosity syndrome, all symptoms disappeared (Bone, 1996). Studies on compound Salvia tablets (ingredients include dan shen, *Panax notoginseng*, and borneol) found that they were an effective treatment for chronic stable angina (Wang et al., 2004; Wang et al., 2006).
- Hepatoprotective: the decoction of the herb decreased elevated levels of serum glutamic-pyruvic transaminase (SGPT) and pathologic changes in rabbits with acute liver damage caused by carbon tetrachloride. The herb also restored normal liver function and prevented liver fibrosis in clinical studies (You-ping, 1998).
- May be useful in protecting the kidney from renotoxic drugs and the effects of continuous hemodialysis (Pu et al., 2006).
- Increases maturation of osteoblasts and fibroblasts; may be useful in promoting healing of fractures.
- A combination of dan shen and turkeytail mushroom (*Coriolus versicolor*) improve immune function in post-treatment breast cancer patients. This formula enhanced T-helper lymphocytes, cytotoxic lymphocytes, and B-lymphocytes and improved the levels of T-helper and T-suppressor cells (Wong et al., 2005).

Available Forms, Dosage, and Administration Guidelines

Preparations: Dried herb, capsules, tea, tincture
Typical Dosage
- *Dried root:* 2 to 6 g a day
- *Capsules:* Two 500-mg capsules, one to three times a day

- *Tea:* 1 tsp dried root in 8 oz hot water, decoct 10 minutes, steep 30 minutes; take two cups a day
- *Tincture* (1:5, 35% alcohol): 30 to 80 gtt (1.5–4 mL) three times a day

Pharmacokinetics—If Available (form or route when known): Not known

Toxicity: Intraperitoneal and intragastric administration in mice in substantial doses showed no toxicity.

Contraindications: Bleeding disorders, pregnancy

Side Effects: A few patients taking this herb may experience dry mouth, dizziness, numbness of the hands, and GI disturbance. These symptoms usually disappear without disrupting treatment.

Long-Term Safety: Safe in normal therapeutic dosages

Use in Pregnancy/Lactation/Children: Avoid in pregnancy and lactation; use in older children with professional supervision

Drug/Herb Interactions and Rationale (if known): Dan shen affects CYP450 activity and in one animal study increased diazepam excretion (Jinping et al., 2003), while in a second study, it significantly increased blood levels of warfarin (Chan et al., 1995). Avoid concurrent use with sedatives, warfarin, and aspirin (Brinker, 2001).

Special Notes
- Much of the research done on dan shen has been with isolated constituents and with injectable forms of the drug. These studies have little relevance to oral use of this herb.
- As with most Chinese herbs, this herb is rarely used by itself. It is almost always combined with other herbs based on traditional Chinese formulas.

BIBLIOGRAPHY

Bone K. (1996). *Clinical Applications of Ayurvedic and Chinese Herbs* (pp. 62–68). Queensland, Australia: Phytotherapy Press.

Brinker F. (2001). *Herb Contraindications and Drug Interactions* (pp. 78–79). Sandy, OR: Eclectic Medical Publications.

Chan K, et al. (1995). The effects of danshen (*Salvia miltiorrhiza*) on warfarin pharmacodynamics and pharmacokinetics of warfarin enantiomers in rats. *Journal of Pharmacy and Pharmacology*. May;47(5):402–406.

Chen J, Chen T. (2004). *Chinese Medical Herbology and Pharmacology*. (pp. 636–640). City of Industry, CA. Art of Medicine Press.

Franek KJ, et al. (2005). In vitro studies of baicalin alone or in combination with *Salvia miltiorrhiza* extract as a potential anti-cancer agent. *International Journal of Oncology*. Jan;26(1):217–224.

Hu L, et al. (1996). Experimental study of the protective effects of astragalus and *Salvia miltiorrhiza* bunge on glycerol-induced acute renal failure in rabbits. *Chung Hua Wai Ko Tsa Chih*. 34(5):311–314.

Jiang RW, et al. (2005). Chemistry and biological activities of caffeic acid derivatives from *Salvia miltiorrhiza*. *Current Medicinal Chemistry*. 12(2):237–246.

Jingping O, et al. (2003). Effects of the aqueous extract from *Salvia miltiorrhiza* Bge on the pharmacokinetics of diazepam and on liver microsomal cytochrome P450 enzyme activity in rats. *Journal of Pharmacy and Pharmacology*. Aug;55(8):1163–1167.

Lam FF, et al. (2006). Salvianolic acid B, an aqueous component of danshen (*Salvia miltiorrhiza*), relaxes rat coronary artery by inhibition of calcium channels. *European Journal of Pharmacology*. Dec 28; 553(1–3):240–245. Epub 2006 Sep 23.

Pu C, et al. (2006). Effects of *Salvia miltiorrhiza* on oxidative stress and microinflammatory state in patients undergoing continuous hemodialysis. *Zhongguo Zhong Xi Yi Jie He Za Zie*. Sep;26(9):791–794.

Suh SJ, et al. (2006). Cryptotanshinone from *Salvia miltiorrhiza* BUNGE has an inhibitory effect on TNF-alpha-induced matrix metalloproteinase-9 production and HASMC migration via down-regulated NF-kappaB and AP-1. *Biochemical Pharmacology*. Dec 15; 17(12) 1680–1689.

Tang W, Eisenbrand G. (1992). *Chinese Drugs of Plant Origin* (pp. 891–902). Berlin: Springer-Verlag.

Wang G, et al. (2006). Compound salvia pellet, a traditional Chinese medicine, for the treatment of chronic stable angina pectoris compared with nitrates: A meta-analaysis. *Medical Science Monitor*. Jan;12(1):SR1–SR7.

Wang L, et al. (2004). Systematic assessment on randomized controlled trials for treatment of stable angina pectoris by compound salvia pellet. *Zhongguo Zhong Xi Yi Jie He Za Zhi*. Jun;24(6):500–504.

Wang X, et al. (2007). New developments in the chemistry and biology of the bioactive constituents of Tanshen. *Med Res Rev*. Jan;27(1):133–148. Epub 2006 Aug 3.

Wasser S, et al. (1998). *Salvia miltiorrhiza* reduces experimentally-induced hepatic fibrosis in rats. *Journal of Hepatology*. 29(5):760–771.

Wong CK, et al. (2005). Immunomodulatory activities of yunzhi and danshen in post-treatment breast cancer patients. *American Journal of Chinese Medicine.* 33(3):381–395.

Wu YJ, et al. (1998). Increase of vitamin E content in LDL and reduction of atherosclerosis in cholesterol-fed rabbits by a water-soluble antioxidant-rich fraction of *Salvia miltiorrhiza.* *Arteriosclerosis and Thrombosis Vascular Biology.* 18(3):481–486.

You-ping Z. (1998). *Chinese Materia Medica: Chemistry, Pharmacology and Applications* (pp. 557–570). Amsterdam: Harwood.

 NAME: Devil's Claw (*Harpagophytum procumbens*)

Common Names: Grapple plant, wood spider

Family: *Pediliaceae*

Description of Plant: Shrubby vine native to southwest Africa; fruit has grapples that attach to animal fur

Medicinal Part: Root

Constituents and Action (if known)
- Iridoid glucosides (0.5%–3%)
  - Harpagoside is found in twice the concentration in secondary roots: anti-inflammatory activity (Vanhaelen et al., 1981; Whitehouse et al., 1983), negative chronotropic and positive inotropic effects by altering calcium influx into smooth muscle
  - Inhibits NF-kappaB activation, cyclo-oxygenase-2 and nitric oxide, limiting downstream inflammation and pain (Huang et al., 2006).
- Procombide (Bendall et al., 1979)
- Harpagide

Nutritional Ingredients: None known

Traditional Use
- Internal: bitter tonic for indigestion; for type 2 diabetes; reduces fever; used as blood purifier; relieves rheumatic and arthritic pain, low back pain, and headaches
- External: treats boils, sores, ulcers

Current Use

- Anti-inflammatory for osteoarthritis of the hip or knee (Chrubasik et al., 1996; Chrubasik et al., 2002; Chantre et al., 2000), tendinitis (Bradley, 1992), and chronic back pain (Laudahn & Walper, 2001). A year-long study using a proprietary extract of the root found that it was well tolerated and as effective as the COX-2 inhibitor rofecoxib (Chrubasik et al., 2005).
- Improves appetite, decreases indigestion and heartburn (ESCOP, 2003)

Available Forms, Dosage, and Administration Guidelines

Preparations: Dried secondary tubers, tea, capsules, tablets, tinctures. Some products are standardized to harpagoside content.

Typical Dosage

- *Capsules:* Up to six 400- to 500-mg capsules a day
- *Tea:* For indigestion, steep 0.25 tsp of dried powdered tuber in 8 oz of hot water for 10 to 15 minutes; take 2 to 4 oz before meals.
- *Tincture* (1:5, 25% alcohol): 20 to 40 gtt (1–2 mL) three times a day
- Or follow manufacturer or practitioner recommendations

Pharmacokinetics—If Available (form or route when known): In human studies, the maximum concentration of harpagosides in the blood was found at 1.3 hours with a rapid decline afterward. The elimination half-life was 5.6 hours (Loew et al., 2001).

Toxicity: None known

Contraindications: Gastric and duodenal ulcers

Side Effects: Mild and infrequent gastrointestinal symptoms and headaches

Long-Term Safety: In studies up to a year, no significant adverse effects have been observed. In animal studies, both acute and subacute studies have shown very low levels of toxicity (ESCOP, 2003).

Use in Pregnancy/Lactation/Children: Unknown; should be used under a practitioner's guidance. Self-medication during pregnancy or breast-feeding is not advised.

Drug/Herb Interactions and Rationale (if known):
Theoretical possibility of interaction with antiarrhythmic
medications

Special Notes: Current research suggests anti-inflammatory
and analgesic activity.

BIBLIOGRAPHY

Bendall M, et al. (1979). The structure of procumbide. *Australian
Journal of Chemistry.* 32(9):2085.

Blumenthal M, et al. (2000). *Herbal Medicine, Expanded Commission
E Monographs* (pp. 84–87). Austin, TX: American Botanical
Council.

Bradley P. [Ed.]. (1992). *British Herbal Compendium*, Vol. I. (pp.
78–80). Bournemouth: British Herbal Medicine Association.

Chantre P, et al. (2000). Efficacy and tolerance of *Harpagophytum
procumbens* versus diacerhein in treatment of osteoarthritis.
Phytomedicine. Jun;7(3):177–183.

Chrubasik S, et al. (1996). Effectiveness of *Harpagophytum
procumbens* in treatment of acute low back pain. *Phytomedicine.*
3(1):1–10.

Chrubasik S, et al. (2002). Comparison of outcome measure during
treatment with the proprietary *Harpagophytum* extract Doloteffin in
patients with pain in the lower back, knee, or hip. *Phytomedicine.*
Apr;9(3):181–194.

Chrubasik S, et al. (2005). A 1-year follow-up after a pilot study with
Doloteffin for low back pain. *Phytomedicine.* Jan;12(1–2):1–9.

European Scientific Cooperative on Phytotherapy. (2003). *ESCOP
Monographs* (pp. 233–240). New York: Thieme.

Huang TH, et al. (2006). Harpagoside suppresses lipopolysaccharide-
induced iNOS and COX-2 expression through inhibition of NF-
kappa B activation. *Journal of Ethnopharmacology.* Mar
8;104(1–2):149–155.

Laudahn D, Walper A. Efficacy and tolerance of *Harpagophytum*
extract L1 174 in patients with chronic non-radicular back pain.
Phytotherapy Research. Nov;15(7):621–624.

Loew D, et al. (2001). Investigations on the pharmacokinetic
properties of *Harpagophytum* extracts and their effects on eicosanoid
biosynthesis in vitro and ex vivo. *Clinical Pharmacology and
Therapeutics.* May;69(5):356–364.

Mahomed IM, et al. (2004). Analgesic, antiinflammatory, and
antidiabetic properties of *Harpagophytum procumbens* DC
(Pedaliaceae) secondary root aqueous extract. *Phytotherapy Research.*
Dec;18(12):982–989.

Vanhaelen M, et al. (1981). Biological activity of *Harpagophytum procumbens* D.C. Part 1: Preparation and structure of harpagogenin. *Journal Pharmacie Belgique.* 36:38.

Wegener T, et al. (2003). Treatment of patients with arthrosis of hip or knee with an aqueous extract of devil's claw *(Harpagophytum procumbens* DC). *Phytotherapy Research.* Dec;17(10):1165–1172.

Wegner T. (1999). Therapy of degenerative diseases of the musculoskeletal system with South African devil's claw. *Wiener Medizinische Wochenschrift.* 149(8–10):254–257.

Whitehouse LW, et al. (1983). Devil's claw *(Harpagophytum procumbens)*: No evidence for anti-inflammatory activity in the treatment of arthritic disease. *Canadian Medical Association Journal.* 129(3):249.

 NAME: Dong Quai *(Angelica sinensis)*

Common Names: Tang kuei, Chinese angelica, dang-gui

Family: *Apiaceae*

Description of Plant: An aromatic member of the parsley family; it thrives in cool, shaded mountain woods in southern and western China

Medicinal Part: Processed root

Constituents and Action (if known)

- EO (0.2%–0.65%)
  - *N*-butylidene phthalide: antispasmodic effect on uterus, vasodilatory action lowers blood pressure but duration of action is short
  - *Z*-ligustilide: antiasthmatic and antispasmodic activity in vivo (Tang & Eisenbrand, 1992); antiproliferative activity in vitro (Mills & Bone, 2000)
  - Ferulic acid: inhibited rat platelet aggregation and serotonin release in vivo and in vitro (Tang & Eisenbrand, 1992)
- Coumarins (osthol, psoralen, bergapten, flurcoumarin, angelol, angelicone): vasodilatory and antispasmodic properties, central nervous system stimulant, increases spleen function, anti-inflammatory, analgesic, antipyretic activity, uterine stimulant

- Psoralens: increases sensitivity to sun
- Other actions: oral administration of *A. sinesis* root powder decreased blood lipids in rats and rabbits (You-Ping, 1998)

Nutritional Ingredients: Vitamin B_{12} and folinic acid (the active form of folic acid); increases oxygen use in liver and glutamic acid and cysteine oxidation

Traditional Use

- One of the most frequently used women's herbs in the world. Has been used in China for thousands of years as a tonic for the female reproductive system, the blood, liver, and the heart.
- Used to nourish the blood and increase circulation. Blood (*xue*) deficiency syndromes include symptoms such as a pale complexion, pale tongue and nails, dizziness, palpitations, feeling cold, and anemia.
- Used in formulas for menstrual, menopausal, and cardiac conditions; also used to treat migraines, neuralgia, coughs, constipation, Raynaud's disease, herpes zoster, and arthralgias
- The root is frequently used in liniments for bruises, sprains, poorly healing sores, and muscle pain.

Current Use

- Useful female reproductive tonic; used in combination with herbs such as chaste tree or black cohosh for menopausal symptoms such as formication, muscle pain, and depression. It is also used with licorice, motherwort, and chaste tree for PMS anxiety, amenorrhea, and dysmenorrhea (Winston, 2006).
- Cardiovascular effects: increases number of red blood cells and platelets; stimulates hematopoiesis in the bone marrow; can prolong the refractory period and correct experimentally induced atrial fibrillation. In animal studies (rats and rabbits), dong quai prevented experimental coronary arteriosclerosis (Mills & Bone, 2000).
- Successfully used to treat Buerger's disease and constrictive aortitis. Often combined with dan shen (*Salvia miltiorrhiza*) to treat angina, peripheral vascular insufficiency, and stroke (Bone, 1996).
- Used in TCM, often with astragalus, to treat hematologic immune disorders such as thrombocytopenic purpura

(Mills & Bone, 2000) and to reduce the immunosuppressive effects of cortisone
* Adjunctive therapy for liver disease: reduced thymol turbidity in 88 cases of chronic hepatitis or liver cirrhosis (Bone, 1996). Use with milk thistle, turmeric, or schisandra berry (Winston, 2006).

Available Forms, Dosage, and Administration Guidelines
Preparations: Dried root (whole, sliced, or powdered); capsules, tablets, tinctures, combination products
Typical Dosage
* *Root:* 2 to 6 g a day
* *Capsules:* Up to six 500- to 600-mg capsules a day
* *Tincture* (1:5, 70% alcohol): 40 to 80 gtt (2–4 mL) up to three times a day
* Or follow manufacturer or practitioner recommendations
* *Tea:* 1 tsp dried root in 12 oz water, lightly decoct (covered) for 20 minutes, let steep 1 hour; take 8 oz two or three times a day
* In Chinese and Japanese medicine, dong quai is always used in conjunction with other herbs.

Pharmacokinetics—If Available (form or route when known): None known

Toxicity: Handling the fresh plant may cause photodermatitis in sensitive people.

Contraindications: Do not use with heavy menses (may increase bleeding) or with bleeding disorders, fibroids, or diarrhea. If breast tenderness or soreness occurs, discontinue use.

Side Effects: Possible photosensitization, menorrhagia; may exacerbate diarrhea

Long-Term Safety: Long-term history of safe use; no safety issues expected

Use in Pregnancy/Lactation/Children: Not used in the first trimester; used cautiously in TCM during the remainder of the pregnancy only by trained professionals. There are several case reports of breast-feeding infants developing a rash when their mothers ingested dong quai (Upton, 2003).

Drug/Herb Interactions and Rationale (if known): With warfarin and other anticoagulant drugs, dong quai may increase the bleeding time. If using concurrently, obtain prothrombin time and International Normalized Ratio (INR) to rule out interactions. Dong quai prevented acetaminophen-induced liver damage (Chen & Chen, 2004). In animal studies, dong quai stimulated CYP450 activity, especially CYP2D6 and CYP3A4 (Tang et al., 2006).

Special Notes

- When recently studied alone, dong quai had no effect on reducing menopausal symptoms (Bates, 1997). However, dong quai is never prescribed alone in the Orient but is always administered in combination with other herbs.
- Dong quai does *not* have estrogenic effects (Hirata et al., 1997).
- High-quality root heads have substantially greater concentrations of active constituents. Ligustilide in high-grade roots has been found to be 10 times the level found in normal commercial-grade root heads.

BIBLIOGRAPHY

Bone K. (1996). *Clinical Applications of Ayurvedic and Chinese Herbs* (pp. 3–6). Queensland: Phytotherapy Press.

Chen J, Chen T. (2004). Chinese *Medical Herbology and Pharmacology* (pp. 918–924). City of Industry, CA, Art of Medicine Press.

Hirata JD, et al. (1997). Does dong quai have estrogenic effects in postmenopausal women? A double-blind, placebo-controlled trial. *Fertility and Sterility.* 68(6):981–986.

Mills S, Bone K. (2000). *Principles and Practice of Phytotherapy* (pp. 350–353). Edinburgh: Churchill Livingstone.

Tang JC, et al. (2006). Effect of the water extract and ethanol extract from traditional Chinese medicines *Angelica sinensis* (Oliv.) Diels, *Ligusticum chuanxiong* Hort. and *Rheum palmatum* L. on rat liver cytochrome P450 activity. *Phytotherapy Research.* Dec;20(12):1046–1051.

Tang W, Eisenbrand G. (1992). *Chinese Drugs of Plant Origin* (pp. 113–125). Berlin: Springer-Verlag.

164 ● Echinacea (*Echinacea angustifolia, E. purpurea, E. pallida*)

Upton R. [Ed.]. (2003). *American Herbal Pharmacopoeia and Therapeutic Compendium—Dang Gui Root*. Scotts Valley, CA: AHP.

Winston D. (2006). *Winston's Botanic Materia Medica*. Washington, NJ: DWCHS.

You-Ping Z. (1998). *Chinese Materia Medica: Chemistry, Pharmacology and Applications* (pp. 579–583). Amsterdam: Harwood.

NAME: Echinacea (*Echinacea angustifolia, E. purpurea, E. pallida*)

Common Names: American coneflower, Kansas snake root, purple coneflower, Missouri snake root

Family: *Asteraceae*

Description of Plant
- The Echinacea genus contains nine species and two varieties.
- Perennial herb, part of the daisy family, native to Midwest North America, from Saskatchewan to Texas
- Height 1.5' to 3' tall
- Most species have purple flowers.

Medicinal Part: The fresh root (*E. angustifolia, E. purpurea, E. pallida*) and the cone of *E. purpurea*

Constituents and Action (if known)
- As with many medicinal plants, no active single ingredient has been identified as being responsible for the medicinal value. Echinacea's numerous constituents all contribute to its activity.
- Caffeic acid derivatives: increase phagocytosis (most active in flowering heads of *E. purpurea*)
  - Echinacosides (*E. angustifolia, E. pallida*), antioxidant (Dalby-Brown et al., 2005), chlorogenic acid (*E. angustifolia, E. purpurea*), chicoric acid (*E. purpurea*); antioxidant (Dalby-Brown et al., 2005)
  - Stimulate phagocytosis, increase leukocyte activity (Melchart et al., 1994, 1998; Schoneberger, 1992)
  - May offer photoprotection from sun damage when applied topically (Facino et al., 1995)

- ○ Has weak activity against *Escherichia coli*, *Pseudomonas aeruginosa*, *Staphylococcus aureus*, and *Streptococci* spp.
- ○ Increase macrophage activity, increase T-cell activity and interferon
- ○ Inhibit hyaluronidase activity, thus limiting degenerative inflammatory disease and the spread of viruses (Mills & Bone, 2000)
- Lipophilic components
  - ○ Alkylamides: enhance phagocytosis, inhibit edema, and enhance wound healing (Mills & Bone, 2000)
  - ○ Echinacein (pungent component): a complex isobutylamide
  - ○ *E. angustifolia* roots or *E. purpurea* flower heads contain unsaturated alkyl ketones or isobutylamides: inhibit leukemic cells. Chewing the cone of *E. purpurea* or the root of *E. angustifolia* causes tingling and numbing of the lips and tongue. Downregulates inflammatory cytokines (Woelkart et al., 2006).
- Polyacetylenes (polyynes) found in *E. pallida* roots: ketoalkynes and ketoalkenes—cytotoxic (Chicca et al., 2007), inhibits inflammatory cytokines (Senchina et al., 2006)
- *D*-acidic arabinogalactan polysaccharide
  - ○ As an injectable, stimulates B-lymphocyte proliferation, T lymphocytes, beta-interferon, and tumor necrosis factor; particularly high in roots of *E. purpurea*; is probably not active orally (Parnham, 1996)
  - ○ Decreases activity of herpes simplex virus-1 and influenza virus A

Nutritional Ingredients: None known

Traditional Use
- Native Americans used echinacea to treat wounds, burns, abscesses, insect bites, sore throats, toothaches, and joint pains and as an antidote for poisonous snake bites.
- In 1870, it was introduced as "Meyer's Blood Purifier" for all matter of ailments. Eclectic physician John King and pharmacist John Uri Lloyd reluctantly tested this patent medicine and were surprised to discover a valuable and active medicine.

- Eclectic physicians used echinacea for patients with blood dyscrasias, a tendency toward infections, sepsis, boils, staphylococcal infections, and putrid sore throat.

Current Use

- To prevent and treat the common cold (may decrease the chances of getting a cold and decrease its severity). Echinacea has been officially approved in Germany for treating colds, influenza, and upper respiratory infections. The last decade has seen a number of studies on the effectiveness of echinacea for treating colds, upper respiratory tract infections, and influenza. The results are contradictory and confusing. Some studies (Goel et al., 2005; Goel et al., 2004; Lindenmuth & Lindenmuth, 2000; Naser et al., 2005) show a reduction in symptoms, severity, or the length of time the patient was ill. Other studies (Barrett et al., 2002; Turner et al., 2005; Weber et al., 2005; Yale & Liu, 2004) show no detectable benefits (or harm) from echinacea. The discrepancy may have to do with the products tested and dosage. In the Barrett study (2002), the product tested was made up of dried, powdered *E. angustifolia* root and *E. purpurea* root and herb. Most clinical herbalists strongly believe that dried echinacea has little activity. In Yale & Liu (2004), a freeze-dried leaf juice was used—again, most clinicians familiar with this plant use products made from the fresh roots or flower cones. In the Turner study (2005), the dosage given was only one-fourth to one-third of the usual clinical dose. The long history of the plant's use for enhancing immunity and shortening the duration of bacterial and viral illnesses, plus the positive studies, suggest that it is premature to declare that echinacea is not effective for colds and respiratory tract infections.
- A product combining echinacea, baptisia, and thuja was found to be effective for treating colds (Naser et al., 2005).
- As a supportive treatment for otitis media, sinusitis, bronchitis, cystitis, prostatitis, tonsillitis, and laryngitis (Upton, 2004).
- In a human study, *E. purpurea*, astralagus, and licorice, individually and in combination, stimulated CD69 expression on CD4 and CD8 T cells (Brush et al., 2006).
- To enhance wound healing (topically)

- Used in Germany along with chemotherapy in the treatment of cancer. In vitro and in vivo (animal studies) suggest that echinacea may offer some benefit for enhancing immune function (Brush et al., 2006) and inhibiting cancers (Chicca et al., 2007). It also may enhance white blood cell count in persons undergoing chemotherapy.

Available Forms, Dosage, and Administration Guidelines

- Research needs to be done to determine the most effective preparations, differences between the species, and the parts of the plant to use.
- Take at first sign of infection (may need to take 1 g three times a day).

Preparations

- Fresh or dried root; capsules, tablets, expressed juice of fresh flowering plant, tinctures
- Some products are standardized to echinacoside, although the compound has not been found to stimulate the immune system nor does it represent the therapeutic activity of the plant.
- The most research has been done in Germany with a product now available in the United States under the brand name Echinaguard (Nature's Way).
- Look for tinctures made with a 50% alcohol content, because active constituents are better extracted in this menstruum.

Typical Dosage

- *Capsules:* Up to nine 300- to 400-mg capsules a day
- *Tincture* (1:2, 50% alcohol): 60 to 90 gtt (3–5 mL) four to six times a day. Use as needed at the onset of symptoms of cold or flu.
- *Freeze-dried plant:* 325 to 650 mg three times a day
- *Juice* (of aerial portion of *E. purpurea* stabilized in 22% ethanol): 0.75 to 1.25 tsp (4–6 mL) three times a day
- *Powdered extract* (6.5:1): 300 mg three times a day

Pharmacokinetics—If Available (form or route when known): Echinacea isbutylamides are detectable in the bloodstream within 30 to 45 minutes after ingestion. Twenty-three hours after ingestion, there was a significant downregulation of inflammatory cytokines (Woelkart et al., 2006).

Toxicity: None known

Contraindications

- Possibly, there are contraindications with autoimmune diseases such as multiple sclerosis and rheumatoid arthritis. This is based on the speculation that stimulating an overactive immune system will worsen symptoms, but there is no research evidence to confirm this. In fact, the herb is commonly used by British and Australian herbalists to treat autoimmune diseases as an immune amphoteric. Recent research indicates that echinacea inhibits inflammatory cytokines and chemokines and modulated rather than stimulated immune response (Sharma et al., 2006).

- If patients have allergies to *Asteraceae* family pollen (chrysanthemum, chamomile, ragweed, daisy), avoid products made from echinacea flowers. The leaf juice or root products should not provoke an allergic response.

Side Effects: Transitory tingling or numbing of the mouth, throat, and lips

Long-Term Safety: Safe

Use in Pregnancy/Lactation/Children: Regular use in Germany by millions of people, including pregnant and breast-feeding women and children, has not produced any known side effects or toxicity. Echinacea is non-teratogenic, and a prospective cohort study found that it is safe during pregnancy and lactation (Perri et al., 2006).

Drug/Herb Interactions and Rationale (if known): None

Special Notes

- In North America, *E. angustifolia* is the most popular species of echinacea, even though there is much more research showing effectiveness for *E. purpurea* and *E. pallida*.

- Echinacea species are being overharvested in the wild. Use products made from the cultivated herb root.

- Most effective when started at first sign of infection. Take in sufficient amounts; split total daily dosage into four to six doses a day.

- Recent research showed no benefit when taken for a 3-month period to prevent colds, but cold symptoms and duration were reduced when taken at the start of a cold (Melchart et al., 1995).

- Some authors have erroneously stated that echinacea can cause liver damage. Echinacea does contain minute amounts of pyrrolizidine alkaloids, but they are the nontoxic (saturated) variety. There is no evidence or known possibility of hepatic damage resulting from the use of this herb.
- Another echinacea myth is that it is best or works only when taken short term (7–14 days). This is due to a mistranslated German study that showed that the effects gradually wear off if you stop taking echinacea. Unfortunately, the improper translation stated that the effects wear off if you continue to take echinacea. The eclectic physicians who introduced echinacea into Western clinical practice and used this medicine extensively for 50 years believed that it was more effective the longer it was used (Bergner, 1994).

BIBLIOGRAPHY

Barnes J, et al. (2005). Echinacea species (*Echinacea angustifolia* (DC) Hell., *Echinacea pallida* (Nutt.), Nutt., *Echinacea purpurea* (L.), Moench): A review of their chemistry, pharmacology and clinical properties. *Journal of Pharmacy and Pharmacology.* Aug;57(8): 929–954.

Barrett BP, et al. (2002). Treatment of the common cold with unrefined echinacea. A randomized, double-blind, placebo-controlled trial. *Annals of Internal Medicine.* Dec 17;137(12):939–946.

Bergner P. (1994). Echinacea myth: Phagocytosis is not diminished after ten days. *Medical Herbalism.* 6(1):1.

Bodinet C, et al. (1993). Host resistance-increasing activity of root extracts from Echinacea species. *Planta Medica.* 59:A672–A673.

Bone K. (1997). Echinacea: What makes it work? *Modern Phytotherapist.* 3(2):19–23.

Braunig B, et al. (1992). *Echinacea pupurea* radix for strengthening the immune response in flu-like infections. *Zeitschrift fur Phytotherapie.* 13:7–13.

Brush J, et al. (2006). The effect of *Echinacea pupurea, Astralagus membranaceus* and *Glycyrrhiza glabra* on CD69 expression and immune cell activation in human. *Phytotherapy Research.* Aug;20(8):687–695.

Burger RA, et al. (1997). Echinacea-induced cytokine production by human macrophages. *International Journal of Immunopharmacology.* 19(7):371–379.

Chicca A, et al. (2007). Cytotoxic effects of echinacea root hexanic extracts on human cancer cell lines. *Journal of Ethnopharmacology*. Mar 1;110(1):148–153.

Dalby-Brown L, et al. (2005). Synergistic antioxidative effects of alkamides, caffeic acid derivatives, and polysaccharide fractions from *Echinacea pupurea* on in vitro oxidation of human low-density lipoproteins. *Journal of Agricultural and Food Chemistry*. Nov 30;53(24):9413–9423.

Dorn M, et al. (1997). Placebo-controlled, double-blind study of *Echinaceae pallidae* radix in upper respiratory tract infections. *Complementary Therapeutic Medicine*. 3:40–42.

Facino R. (1995). Echinacea in preventing skin damage. *Planta Medica*. 61:510–514.

Facino RM, et al. (1995). Echinacoside and caffeoyl conjugates protect collagen from free radical-induced degradation. A potential use of Echinacea extracts in the prevention of skin photodamage. *Planta Medica*. 61(6):510–514.

Goel V, et al. (2004). Efficacy of a standardized echinacea preparation (Echinilin) for the treatment of the common cold: A randomized, double-blind, placebo-controlled trial. *Journal of Clinical Pharmacy and Therapeutics*. Feb;29(1):75–83.

Goel V, et al. (2005). A proprietary extract from the echinacea plant (*Echinacea purpurea*) enhances systemic immune response during a common cold. *Phytotherapy Research*. Aug;19(8):689–694.

Lindenmuth GF, Lindenmuth EB. (2000). The efficacy of echinacea compound herbal tea preparation on the severity and duration of upper respiratory and flu symptoms: A randomized, double-blind placebo-controlled study. *Journal of Alternative and Complementary Medicine*. Aug;6(4):327–334.

Matthias A, et al. (2005). Echinacea alkamide disposition and pharmacokinetics in humans after tablet ingestion. *Life Sciences*. Sep 2;77(16):2018–2029.

Melchart D, et al. (1994). Immunomodulation with *Echinacea*: A systematic review of controlled clinical trials. *Phytomedicine*. 1:245–254.

Melchart D, et al. (1995). Results of five randomized studies on the immunomodulatory activity of preparations of Echinacea. *Journal of Alternative and Complementary Medicine*. 1:145–160.

Melchart D, et al. (1998). Echinacea root extracts for the prevention of upper respiratory tract infections: A double-blind, placebo-controlled randomized trial. *Archives of Family Medicine*. 6:541–545.

Mills S, Bone K. (2000). *Principles and Practice of Phytotherapy* (pp. 354–362). Edinburgh: Churchill Livingstone.

Myers S, Wohlmuth H. (1998). Echinacea-associated anaphylaxis. *Medical Journal of Australia.* 168(11):583–584.

Naser B, et al. (2005). A randomized, double-blind, placebo-controlled, clinical dose-response trial of an extract of Baptisia, Echinacea and Thuja for the treatment of patients with common cold. *Phytomedicine.* Nov;12(10):715–722.

Parnham MJ. (1996). Benefit-risk assessment of the squeezed sap of the purple coneflower (*Echinacea purpurea*) for long-term oral immunostimulation. *Phytomedicine.* 3(1):95–102.

Perri D, et al. (2006). Safety and efficacy of echinacea (*Echinacea angustafolia, E. purpurea*, and *E. pallida*) during pregnancy and lactation. *Canadian Journal of Clinical Pharmacology.* 13(3):e262–e267.

Schoneberger D. (1992). The influence of immune stimulating effects of pressed juice from *Echinacea purpurea* on the course and severity of colds. *Forum Immunologie.* 8:2–12.

Senchina DS, et al. (2006). Year-and-a-half old, dried Echinacea roots retain cytokine-modulating capabilities in an in vitro human older adult model of influenza vaccination. *Planta Medica.* Oct; 72(13): 1207–1215.

Sharma M, et al. (2006). Echinacea extracts modulate the pattern of chemokines and cytokine secretion in rhinovirus-infected and uninfected epithelial cells. *Phytotherapy Research.* 20:147–152.

Turner RB, et al. (2005). An evaluation of *Echinacea angustifolia* in experimental rhinovirus infections. *New England Journal of Medicine.* Jul 28;353(4):341–348.

Upton R. [Ed.]. (2004). American Herbal Pharmacopoeia and Therapeutic Compendium—*Echinacea purpurea* Root. Scotts Valley, CA: AHP.

Weber W, et al. (2005). *Echinacea purpurea* for prevention of upper respiratory tract infections in children. *Journal of Alternative and Complementary Medicine.* Dec;11(6):1021–1026.

Woelkart K, et al. (2006). Bioavailability and pharmacokinetics of *Echinacea purpurea* preparations and their interaction with the immune system. *International Journal of Clinical Pharmacology and Therapeutics.* Sep;44(9):401–408.

Yale SH, Liu K. (2004). *Echinacea pupurea* therapy for the treatment of the common cold: A randomized, double-blind, placebo-controlled trial. *Archives of Internal Medicine.* Jun 14;164(11): 1237–1241.

NAME: Elderberry (*Sambucus nigra, S. canadensis*)

Common Names: Black elder, elder bloom, European elder

Family: *Caprifoliaceae*

Description of Plant
- It is a small shrubby tree that prefers damp areas and partial shade.
- It has large clusters of fragrant white flowers in the early summer, followed by purplish-black berries in the late summer.

Medicinal Part: Berry, flower

Constituents and Action (if known)
Fruit
- Monomeric anthocyanins: antiviral, anti-inflammatory (Duke, 2006), antioxidant (Wu et al., 2004)
- Nontoxic type 2 ribosome-inactivating proteins (RIPs)-SNA-I, SNAIVF, SNA-V, SNRP: antiviral (Vandenbussche et al., 2004)
- Vitamin C: antioxidant, antiviral (Duke, 2006)
- Malic acid: antiarteriosclerotic, antioxidant, antifungal (Duke, 2006)

Flowers
- Flavonoids
  - Kaempferol: inhibits estrogen-related cancers (Oh, 2006), antiallergic, antibacterial, anti-inflammatory, antioxidant, antiviral (Duke, 2006), antiosteoclastogenic (Pang et al., 2006)
  - Quercetin: anticancer (Jin et al., 2006), antioxidant (Gabrielska et al., 2006), anti-inflammatory (Jackson et al., 2006)
  - Rutin: antiallergic, antibacterial, anti-inflammatory (Duke, 2006), antioxidant (Karthick et al., 2006)
- Chlorogenic acid: antioxidant, anti-inflammatory, hypotensive (Suzuki et al., 2006)
- Cycloartenol: antibacterial, anti-inflammatory (Duke, 2006)

Nutritional Ingredients: Elderberries have been used to make wine, jellies, and preserves. The flowers can be dipped in batter and used to make tempura.

Traditional Use

- The berries were traditionally made into syrups (electuaries) used for constipation, arthritis, fevers, coughs, and colds.
- The flowers were more commonly used in traditional medicine for their antiviral, diaphoretic, diuretic, and emollient activity.
- Elder flower and peppermint is a common formula for children's fevers caused by colds, influenza, measles, chicken pox, and fifth disease.
- The Eclectic physicians used elder flowers for indolent ulcers with boggy borders. The tissue is edemic, and the epidermis has abundant serous discharge and forms crusts (impetigo) (Felter & Lloyd, 1986). It is used topically and orally with yellow dock root and burdock seed.
- The flowers were also used in the famous Queen of Hungary water, which softens skin and relieves dryness and itching.

Current Use

- Elderberry syrups have become a popular remedy for treating colds, influenza, viral bronchitis, and sinusitis. Several studies (Barak et al., 2002; Zakay-Rones et al., 1995; Zakay-Rones et al., 2004) show that elderberries enhance immunostimulatory cytokines and shortens the duration of influenza A and B infections by interfering with viral replication.
- Elderberry extracts (Sambucol) have also been shown to inhibit herpes simplex virus (Anonymous, 2005).
- The antioxidant anthocyanins found in elderberry have shown the ability to reduce oxidation of blood lipids (Murkovic, 2005) and protect against reactive oxygen species (ROS)–related cell damage (Youdim, 2000). Various diseases that are caused or exacerbated by oxidative stress, such as atherosclerosis, age-related macular degeneration, cognitive decline, diabetic retinopathy, peripheral neuropathy, and arthritis, may be benefited by regular consumption of concentrated elderberry extracts.
- Elder flowers are still used with peppermint (for children) or yarrow (for adults) to stimulate sweating and lower a

fever. Recent studies have also found the flowers inhibit *Porphyromonas gingivalis* and *Actinobacillus actinomycetemcomitans*, which are two bacteria that cause periodontal disease, and it potently inhibits the bacteria's proinflammatory activity (Harokopakis et al., 2006).

Available Forms, Dosage, and Administration Guidelines

Preparations: Berries: syrup, tincture, capsules; flowers: tea, tincture

Typical Dosage

Berries

- *Syrup:* 15 mL three times a day
- *Tincture* (1:2, 25% alcohol): 80 to 120 gtt (4–6 mL) four to six times a day
- *Capsules:* Two to three 500-mg capsules a day

Flowers

- *Tea:* 1 tsp dried flowers to 8 oz hot water, steep 20 to 30 minutes; take two to three cups a day
- *Tincture* (1:2 or 1:5, 30% alcohol): 40 to 80 gtt (2–4 mL) four times a day

Pharmacokinetics—If Available (form or route when known): Elderberry anthocyanins have a low urinary excretion rate (1%), which indicates that a large proportion of these antioxidant compounds are metabolized before entry into circulation (Frank et al., 2005).

Toxicity: The fresh berries (actually the seeds) contain small amounts of cyanogenic glycosides, which can cause nausea and diarrhea when eaten in large amounts. The dried and cooked berries and flowers are nontoxic.

Contraindications: None known

Side Effects: None known

Long-Term Safety: Safe

Use in Pregnancy/Lactation/Children: Avoid eating the fresh berries. The dried, cooked, or processed berries are safe, as are the flowers.

Drug/Herb Interactions and Rationale (if known): None known

Special Notes: Lectins extracted from elder bark have also been studied for antiviral and antitumor activity. In traditional European folk medicine, the bark was used as a diuretic, a purgative, and for seizures.

BIBLIOGRAPHY

Anonymous. (2005). Alternative Medicine Review: *Sambucus nigra*, March;10(1):51–54.

Barak V, et al. (2002). The effect of herbal remedies on the production of human inflammatory and anti-inflammatory cytokines. *Israel Medical Association Journal.* Nov;4[11 Suppl.]:919–922.

Duke J. Dr. Duke's phytochemical and ethnobotanical databases. Retrieved September 22 2006, from www.ars-grin.gov/cgi-bin/duke/chemactivities.

Felter HW, Lloyd JU. (1986). *King's American Dispensatory* (19th ed.; pp. 1706–1708). Sandy, OR: Eclectic Medical Publications.

Frank T, et al. (2005). Urinary pharmacokinetics of cyanidin glycosides in healthy young men following consumption of elderberry juice. *International Journal of Clinical Pharmacology Research.* 25(2):47–56.

Gabrielska J, et al. (2006). Antioxidative effect of quercetin and its equimolar mixtures with phenyltin compounds on liposome membranes. *Journal of Agricultural and Food Chemistry.* Oct 4;54(20):7735–7746.

Grieve M. (1973). The Modern Herbal (pp. 265–276). New York: Dorset Press.

Harokopakis E, et al. (2006). Inhibition of proinflammatory activities of major periodontal pathogens by aqueous extracts from elder flower (*Sambucus nigra*). *Journal of Periodontology.* Feb;77(2):271–279.

Jackson JK, et al. (2006). The antioxidants curcumin and quercetin inhibit inflammatory processes associated with arthritis. *Inflammation Research.* Apr;55(4):168–175.

Jin NZ, et al. (2006). Preventive effects of quercetin against benzo[a]pyrene-induced DNA damages and pulmonary precancerous pathologic changes in mice. *Basic and Clinical Pharmacology and Toxicology.* Jun;98(6):593–598.

Karthick M, Stanely Mainzen Prince P. (2006). Preventive effect of rutin, a bioflavonoid, on lipid peroxides and antioxidants in isoproterenol-induced myocardial infarction in rats. *Journal of Pharmacy and Pharmacology.* May;58(5):701–707.

Murkovic M, et al. (2004). Effects of elderberry juice on fasting and postprandial serum lipids and low-density lipoprotein oxidation in healthy volunteers: a randomized, double blind, placebo-controlled study. *European Journal of Clinical Nutrition.* Feb;58(2):244–249.

Oh SM, et al. (2006). Biphasic effects of kaempferol on the estrogenicity in human breast cancer cells. *Archives of Pharmacal Research.* May;29(5):354–362.

Pang JL, et al. (2006). Different activity of kaempferol and quercetin in attenuating tumor necrosis factor receptor family signaling in bone cells. *Biochemical Pharmacology.* Mar 14;71(6):818–826.

Suzuki A, et al. (2006). Chlorogenic acid attenuates hypertension and improves endothelial function in spontaneously hypertensive rats. *Journal of Hypertension.* Jun;24(6):1065–1073.

Vandenbussche F, et al. (2004). Analysis of the in planta antiviral activity of elderberry ribosome-inactivating proteins. *European Journal of Biochemistry.* Apr;271(8):1508–1515.

Winston D. (2006). *Winston's Botanic Materia Medica.* Washington, NJ: DWCHS.

Wu X, et al. (2004). Characterization of anthocyanins and proanthocyanidins in some cultivars of Ribes, Aronia, and Sambucus and their antioxidant capacity. *Journal of Agricultural and Food Chemistry.* Dec 29;52(26):7846–7856.

Youdim KA, et al. (2000). Polyphenolics enhance red blood cell resistance to oxidative stress: in vitro and in vivo. *Biochem Biophys Acta.* Sep 1;1523(1):117–122.

Zakay-Rones Z, et al. (1995). Inhibition of several strains of influenza virus in vitro and reduction of symptoms by an elderberry extract (*Sambucus nigra* L.) during an outbreak of influenza B Panama. *Journal of Alternative and Complementary Medicine.* Winter;1(4):361–369.

Zakay-Rones Z, et al. (2004). Randomized study of the efficacy and safety of oral elderberry extract in the treatment of influenza A and B virus infections. *Journal of International Medical Research.* Mar–Apr;32(2):132–140.

 NAME: Eucalyptus Leaf (*Eucalyptus globulus*)

Common Names: Blue Gum tree

Family: *Myrtaceae*

Description of Plant

- Eucalyptus is a fast-growing weedy tree with highly aromatic, leathery leaves.

- This tree was widely planted in wetlands to dry them up. It has now become a major weed in the Everglades and California.

Medicinal Part: Dried leaves, EO

Constituents and Action (if known)

- Essential oil (EO)
  - 1,8-cineole (Eucalyptol) 70%: pediculoside (Yang et al., 2004)
  - α-pinine: antibacterial, expectorant (Duke, 2006), cytokine inhibitor (Juergens et al., 1998), anti-inflammatory (Juergens et al., 2003)
  - L-phellandrene

Other Actions:

- Anti-inflammatory, analgesic (Silva et al., 2003), antiviral (ESCOP, 2003), antibacterial (Takahashi et al., 2004)
- Flavonoids
  - Quercetin: anticancer (Jin et al., 2006), antioxidant (Gabrielska et al., 2006), anti-inflammatory (Jackson et al., 2006)
  - Rutin: antiallergic, antibacterial, anti-inflammatory (Duke, 2006), antioxidant (Karthick et al., 2006)
  - Tannins: astringent (Skenderi, 2003), antioxidant, antibacterial, hepatoprotective (Duke, 2006)

Nutritional Ingredients: Eucalyptus is used in many cough drops and in some candies mixed with mint or chocolate.

Traditional Use

- Antibacterial, antifungal, anti-inflammatory, antipuretic, antiviral, antioxidant, astringent, carminative, diuretic, expectorant
- The Australian Aborigines used eucalyptus as a wash for joint pain and arthritis pain. The tea is used for nasal congestion, fevers, and weakness caused by colds and influenza (Aboriginal communities, 1990).
- The Eclectic physicians used this herb as a urinary antiseptic for prostatitis, nephritis, and for gonorrhea. They also used it for malarial fevers, typhoid, and diptheria (Felter & Lloyd, 1986).

Current Use

- Eucalyptus still enjoys significant popularity for respiratory tract infections, sinus congestion, coughs, colds, and sore throats. An in vitro study using *Staphylococcus aureus*, *Streptococcus pyogenes*, *Streptococcus pneumoniae*, and *Haemophilus influenzae* isolated from patients with respiratory tract disorders found that this herb had significant inhibitory effects on each of these bacteria (Salari et al., 2006). A second in vitro study found that eucalyptus extracts strongly inhibited gram-positive bacteria (*S. aureus*, MRSA, *Bacillus cereus*, *Enterococcus faecalis*, *Alicyclobacillus acidoterrestris*, *Propionibacterium acnes*) and a fungi (*Trichophyton mentagrophytes*). An animal study found that eucalyptus EO reduced bronchial inflammation and mucin hypersecretion caused by lipopolysaccharide-induced chronic bronchitis (Lu et al., 2004).
- Eucalyptus EO and the major constituent of the EO, 1,8-cineole (Eucalyptol), have been shown to have anti-inflammatory, antiviral (herpes simplex types I and II), analgesic, bronchodilator, and expectorant effects. 1,8-Cineole has been used successfully in double-blind trials to increase respiratory function in patients with steroid-dependent bronchial asthma (Juergens et al., 2003), chronic obstructive pulmonary disorder (ESCOP, 2003), and chronic bronchitis and emphysema (ESCOP, 2003).
- Several human studies have shown that the EO of eucalyptus (the pure oil as well as concentrations of 50% and 75%) is effective for treating scabies (Morsy et al., 2003) and head lice (Yang et al., 2004).
- The diluted EO is commonly used in liniments and salves for topical use as an analgesic for muscle pain and headaches and to reduce bronchial congestion (Winston, 2006).

Available Forms, Dosage, and Administration Guidelines
Preparations: Tea, tincture, capsules, EO
Typical Dosage
- *Tea:* 1 tsp dried leaf to 8 oz hot water, steep covered for 15 to 20 minutes; take 4 oz three times a day
- *Tincture* (1:5, 65% alcohol): 10 to 20 gtt (0.5–1.0 mL) three times a day

- *Capsules:* 200 to 300 mg of the dried herb two to three times a day
- *EO:* 0.05 to 0.20 mL per dose, 0.3 to 0.6 mL daily (ESCOP, 2003)

Pharmacokinetics—If Available (form or route when known): Inhalation of the major constituent of the EO, 1,8-cineole, had a plasma half-life of 35.8 minutes (ESCOP, 2003).

Toxicity: Overdose of the EO can cause nausea, vomiting, irritation of the kidneys or stomach, difficulty breathing, and CNS depression. There are reports of ingestion of 3:5–5 mL of the EO causing death. There are also reports of people surviving and recovering from ingestion of much larger amounts of the EO (De Vincenzi et al., 2002).

Contraindications: Avoid use in patients with liver disease, kidney, gallbladder, or GI irritation (ESCOP, 2003).

Side Effects: The use of eucalyptus-based nasal inhalers for sinus congestion can cause a rebound effect.

Long-Term Safety: Safe in normal doses but best used short-term as needed.

Use in Pregnancy/Lactation/Children: Avoid internal use in pregnancy and while lactating. Avoid use of undiluted EO on the skin, especially on the face of infants and young children.

Drug/Herb Interactions and Rationale (if known): Eucalyptus should not be given along with herbs containing pyrrolizidine alkaloids (coltsfoot, butterbur, comfrey, pulmonaria, etc.), as it may increase their hepatotoxicity (White et al., 1983). It also stimulates CYP-450 activity and may increase clearance of some medications, including amphetamines, aminopyrine, and pentobarbital (Brinker, 2001).

Special Notes: A novel use of eucalyptus for inhibiting fructose absorption and reducing weight has been studied in rats (Sugimoto et al., 2005). It is unclear whether eucalyptus would be effective or safe to use this way in humans.

BIBLIOGRAPHY

Aboriginal Communities of the Northern Territory of Australia. (1990). *Traditional Bush Medicines, an Aboriginal Pharmacopoeia.* Northern Territory of Australia.

Brinker F. (2001). *Herb Contraindications & Drug Interactions* (3rd ed.; p. 91). Sandy, OR: Eclectic Medical Publications.

De Vincenzi M, et al. (2002). Constituents of aromatic plants: Eucalyptol. *Fitoterapia.* Jun;73(3):269–275.

Duke J. Dr. Duke's phytochemical and ethnobotanical databases. Retrieved September 23 2006, from www.ars-grin.gov/ cgi-bin/duke/chemactivities.

European Scientific Cooperative on Phytotherapy. (2003). *ESCOP Monographs.* (2nd ed.; pp. 150–156*).* Stuttgart: Thieme.

Felter HW, Lloyd JU. (1986). King's American Dispensatory (19th ed.; pp. 733–736). Sandy, OR: Eclectic Medical Publications.

Gabrielska J, et al. (2006). Antioxidative effect of quercetin and its equimolar mixtures with phenyltin compounds on liposome membranes, *Journal of Agricultural and Food Chemistry.* Oct 4;54(20):7735–7746.

Jackson JK, et al. (2006). The antioxidants curcumin and quercetin inhibit inflammatory processes associated with arthritis. *Inflammation Research.* Apr;55(4):168–175.

Jin NZ, et al. (2006). Preventive effects of quercetin against benzo[a]pyrene-induced DNA damages and pulmonary precancerous pathologic changes in mice. *Basic and Clinical Pharmacology and Toxicology.* Jun;98(6):593–598.

Juergens UR, et al. (1998). Inhibition of cytokine production and arachidonic acid metabolism by eucalyptol (1.8-cineole) in human blood monocytes in vitro. *European Journal of Medical Research.* Nov 17;3(11):508–510.

Juergens UR, et al. (2003). Anti-inflammatory activity of 1.8-cineol (eucalyptol) in bronchial asthma: A double-blind placebo-controlled trial. *Respiratory Medicine.* Mar;97(3):250–256.

Karthick M, Stanely Mainzen Prince P. (2006). Preventive effect of rutin, a bioflavonoid, on lipid peroxides and antioxidants in isoproterenol-induced myocardial infarction in rats. *Journal of Pharmacy and Pharmacology.* May;58(5):701–707.

Lu XO, et al. (2004). Effect of *Eucalyptus globules* oil on lipopolysaccharide-induced chronic bronchitis and mucin hypersecretion in rats. *Zhongguo Zhong Yao Za Zhi.* Feb;29(2):168–171.

Morsy TA, et al. (2003). *Eucalyptus globules* (camphor oil) against the zoonotic scabies, *Sarcoptes scabiei. Journal of the Egyptian Society of Parasitology.* Apr;33(1):47–53.

Salari MH, et al. (2006). Antibacterial effects of *Eucalyptus globulus* leaf extract on pathogenic bacteria isolated from specimens of patients with respiratory tract disorders. *Clinical Microbiology and Infection.* Feb;12(2):194–196.

Silva J, et al. (2003). Analgesic and anti-inflammatory effects of essential oils of eucalyptus. *Journal of Ethnopharmacology.* Dec;89(2–3):277–283.

Skenderi G. (2003). *Herbal Vade Mecum* (pp. 147–148). Rutherford, NJ: Herbacy Press.

Sugimoto K, et al. (2005). Eucalyptus leaf extract inhibits intestinal fructose absorption, and suppresses adiposity due to dietary sucrose in rats. *British Journal of Nutrition.* Jun;93(6):957–963.

Takahashi T, et al. (2004). Antimicrobial activities of eucalyptus leaf extracts and flavonoids from *Eucalyptus maculata. Letters in Applied Microbiology.* 39(1):60–64.

White RD, et al. (1983). Effects of microsomal enzyme induction on the toxicity of pyrrolizidine (senecio) alkaloids. *Journal of Toxicology and Environmental Health.* Oct-Dec;12(4–6):633–640.

Winston D. (2006). *Winston's Botanic Materia Medica.* Washington, NJ: DWCHS.

Yang YC, et al. (2004). Ovicidal and adulticidal activity of *Eucalyptus globules* leaf oil terpenoids against *Pediculus humanus* capitis (Anoplura: Pediculidae). *Journal of Agricultural and Food Chemistry.* May 5;52(9):2507–2511.

 NAME: Evening Primrose (*Oenothera biennis*)

Common Names: King's cure-all

Family: *Onagraceae*

Description of Plant: It is native to North America and naturalized in the United Kingdom. The plant is a weedy, yellow-flowered, biennial herb growing up to 4.5' tall.

Medicinal Part: Oil from seeds, dried leaf, flower, and root bark

Constituents and Action (if known)
- Essential fatty acids
  - Gamma-linolenic acid (GLA): reduces inflammation by reducing prostaglandin E_1 (Fan & Chapkin, 1998), reduces hypertension and platelet aggregation (Skenderi, 2003)
  - May enhance oxygen free radical production and lipid peroxidation in glioma tumor cells, thus slowing their growth (Das et al., 1995)

- ○ Linoleic acid (LA): cannot be produced by the human body; body must convert LA to GLA. Deficiencies of LA are associated with diabetes, cancer, viral infections, and hypercholesterolemia and affect prostaglandin E_1 and E_2 synthesis.
- ○ Oleic acid
- ○ Palmitic acid
- ○ Stearic acid

Other Actions: EPO seed extracts are antioxidant (Birch et al., 2001).

Nutritional Ingredients: Seeds were used for food by Native Americans and are high in omega-6 oils. Root and young leaves may be used as a vegetable, but they have a peculiar and somewhat unpleasant bitter flavor.

Traditional Use
- The whole plant has been used as poultice for bruises.
- Leaf, flower, and root bark used for spastic coughs, IBS, and GI-based depression (along with hypericum and culver's root)
- There is no traditional medicinal use for the seed oil.

Current Use
Seed Oil
- Reduces symptoms of bronchial asthma (Skenderi, 2003)
- Reduces inflammation in arthritis, but no evidence that it can modify disease (Belch & Hill, 2000; Darlington & Stone, 2001)
- Decreases premenstrual symptoms (O'Brien & Massil, 1990; Skenderi, 2003)
- The oil, applied topically, softens the cervix; start using in the last 3 weeks of pregnancy.
- Reduces symptoms of uremic pruritus (Yoshimoto-Furuie et al., 1999)
- Increases fat content of breast milk when taken during lactation (Cant et al., 1991)
- Reduces symptoms of atopic dermatitis and eczema (McCaleb et al., 2000). Especially effective for severe noninflammatory atopic dermatitis (Yoon et al., 2002).
- Preliminary research shows a reduction of symptoms in diabetic neuropathy (Keen et al., 1993)

- May reduce hyperactivity in children with ADHD, but large doses are necessary (Arnold et al., 1989)
- May be lethal to cancer cells (high levels of fatty acids) but not normal cells. More research is needed.
- A combination of isoflavones, EPO, and vitamin E significantly reduced menopausal symptoms (Cancelo Hidalgo et al., 2006).

Available Forms, Dosage, and Administration Guidelines

Preparations: Expressed oil from seeds; capsules
Typical Dosage
- Dosage is based on a GLA content of 8%.
- *Capsules:* Up to 12 gel-caps of the oil a day (3–6 g a day)
- *Oil:* 0.5 tsp a day
- Or follow manufacturer or practitioner recommendations
- For ADHD, 5 to 8 g a day in divided doses

Pharmacokinetics—If Available (form or route when known): None known

Toxicity: None known

Contraindications: Seizure disorder; may exacerbate seizures

Side Effects: A few patients taking large doses experienced abdominal discomfort, nausea, or headache.

Long-Term Safety: Safe for long-term use when used appropriately

Use in Pregnancy/Lactation/Children
- Safe oral doses do not start or affect labor.
- Children: use only under supervision of a qualified practitioner

Drug/Herb Interactions and Rationale (if known): Do not use concurrently with phenothiazines: may increase risk of seizures.

Special Notes
- Research on six healthy volunteers could not determine any change in prostaglandin levels (Martens-Lobenhoffer & Meyer, 1998).

- Black currant seed oil and borage seed oil contain greater quantities of GLA at a lower cost, but research on the usefulness of these oils is lacking.
- Patients taking omega-6 supplements should also supplement their intake of omega-3 fatty acids (fish or flaxseed oil). Omega-6 fatty acids in excess can contribute to inflammatory processes and impede absorption of omega-3 fatty acids. A good ratio is 4:1 (omega-6 fatty acids to omega-3 fatty acids).

BIBLIOGRAPHY

Arnold LE, et al. (1989). Gamma-linoleic acid for attention-defiicit hyperactivity disorder: Placebo-controlled comparison to D-amphetamine. *Biological Psychiatry*. Jan 15;25(2):222–228.

Belch JJ, Hill A. (2000). Evening primrose oil and borage oil in rheumatologic conditions. *American Journal of Clinical Nutrition*. Jan;71[1 Suppl.]:352S–356S.

Birch AE, et al. (2001). Antioxidant properties of evening primrose seed extracts. *Journal of Agricultural and Food Chemistry*. Sep;49(9):4502–4507.

Cancelo Hidalgo JJ, et al. (2006). Effect of a compound containing isoflavones, primrose oil, and vitamin E in two different doses on climacteric symptoms. *Journal of Obstetrics and Gynaecology*. May;26(4):344–347.

Cant A, et al. (1991). The effect of maternal supplementation with linoleic and gamma-linolenic acids on the fat composition and content of human milk: A placebo-controlled trial. *Journal of Nutritional Science and Vitaminology (Tokyo)*. Dec;37(6):573–579.

Darlington LG, Stone TW. (2001). Antioxidants and fatty acids in the amelioration of rheumatoid arthritis and related disorders. *British Journal of Nutrition*. Mar;85(3):251–269.

Das UN, et al. (1995). Local application of gamma-linolenic acid in the treatment of human gliomas. *Cancer Letters*. 94:147–155.

Fan YY, Chapkin RS. (1998). Importance of dietary gamma-linolenic acid in human health and nutrition. *Journal of Nutrition*. 128(9):1411–1414.

Keen H, et al. (1993). Treatment of diabetic neuropathy with gamma-linolenic acid. *Diabetes Care*. 16(1):8–15.

Martens-Lobenhoffer J, Meyer FP. (1998). Pharmacokinetic data of gamma-linolenic acid in healthy volunteers after the administration of evening primrose oil (Epogam). *International Journal of Clinical Pharmacology and Therapeutics*. 36(7):363–366.

McCaleb R, et al. (2000). *Encyclopedia of Popular Herbs* (pp. 148–156). Roseville, CA: Prima Publishers.

O'Brien PM, Massil H. (1990). Premenstrual syndrome: Clinical studies on essential fatty acids. In: Horrobin DF. [Ed.]. *Omega 6 Essential Fatty Acids: Pathophysiology and Role in Clinical Medicine*. New York: Wiley-Liss.

Skenderi G. (2003). Herbal Vade Mecum (pp. 149–150). Rutherford, NJ: Herbacy Press.

Yoon S, et al. (2002). The therapeutic effect of evening primrose oil in atopic dermatitis patients with dry scaly skin lesions is associated with the normalization of serum gamma-interferon levels. *Skin Pharmacology and Applied Skin Physiology*. Jan-Feb;15(1):20–25.

Yoshimoto-Furuie K, et al. (1999). Effects of oral supplementation with evening primrose oil for six weeks on plasma essential fatty acids and uremic skin symptoms in hemodialysis patients. *Nephron*. 81(2):151–159.

 NAME: Eyebright (*Euphrasia officinale*)

Common Names: Red eyebright

Family: *Scrophulariaceae*

Description of Plant: Annual; grows about 4″ to 1′ tall, blooms from July to September; partially parasitic on grasses, grows in northern regions (Canada, northern Europe, Maine)

Medicinal Part: Fresh or dried herb (preparations made from the fresh herb are vastly superior)

Constituents and Action (if known)

- Iridoid glycosides: aucubin (anti-inflammatory [Recio et al., 1994]), catalpol, euphroside, ixoroside, aucubigenin (aglycone of aucubin): antibacterial activity against *Micrococcus aureus*, *Escherichia coli*, *Bacillis subtilis*, *Mycobacterium phlei*, and to a lesser degree antifungal, with the greatest activity against *Penicillium italicum* (Mills & Bone, 2000). Antiviral activity: hepatitis B and hepatoprotective activity (Chang & Yamaura, 1993; Mills & Bone, 2000).
- Tannins: astringent, anti-inflammatory (Duke, 2006)
- Flavonoids (quercetin, apigenin): anti-inflammatory (Duke, 2006)
- Volatile oils

Nutritional Ingredients: None known

Traditional Use

- To treat allergic rhinitis, postnasal drip, sinus headaches, sinusitis, otitis media, and red, itchy eyes associated with hay fever (Winston, 2006).
- Part of British herbal tobacco smoked for chronic bronchial infections and colds
- To treat coughs and sore throats
- Topical: eye fatigue, conjunctivitis (homeopathic remedy) (Wichtl & Bisset, 1994)

Current Use

- Fresh eyebright tincture is very effective when used orally for hypersecretory acute or chronic sinusitis, allergic rhinitis, serous otitis media, and postnasal drip, especially when combined with echinacea (Winston, 2006).
- Eyedrops made with this herb effectively treated inflammatory or catarrhal conjunctivitis (Stoss et al., 2000).

Available Forms, Dosage, and Administration Guidelines

Preparations: Dried herb, whole, cut and sifted, or powdered; capsules, tablets, fresh plant tinctures, eye wash, other preparations

Typical Dosage

- *Capsules:* Up to five 400- to 500-mg capsules a day
- *Tea:* Steep 1 to 2 tsp in a cup of hot water for 10 to 15 minutes; take three times a day.
- May be used externally as an eye wash or compress
- *Fresh plant tincture* (1:2, 35% alcohol): 30 to 40 gtt (1.5–2 mL) up to four times a day
- Or follow manufacturer or practitioner recommendations

Pharmacokinetics—If Available (form or route when known): None known

Toxicity: None known

Contraindications: None known

Side Effects: None

Long-Term Safety: Unknown; no adverse effects expected

Use in Pregnancy/Lactation/Children: No research available; no adverse effects expected

Drug/Herb Interactions and Rationale (if known): None known

Special Notes

- Topical ophthalmic preparations should be made into sterile saline solutions.
- Only one controlled study is available to determine efficacy for its topical use. No studies exist to document its internal use. Long-term clinical use by Eclectic and naturopathic physicians and herbalists and the astringent, anti-inflammatory, antiviral, and antibacterial activity of its constituents suggest efficacy.
- Many popular books recommend the herb (orally) for glaucoma, cataracts, and other serious eye problems. It is unlikely to have any activity for these conditions.

BIBLIOGRAPHY

Chang IM, Yamaura Y. (1993). Aucubin: A new antidote for poisonous Amanita mushrooms. *Phytotherapy Research*. 7:53–56.

Der Marderosian A, Beutler J. [Eds.]. (1996). *The Review of Natural Products*. St. Louis, MO: Facts and Comparisons.

Duke J. Dr. Duke's phytochemical and ethnobotanical databases. Retrieved September 22 2006, from www.ars-grin.gov/cgi-bin/duke/chemactivities.

Mills S, Bone K. (2000). *Principles and Practice of Phytotherapy* (pp. 374–377). Edinburgh: Churchill Livingstone.

Recio M, et al. (1994). Structural considerations on the iridoids as antiinflammatory agents. *Planta Medica*. 60:232–234.

Stoss M, et al. (2000). Prospective cohort trial of Euphrasia single-dose eye drops in conjunctivitis. *Journal of Alternative and Complementary Medicine*. Dec;6(6):499–508.

Wichtl M, Bisset NG. [Eds.]. (1994). *Herbal Drugs and Phytopharmaceuticals*. Stuttgart: Medpharm Scientific Publishers.

Winston D. (2006). *Winston's Botanic Materia Medica*. Washington, NJ: DWCHS.

F

 NAME: False Unicorn (*Chamaelirium luteum*)

Common Names: Helonias root, devil's bit, blazing star, fairy-wand

Family: *Liliaceae*

Description of Plant: It is a small perennial native to the United States. The male and female flowers bloom on separate plants. It is a threatened species because of overharvesting and loss of habitat.

Medicinal Part: Root, collected in autumn

Constituents and Action (if known)

- Steroidal saponins
  - Chamaelirin
  - Diosgenin
- Fatty acids: oleic, linoleic, stearic acid (Cataline et al., 1942)
- Other actions: may act by increasing human chorionic gonadotropin (Brandt, 1996)

Nutritional Ingredients: None known

Traditional Use

- It has been used as a uterine and female reproductive tonic by Native Americans, Eclectic physicians, naturopaths, and clinical herbalists. It is indicated for amenorrhea, dysmenorrhea (with pelvic congestion and a feeling of fullness), infertility, morning sickness; was an ingredient in a well-known Eclectic formula called "mother's cordial." This formula was given in the last 2 to 3 weeks of pregnancy to promote a healthy delivery.
- Bitter tonic to stimulate appetite
- Diuretic

Current Use

- It is used as a female reproductive amphoteric to restore hormonal balance, especially in women who have mild elevations of androgens or those discontinuing contraceptive pills (Winston, 2006).
- Menstrual and uterine problems, such as premenstrual symptoms, amenorrhea, dysmenorrhea, menorrhagia
- Infertility with anovulatory cycles
- In an animal study, false unicorn inhibited growth of prostate tumor xenografts by 81%. Researchers speculate that the herb has an antiandrogenic effect and may be preventative for prostate cancer (Ng & Figg, 2003).

Available Forms, Dosage, and Administration Guidelines
Preparations: Dried root, decoction, capsule, tincture
Typical Dosage
- *Tincture* (1:5, 60% alcohol): 20 to 30 gtt (1–1.5 mL) three or four times a day
- *Decoction:* 0.5 tsp dried root to 8 oz boiling water, gently decoct 15 minutes, steep 45 minutes; take 4 oz (half-cup) twice a day

Pharmacokinetics—If Available (form or route when known): None known

Toxicity: None reported

Contraindications: None known

Side Effects: Large doses may cause nausea and vomiting.

Long-Term Safety: No adverse effects expected

Use in Pregnancy/Lactation/Children: Traditionally used during pregnancy, but safety cannot be confirmed. No research on use during breast-feeding, so avoid.

Drug/Herb Interactions and Rationale (if known): None known

Special Notes
- Because of its threatened status, this plant should be used only when absolutely indicated. Other herbs such as chaste tree, shatavari, or dong quai can be used for many of the same complaints.
- Often adulterated in commerce with true unicorn root (*Aletris farinosa*), which has a decidedly different activity.

BIBLIOGRAPHY
Brandt D. (1996). A clinician's view. *HerbalGram*. 36:75.
Cataline EL, et al. (1942). The phytochemistry of Helonias I. Preliminary examination of the drug. *Journal of the American Pharmaceutical Association*. 31:519.
Der Marderosian A, Beutler J. [Eds.]. (2004). *The Review of Natural Products*. St. Louis, MO: Facts and Comparisons.
Grieve M. (1996). *A Modern Herbal* (pp. 823–824). New York: Barnes & Noble, Inc.

Mills S, Bone K. (2000). *Principles and Practice of Phytotherapy* (pp. 242–244). Edinburgh: Churchill Livingstone.

Ng SS, Figg WD. (2003). Antitumor activity of herbal supplements in human prostate cancer xenografts implanted in immunodeficient mice. *Anticancer Research.* Sep-Oct;23(5A):3585–3590.

Winston D. (2006). *Winston's Botanic Materia Medica.* Washington, NJ: DWCHS.

 NAME: Fenugreek (*Trigonella foenum-graecum*)

Common Names: Bird's foot, Greek hayseed, trigonella

Family: *Fabeaceae*

Description of Plant: Member of the pea family. Annual native to the Mediterranean region and India; now commonly cultivated in India, Morocco, Turkey, Ukraine, and China.

Medicinal Part: Dried ripe seeds

Constituents and Action (if known)

- Galactomannans: mucilagin coats stomach and can relieve constipation because it adds fiber; may also be responsible for lowering cholesterol
- Pyridine alkaloids: trigonelline, gentianine, and carpaine can be degraded to nicotinic acid during roasting. This change is associated with the flavor of the seed and may also lower cholesterol (Bordia et al., 1997).
- Steroidal sapogenins
  - Diosgenin: inhibits abnormal crypt foci formation in rats and induces apoptosis in HT-29 human colon cancer cells (Raju et al., 2004), yamogenin, tigogenin, neotigogenin, sarsasapogenin, and yuccagen can lower plasma cholesterol, glucose, and glucagon levels; may increase food consumption (Khosla et al., 1995)
  - Graecunins—saponins (actual glycosides of diosgenin, gitogenin, and trigogenin, fenugrin B, and coumarin compounds): may cause side effect of bleeding (Petit et al., 1995; Sauvaire et al., 1991)
  - Fenugreekine, a saponin, may possess cardiotonic, diuretic, antiviral, and antihypertensive properties (Dinesh et al., 1994a).

- Flavonoids
  - Vitexin, isovitexin, apigenin, luteolin, orientin, quercetin: anti-inflammatory, antioxidants
  - Protein (20%–30%) and free amino acids (lysine, tryptophan, histidine, arginine)
  - Minerals and lipids

Nutritional Ingredients: Vitamins A, B_1, C; minerals (calcium, iron). Seeds are rich in protein and have been used as animal forage. Used as a flavoring for maple syrup substitutes. Used for centuries as a cooking spice (curries in India, bread in Egypt, coffee substitute in Africa).

Traditional Use
- Demulcent, emollient, nutritive, hypoglycemic agent, galactogogue, digestive stimulant
- For chronic coughs, bronchitis
- To stimulate milk flow in nursing mothers
- As a tea for gastric irritation (gastritis, ulcers) and digestive upset (gas, biliousness, dyspepsia)
- Used topically to treat boils, cellulitis, leg ulcers, eczema

Current Use
- Lowers glucose levels in type 2 diabetes, increases glycemic control and decreases insulin resistance (Gupta et al., 2001; Kochlar & Nagi, 2005; Sharma et al., 1996)
- Lowers cholesterol levels, triglycerides, LDL cholesterol, and total cholesterol (Bordia et al., 1997)
- Decreases symptoms of gastritis (tea is particularly soothing) and lack of appetite (Blumenthal et al., 2000)
- In vitro and animal studies suggest several novel uses for fenugreek. The seeds have chemopreventative effects against breast and colon cancer (Amin et al., 2005; Raju et al., 2004). Fenugreek also decreased serum concentrations of T3 and T4 in hyperthyroid rats (Tahiliani & Kar, 2003).

Available Forms, Dosage, and Administration Guidelines
Preparations: Seed, whole or powdered; capsules, tablets, tinctures, tea
Typical Dosage
- *Seed:* 1.5 tsp a day
- *Capsules:* Up to six 600- to 700-mg capsules a day

- *Tea:* 1 to 2 tsp freshly powdered seed to 8 oz hot water, steep 1 hour; take two or three cups a day
- *Tincture* (1:5, 30% alcohol): 60 to 120 gtt (3–6 mL) three times a day
- *External use:* Soak 10 tsp powdered seed in hot water to make a poultice.
- Or follow manufacturer or practitioner recommendations

Pharmacokinetics—If Available (form or route when known): None known

Toxicity: None

Contraindications: None known

Side Effects: Intestinal gas and diarrhea; possible hypoglycemia; repeated topical applications may cause rashes. Fenugreek causes the urine to smell like maple syrup, which can be mistaken for pseudo–maple syrup urine disease (Korman et al., 2001).

Long-Term Safety: Used as a spice in the Middle East; no adverse effects expected

Use in Pregnancy/Lactation/Children: Do not use in pregnancy; may stimulate uterus. Traditionally used to promote milk flow in nursing mothers. Safety data unavailable.

Drug/Herb Interactions and Rationale (if known): May potentiate antidiabetic medications. If given concurrently, monitor blood sugar levels. Separate all drugs by 2 hours to prevent binding by fenugreek's mucilage content. May potentiate effects of anticoagulants; monitor International Normalized Ratio (INR) and PT if given concurrently.

Special Notes: In persons with diabetes, fenugreek seems to lower cholesterol and blood glucose levels. It does not seem to strongly affect blood sugar levels in nondiabetics.

BIBLIOGRAPHY

Amin A, et al. (2005). Chemopreventive activites of *Trigonella foenum-graecum* (fenugreek) against breast cancer. *Cell Biology International.* Aug;29(8):687–694.

Blumenthal M, et al. (2000). *Herbal Medicine: Expanded Commission E Monographs* (pp. 130–133). Austin, TX: American Botanical Council.

Bordia A, et al. (1997). Effect of ginger (*Zingiber officinale* Rosc.) and fenugreek (*Trigonella foenum graecum* L.) on blood lipids, blood sugar and platelet aggregation in patients with coronary artery disease. *Prostaglandins, Leukotrienes and Essential Fatty Acids.* 58(5):379–384.

Dinesh P, et al. (1994a). Hypocholesterolemic effect of hypoglycaemic principle of fenugreek (*Trigonella foenum graecum*) seeds. *Indian Journal of Clinical Biochemistry.* 9:13–16.

Dinesh P, et al. (1994b). Effects of the hypoglycemic principle from *Trigonella foenum graecum.* Proceedings of the XVIth International Congress of Biochemistry and Molecular Biology, New Delhi, 1994.

Gupta A, et al. (2001). Effect of *Trigonella foenum-graecum* (fenugreek) seeds on glycaemic control and insulin resistance in type 2 diabetes mellitus: A double blind placebo controlled study. *Journal of the Association of Physicians of India.* Nov;49:1057–1061.

Khosla P, et al. (1995). Effect of *Trigonella foenum graecum* (fenugreek) on blood glucose in normal and diabetic rats. *Indian Journal of Physiology and Pharmacology.* 39(2):173.

Kochhar A, Nagi M. (2005). Effect of supplementation of traditional medicinal plants on blood glucose in non-insulin dependent diabetics: A pilot study. *Journal of Medicinal Food.* Winter;8(4):5445–5449.

Korman SH, et al. (2001). Pseudo-maple syrup urine disease due to maternal prenatal ingestion of fenugreek. *Journal of Paediatrics and Child Health.* Aug;38(4):403–404.

Petit PR, et al. (1995). Steroid saponins from fenugreek seeds: Extraction, purification, and pharmacological investigation on feeding behavior and plasma cholesterol. *Steroids.* 60(10):674.

Raju J, et al. (2004). Diosgenin, a steroid saponin of *Trigonella foenum-graecum* (fenugreek), inhibits azoxymethane-induced aberrant crypt foci formation in F344 rats and induces apoptosis in HT-29 human colon cancer cells. *Cancer Epidemiology, Biomarkers and Prevention.* Aug;13(8):1392–1398.

Sauvaire Y, et al. (1991). Implication of steroid saponins and sapogenins in the hypocholesterolemic effect of fenugreek. *Lipids.* 26(3):191.

Sharma RD, et al. (1996). Hypolipidaemic effect of fenugreek seeds: A chronic study in non-insulin dependent diabetic patients. *Physiotherapy Research.* 10:332–334.

Tahiliani P, Kar A. (2003). The combined effects of Trigonella and Allium extracts in the regulation of hyperthyroidism in rats. *Phytomedicine.* Nov;10(8):665–668.

Vijayakumar MV, et al. The hypoglycemic activity of fenugreek seed extract is mediated through the stimulation of an insulin signalling pathway. *British Journal of Pharmacology.* Sep;146(1):41–48.

NAME: Feverfew (*Tanacetum parthenium*)

Common Names: Featherfew, bachelor's button, midsummer daisy

Family: *Asteraceae*

Description of Plant: A member of the daisy family native to central and southern Europe. Short bushy perennial that grows 1' to 3' tall. Commonly cultivated in England, North America, and Latin America. Flowers are daisy-like, with a yellow center and 10 to 20 white rays; blooms July to October.

Medicinal Part: Leaves and flowers (fresh or dried)

Constituents and Action (if known)

- Sesquiterpene lactones
  - Parthenolides (which are very unstable in feverfew) lower serotonin levels (Heptinstall et al., 1992; Johnson et al., 1985; Murphy et al., 1988): antileishmanial (Tiuman et al., 2005).
  - Parthenolides were believed to be the sole active constituents, but research has shown this to be untrue (Awang, 1998a).
  - They interact with the protein kinase C pathway, inhibiting granule secretion from platelets, which causes an antimigraine effect, and from polymorphs, which has an antiarthritic activity (Mills & Bone, 2000).
  - Pathenolides have shown in vitro and in vivo antitumor and antiangiogenic activity (Curry et al., 2004). In human studies, adequate blood levels of this compound were not achievable by oral administration (Curry et al., 2004).
  - 3 beta-hydroxyparthenolide
- Flavonoids (Knight, 1995): luteolin, apigenin
- Eudesmanolides: antibacterial activity; inhibited *Staphylococcus aureus*, *Escherichia coli*, *Salmonella* spp.
- Monoterpenes (trans chrysanthenyl): possible anti-inflammatory activity (Awang, 1998b), insecticidal activity (Hobbs, 1990)
- EOs: bactericidal, fungicidal (Winston, 2006)
- Other actions: anti-inflammatory; inhibits platelet phospholipase A, which prevents the release of arachidonic

acid activity (Groenewegen & Heptinstall, 1992; Mills & Bone, 2000); inhibits histamine release; inactivates polymorphonuclear leukocytes; inhibits leukotrienes, prostaglandins, and histamine secretion; inhibits 5-hydroxytryptamine-mediated contractile responses (Hoffmann, 2003).

Nutritional Ingredients: None known

Traditional Use
- Anthelmintic, antipyretic, anti-inflammatory, bitter tonic, emmenagogue (high doses)
- Use dates back thousands of years (Greeks and early Europeans) for the treatment of headaches (including migraines), arthritis, menstrual cramps, digestive upsets, and respiratory conditions such as asthma.
- Antipyretic: hot tea used to break high fevers
- Topical use for insect bites

Current Use
- Beneficial in migraine headaches (reduces severity and frequency) (Diener et al., 2005; Palevitch et al., 1997)
- Is approved in Canada for migraine prevention as long as it contains 0.2% parthenolide (this is not a guarantee of therapeutic activity). It is most effective for vasodilative migraines (Winston, 2006).
- A sublingual preparation with feverfew and ginger was effective for treating migraines during the early pain phase (Cady et al., 2005).
- Reduces inflammation in arthritis if taken regularly (Pattrick et al., 1989)
- Possible benefit for psoriasis and arthritis (Mills & Bone, 2000), Ménière's disease, and vertigo (Bartram, 1995) as well as menstrual pain.

Available Forms, Dosage, and Administration Guidelines
Preparations: Fresh or dried leaves; capsules, tablets, tinctures. Some products are standardized to 0.2% parthenolide, even though other constituents may be responsible for the herb's activity.

Typical Dosage

- *Capsules:* Capsules with 25 mg of freeze-dried leaves
- *Fresh herb:* Eat two average-sized leaves a day
- *Tincture* (1:2 or 1:5, 30% alcohol): 20 to 40 gtt (1–2 mL) three times a day
- Or follow manufacturer or practitioner recommendations
- Need to take for 1 to 2 weeks before result is seen

Pharmacokinetics—If Available (form or route when known): None known

Toxicity: None known

Contraindications: Hypersensitivity to members of the *Asteraceae* family (ragweed, chamomile, chrysanthemums, etc.)

Side Effects

- With regular use, rebound migraine headaches and joint stiffness may occur after stopping: "post-feverfew syndrome" (de Weerdt et al., 1996; Johnson et al., 1985).
- Mouth ulcerations, sore tongue, and lip swelling have occurred when consuming the fresh leaves.
- Contact dermatitis associated with handling the plant
- Allergic reaction (allergy to *Asteraceae*)

Long-Term Safety: Safe, but when stopped, increased number of headaches may develop

Use in Pregnancy/Lactation/Children: Do not use in pregnancy (may cause uterine contractions), in breast-feeding women, or in children younger than 2 years of age.

Drug/Herb Interactions and Rationale (if known): Use cautiously with anticoagulants; may increase bleeding. Monitor INR and PT.

Special Notes: Long-term use is more effective for reducing the severity and number of migraines. Slow withdrawal may reduce the likelihood and severity of post-feverfew syndrome. Herbalists believe that the plant is most effective when harvested when in flower.

BIBLIOGRAPHY

Awang D. (1998a). Parthenolide: The demise of a facile theory of feverfew activity. *Journal of Herbs, Spices and Medicinal Plants.* 5(4):95–98.

Awang D. (1998b). Prescribing therapeutic feverfew (*Tanacetum parthenium*). *Integrative Medicine*. 1(1):11–13.

Awang DVC. (1993). Feverfew fever. *HerbalGram*. 29:34.

Barsby RWJ, et al. (1993). Feverfew and vascular smooth muscle: Extracts from fresh and dried plants show opposing pharmacological profiles, dependent upon sesquiterpene lactone content. *Planta Medica*. 59:20–25.

Bartram T. (1995). *Encyclopedia of Herbal Medicine* (pp. 182–183). Dorset: Grace Publisher.

Cady RK, et al. (2005). Gelstat migraine (sublingually administered feverfew and ginger compound) for acute treatment of migraine when administered during the mild pain phase. *Medical Science Monitor*. Sep;11(9):P165–P169.

Curry EA 3rd, et al. (2004). Phase I dose escalation trial of feverfew with standardized doses of parthenolide in patients with cancer. *Investigational New Drugs*. Aug;22(3):299–305.

de Weerdt CJ, et al (1996). Randomized double-blind placebo controlled trial of a feverfew preparation. *Phytomedicine*. 3(3):225.

Der Marderosian A, Beutler J. [Eds.]. (2004). *The Review of Natural Products*. St. Louis, MO: Facts and Comparisons.

Diener HC, et al. (2005). Efficacy and safety of 6.25 mg t.i.d. feverfew CO_2-extract (MIG-99) in migraine prevention—A randomized, double-blind, multicentre, placebo-controlled study. *Cephalalgia*. Nov;25(11):1031–1041.

Groenewegen WA, Heptinstall S. (1992). A comparison of the effects of an extract of feverfew and parthenolide, a component of feverfew, on human platelet activity in vitro. *Journal of Pharmacy and Pharmacology*. 43:391–395.

Heptinstall S, et al. (1985). Extracts from feverfew inhibit granule secretion in blood platelets and polymorphonuclear leucocytes. *Lancet*. 8437:1071–1074.

Heptinstall S, et al. (1992). Parthenolide content and bioactivity of feverfew (*Tanacetum parthenium* [L] Schultz-Bip.). Estimation of commercial and authenticated feverfew products. *Journal of Pharmacy and Pharmacology*. 44:391–395.

Hobbs C. (1990). Feverfew. *National Headache Foundation Newsletter*. Winter:10.

Hoffmann D. (2003). Medical Herbalism (p. 587). Rochester, VT: Healing Arts Press.

Johnson ES, et al. (1985). Efficacy of feverfew as prophylactic treatment of migraine. *British Medical Journal*. 291:569.

Knight DW. (1995). Feverfew: Chemistry and biological activity. *Natural Products Report*. 12(3):271–276.

Mills S, Bone K. (2000). *Principles and Practice of Phytotherapy* (pp. 385–393). Edinburgh: Churchill Livingstone.

Murch S, et al. (1997). Melatonin in feverfew and other medicinal plants. *Lancet*. 350:1598–1599.

Murphy JJ, et al. (1988). Randomized double-blind placebo-controlled trial of feverfew in migraine prevention. *Lancet*. 8(601): 189–192.

Palevitch D, et al. (1997). Feverfew (*Tanacetum parthenium*) as a prophylactic treatment for migraine: A double-blind placebo-controlled study. *Phytotherapy Research*. 11:508–511.

Pattrick M, et al. (1989). Feverfew in rheumatoid arthritis: A double-blind, placebo-controlled study. *Annals of Rheumatic Disease*. 48:547.

Tiuman TS, et al. (2005). Antileishmanial activity of parthenolide, a sesquiterpene lactone isolated from *Tanacetum parthenium*. *Antimicrobial Agents and Chemotherapy*. Jan;29(1):176–182.

Vogler BK, et al. (1998). Feverfew as a preventive treatment for migraine: A systematic review. *Cephalalgia*. 18(10):704–708.

Williams CA, et al. (1999). The flavonoids of *Tanacetum partheneum* and *T. vulgare* and their anti-inflammatory properties. *Phytochemistry*. 51(3):417–423.

Winston D. (2006). *Winston's Botanic Materia Medica*. Washington, NJ: DWCHS.

 NAME: Flax (*Linum usitatissimum*)

Common Names: Flaxseed, linseed

Family: *Linaceae*

Description of Plant: One of the world's oldest cultivated plants (8,000–10,000 years). Grown for its fiber (linen), seed oil (linseed oil), and seeds. Cultivated throughout the world (India, China, Turkey, Argentina, Morocco).

Medicinal Part: Seeds and oil

Constituents and Action (if known)

- Essential fatty acids
  - Omega-3, essential fatty acids (linolenic, lenoleic, oleic acids): responsible for anti-inflammatory properties and cholesterol-lowering properties Caughey et al., 1996; Lucas et al., 2002; Mandasescu et al., 2005; Prasad, 1997;

Prasad et al., 1998); lower thrombin-stimulated platelet aggregation (Ferretti & Flanagan, 1996); may slow renal failure and decrease renal transplant rejection (Parbtani & Clark, 2003)

- Lignans, including secoisolariciresinol diglucoside, are phytochemicals shown to have weak estrogenic and antiestrogen properties. They assist with control of menopausal signs and changes (Haggans et al., 1999; Hu et al., 2007). Anticarcinogenic, possibly of benefit in treating SLE, hyperlipidemia, and rheumatoid arthritis. May have anticancer effects by lowering tumor necrosis factor (Caughey et al., 1996; Thompson et al., 1997; Boon et al., 2007).
- Mucilage (3%–10%)

Nutritional Ingredients: Flaxseed is a source of both dietary lignans (phytochemicals) and omega-3 fatty acids. Seed is 25% protein.

Traditional Use
- Emollient, demulcent, bulk laxative
- Seeds used by early Romans for coughs, urinary tract inflammation, lung conditions, and as a laxative
- Poultice of the seeds, mixed with oil or water, applied to inflamed skin, boils, styes, and dry, itching skin
- Decoctions used for sore throats
- Seeds have been used to remove foreign objects from the eye. The seed is placed in the eye, the foreign object adheres to it, and then both are removed.

Current Use
- Flaxseed is an excellent source of soluble fiber; it is a stool softener and bulk laxative for chronic constipation. The moistened seeds decrease transit time, increase stool weight, stimulate peristalsis, and protect and soothe mucosa.
- Laxative-dependent constipation
- May assist in weight loss when taken before meals because it provides a feeling of fullness
- Lowers plasma lipids: cholesterol (9%), triglycerides, low-density lipoproteins (18%) (Cunnane et al., 1993;

Mandasescu et al., 2005), which may reduce the need for statin drugs)
- Decreases pain from inflammatory bowel disease
- Acts as a phytoestrogen to reduce premenstrual symptoms and signs and changes of menopause (Brooks et al., 2004). Flaxseed does not affect bone metabolism in menopausal women (Lucas et al., 2002).
- Reduces pathogenesis of degenerative nephritis in autoimmune disease such as lupus (Clark et al., 2001)
- Decreases platelet stickiness
- Animal studies indicate that it can reduce the incidence and progression of cancer by increasing tumor necrosis factor levels. Dietary flaxseed enhanced the inhibitory effects of tamoxifen in rats with estrogen-sensitive human breast cancer (Chen et al., 2004).
- May reduce risk of breast, ovarian, and prostate cancer if used regularly (Thompson, 1998).
- Dogs fed flax or sunflower seed for 1 month had improved skin and hair coats (Rees et al., 2001).

Available Forms, Dosage, and Administration Guidelines
Preparation: Seed, whole or powdered; expressed oil of seed
Typical Dosage
- *Seed:* Soak 1to 2 tbsp whole or cracked seed in 1 cup water for 1 hour and drink; take up to three times a day.
- *Ground:* Grind flaxseeds in coffee grinder and take 1 tsp twice a day, up to 4 tbsp twice daily. Flaxseeds begin to oxidize in 20 minutes, so use fresh ground. Sprinkle on food or mix in liquid.
- *Soft gel tab:* 1,000 mg four times a day
- *Oil:* 1 to 4 tbsp a day. Very temperature-sensitive, so store in refrigerator, do not heat, and use in recipes that do not require cooking.
- Or follow manufacturer or practitioner recommendations

Pharmacokinetics—If Available (form or route when known): None known

Toxicity: None known

Contraindications: Persons with diverticulosis should not ingest seeds because they can get trapped in the diverticula and cause inflammation. Also contraindicated in persons with small bowel disease and inflammation, colicky bowel conditions, and bowel obstruction.

Side Effects: Seed ingestion can produce diarrhea, flatulence, nausea; allergic reaction.

Long-Term Safety: Safe

Use in Pregnancy/Lactation/Children: In pregnancy, flaxseed is a common food; no adverse effects are expected. For breast-feeding women and children, use appears safe, and no adverse effects are expected.

Drug/Herb Interactions and Rationale (if known)

- Separate from all other drugs by at least 2 hours. Because of its mucilaginous properties, flaxseed can bind with drugs, rendering them unabsorbable (especially cardiac glycosides).
- Avoid concurrent use with laxatives and stool softeners because it may potentiate the laxative effect.

Special Notes: Differences in flaxseed are found in various growing locations, variety, and harvest year. Drink enough fluid to minimize flatulence and prevent constipation. Never ingest immature seeds, because they contain cyanogenic nitrates and glucosides, which may cause unsteady gait, tachycardia, weakness.

BIBLIOGRAPHY

Blumenthal M, et al. (2000). *Herbal Medicine: Expanded Commission E Monographs* (pp. 134–138). Austin, TX: American Botanical Council.

Boon HS, et al., (2007). Trends in complementary/alternative medicine use by breast cancer survivors: comparing survey data from 1998 and 2005. *BMC Womens Health.* Mar 30;7:4.

Brooks JD, et al. (2004). Supplementation with flaxseed alters estrogen metabolism in postmenopausal women to a greater extent than does supplementation with an equal amount of soy. *American Journal of Clinical Nutrition.* Feb;79(2):318–325.

Caughey GE, et al. (1996). The effect on human tumor necrosis factor alpha and interleukin 1 beta production on diets enriched in n-3 fatty acids from vegetable oil or fish oil. *American Journal of Clinical Nutrition.* 63(1):116–122.

Chen J, et al. (2004). Dietary flaxseed enhances the inhibitory effect of tamoxifen on the growth of estrogen-dependent human breast cancer (MCF-7) in nude mice. *Clinical Cancer Research*. Nov 15;10:7703–7711.

Clark WF, et al. (2001). Flaxseed in lupus nephritis: A two-year nonplacebo-controlled crossover study. *Journal of the American College of Nutrition*. Apr;20[2 Suppl.]:143–148.

European Scientific Cooperative on Phytotherapy. (2003). *ESCOP Monographs* (pp. 290–296). New York: Thieme.

Ferretti A, Flanagan VP. (1996). Antithromboxane activity of dietary alpha-linolenic acid: A pilot study. *Prostaglandins Leukotrienes and Essential Fatty Acids*. 54(6):451–455.

Haggans CJ, et al. (1999). Effect of flaxseed consumption on urinary estrogen metabolites in postmenopausal women. *Nutrition and Cancer*. 33(2):188–195.

Haggerty W. (1999). Flax, ancient herb and modern medicine. *HerbalGram*. 45:51–56.

Hu C, et al. (2007). Antioxidant activities of the flaxseed lignan secoisolariciresinol diglucoside, its aglycone secoisolariciresinol and the mammalian lignans enterodiol and enterolactone in vitro. *Food Chem Toxicol*. Jun 2; [Epub ahead of print].

Lucas EA, et al. (2002). Flaxseed improves lipid profile without altering biomarkers of bone metabolism in postmenopausal women. *Journal of Clinical Endocrinology and Metabolism*. Apr;87(4):1527–1532.

Kurzer MS, Xu X. (1997). Dietary phytoestrogens. *Annual Review of Nutrition*. 17:353–381.

Mandasescu S, et al. (2005). Flaxseed supplementation in hyperlipidemic patients. *Revista Medico-Chirurgicala a Societatii de Medici si Naturalisti Din Iasi*. Jul-Sep;109(3):502–506.

Nesbitt PD, et al. (1999). Human metabolism of mammalian lignan precursors in raw and processed flaxseed. *American Journal of Clinical Nutrition*. 69(3):549–555.

Nesbitt PD, Thompson LU. (1997). Lignans in homemade and commercial products containing flaxseed. *Nutrition and Cancer*. 29(3):222–227.

Parbtani A, Clark WF. (2003). Flaxseed and its components in renal disease. In: Thompson L, Cunnane S [Eds.]. *Flaxseed in Human Nutrition*. 2nd ed. Champaign, IL: AOCS Publishing.

Prasad K. (1997). Dietary flaxseed in prevention of hypercholesterolemic atherosclerosis. *Atherosclerosis*. 32(1):69–76.

Prasad K, et al. (1998). Reduction of hypercholesterolemic atherosclerosis by CDC-flaxseed with very low alpha-linolenic acid. *Atherosclerosis*. 136(2):367–375.

Rees, CA, et al. (2001). Effects of dietary flax seed and sunflower seed supplementation on normal canine serum polyunsaturated fatty acids and skin and hair coat condition scores. *Veterinary Dermatology.* Apr;12(2):111–117.

Thompson LU. (1998). Experimental studies on lignans and cancer. *Bailliere's Clinical Endocrinology and Metabolism.* 12(4):691–705.

Thompson LU, et al. (1997). Variability in anticancer lignan levels in flaxseed. *Nutrition and Cancer.* 27(1):26–30.

G

 NAME: Garlic (*Allium sativum*)

Common Names: *Knoblaunch* (German), stinking rose, *da suan* (Chinese)

Family: *Lilliaceae*

Description of Plant

- A pungent member of the lily family that is cultivated worldwide. The largest commercial production of garlic is in central California.
- The odor of garlic is caused mainly by the enzymatic breakdown of alliin into allicin. Once cooked, there is less odor and less physiologic effect.

Medicinal Part: Bulb

Constituents and Action (if known)

- Garlic contains hundreds of constituents, with at least 23 sulphur compounds having been identified.
- Thiosulfanates (sulfur compounds; 1% dry weight)
  - Allicin is one of the most active ingredients, and its breakdown produces other sulphur compounds such as allyl sulphides, ajoenes, oligosulphides, and vinyldithiines. Allicin has extensive antimicrobial activity, inhibiting the growth of many bacteria (*Helicobacter pylori*) and fungus (*Candida albicans*) and localized yeast infections (Jonkers et al., 1999). It interferes with the hepatic metabolism of cholesterol, thus reducing serum cholesterol levels (Berthold et al., 1998; Koscielny et al., 1999). It tends to lower low-density lipoproteins and raise high-density

lipoproteins, which transports cholesterol to the liver (Isaacsohn et al., 1998). It may protect endothelial tissue from oxidized low-density lipoprotein injury (Ide & Lau, 1999; Munday et al., 1999). It reduces serum triglycerides by as much as 13% (Silagy & Neil, 1994a). It reduces blood pressure (Silagy & Neil, 1994b). It improves peripheral arterial disease. It may modestly reduce blood glucose.

○ Ajoene has weak antifungal activity and reduces platelet stickiness but only for a few hours (Legnani et al., 1993). It has antiviral activity against HIV (Shoji et al., 1993).

○ Diallyl sulfide and other sulfur components have antitumor activity and may raise levels of glutathione S-transferase, which contributes to detoxification of carcinogens. It has antiviral properties and inhibits herpes simplex, HIV, and cytomegalovirus in vitro (Tanaka et al., 2006).

• Y-glutamyl-s-trans-propenyl cysteine

Other Actions

• Antioxidant activity
• May mediate nitric oxide synthase activation, which helps restore endothelial function, which in turn improves the elasticity of blood vessels and reduces atherosclerotic heart disease (ASHD) and blood pressure (Williams et al., 2005).
• Inhibits inflammatory prostaglandins

Nutritional Ingredients: Garlic is a common food and spice used in Chinese, French, Thai, Cajun, Italian, and many other world cuisines. Garlic is a minor source of selenium, chromium, potassium, germanium, calcium, iron, and vitamins A, C, and B complex.

History: Sanskrit records document the use of garlic 5,000 years ago. The Chinese have used it for at least 3,000 years. Hippocrates and Aristotle wrote about garlic to treat many medical conditions.

Traditional Use

• Antibacterial and antiviral for the lungs: pneumonia, bronchitis, coughs
• Traditionally, garlic has been and is still used today in Chinese, Ayurvedic, and naturopathic medicine as an

antibacterial and antiviral agent, an expectorant, and a wound dressing. It is used to reduce mildly elevated blood pressure and to treat colds, gastric ulcers, bacterial diarrhea, sinus infections, vaginal yeast infections, and otitis media.

- Louis Pasteur confirmed the antibacterial activity of garlic in 1858.
- Used topically, garlic relieves wasp and bee stings.

Current Use

- Antibacterial and viral properties: fresh garlic is an effective treatment for antibiotic-resistant pneumonia (Dikasso et al., 2002) as well as viral lung and sinus infections and colds (Andrianova et al., 2003). It is also useful for treating *Helicobacter pylori* infections causing gastric or duodenal ulcers and traveler's diarrhea (Ankri & Mirelman, 1999).
- Lowers high blood pressure; used in the treatment of mild hypertension (Andrianova et al., 2003; Blumenthal et al., 2000)
- Reduces ASHD and peripheral arterial vascular disease. Garlic reduced thrombocyte aggregation, decreased erythrocyte aggregation, and increased skin temperature in patients with progressive systemic sclerosis (Rapp et al., 2006). In men with coronary artery disease, garlic improved endothelial function (Williams et al., 2005).
- May prevent blood clots because it inhibits platelet aggregation and thins the blood. It also seems to inhibit sickling of blood cells, helping to reduce the damaging effects of sickle-cell anemia (Takasu et al., 2006).
- Reduces cholesterol and triglyceride levels (hypolipidemia). The majority of more than 100 studies show that garlic can reduce low-density lipoproteins (mean decrease 16%), lower total cholesterol (mean decrease serum cholesterol 10.6%), and reduce triglycerides (average decrease 13.4%) (Durak et al., 2004; Koch & Lawson, 1996).
- Cancer prevention: more than 220 studies have correlated ingestion of garlic (raw and cooked) with lower rates of stomach, intestinal, and other cancers. One study concluded that garlic and other alliums inhibited the formation of

carcinogenic nitroso compounds (Galeone et al., 2006; Lamm & Riggs, 2000). Garlic also inhibits colorectal adenomas in humans (Tanaka et al., 2006).

- Decreases atherosclerosis: garlic is approved in Europe for its cardiovascular effect to lower blood lipids and decrease atherosclerotic heart disease changes in the blood vessels. In a 4-year randomized double-blind clinical trial, patients took either garlic tablets (900 mg a day) or placebo. After 4 years, the garlic group had a 2.6% reduction in plaque volume, and the placebo group had an increase of 15.6% (Blumenthal et al., 2000). In patients concurrently receiving statins, garlic inhibited the progression of coronary calcification (Budoff et al., 2004).

- Children with hepatopulmonary syndrome had increased oxygenation and less dyspnea when given garlic (Najafi Sani et al., 2006).

Available Forms, Dosage, and Administration Guidelines

Preparations: Fresh or dried cloves, capsules, "odorless" tablets, tinctures, aged garlic extracts

Typical Dosage

- *Capsules:* Up to three 500- to 600-mg capsules a day, or follow manufacturer recommendations. Look for products that deliver at least 5,000 micrograms of allicin daily. Do not use the odorless variety; research on its effectiveness is contradictory.

- *Food:* One clove of fresh garlic per day. As for garlic constituents, the whole is greater than any of the parts. Whole fresh garlic is more active than any single constituent. Mince a clove of garlic, let it stand 10 to 15 minutes, and then mix with yogurt, applesauce, honey, or some other carrier agent. Consuming parsley after eating garlic also helps control "garlic breath." One to 1.5 fresh cloves (1.8–2.7 g) equals 10 g fresh garlic, 18 mg garlic oil, or 600- to 900-mg garlic powder. Drying alters the active ingredients of garlic, including allicin (Krest & Keusgen, 1999a).

- Lipid-lowering effect: 600 to 900 mg, 4 g fresh garlic, or 10-mg garlic oil gel caps, 2 to 3 a day

Pharmacokinetics—If Available (form or route when known): Unknown

Toxicity: In average doses, no toxicity. In humans, daily administration of high doses of garlic EO (120 mg), equal to 60 g fresh garlic per day, for a 3-month period, did not produce any abnormal findings.

Contraindications: Some concerns have been raised about the consumption of garlic before surgery. Studies have shown a very transient inhibition of platelet aggregation (only a few hours), so patients need not worry about reduced clotting if they discontinue the use of garlic 4 to 7 days before surgery. Persons with garlic or allium allergies should avoid using garlic.

Side Effects: Heartburn, nausea, flatulence, GI disturbances, allergic reactions, body and breath odor, headache (rare). Topically, may cause skin irritation. May increase bleeding tendencies.

Long-Term Safety: Very safe

Use in Pregnancy/Lactation/Children: Normal doses are fine. Use caution when consuming abnormally large amounts of fresh garlic or garlic preparations. Excessive garlic intake can cause colic in breast-feeding infants.

Drug/Herb Interactions and Rationale (if known)
- Use caution with anticoagulants: may increase risk of bleeding. Five to 20 cloves of garlic are claimed to equal 1 aspirin (650 mg). Garlic does not cause irreversible inhibition of platelets as does aspirin. Check prothrombin time and INR.
- May enhance activity of antiplatelet products; concurrent use not recommended

- In a human study, garlic did not affect CYP2D6 or CYP3A4 (Markowitz et al., 2003), nor did it affect metabolism of rinoavir or gentamicin (Maldonado et al., 2005).

Special Notes: Do not cook at high temperatures or for very long: garlic loses its medicinal value when it loses volatile compounds. When cooking with fresh garlic, cut, chop, or crush the clove 10 to 15 minutes before it is to be used. Alliin, inactive in the whole garlic clove, is activated by the enzyme allinase. Alliin in turn becomes the active ingredient allicin.

BIBLIOGRAPHY

Andrianova IV, et al. (2003). Effect of long-acting garlic tablets "allicor" on the incidence of acute respiratory viral infections in children. *Terapevticheskii Arkhiv.* 75(3):53–56.

Ankri S, Mirelman D. (1999). Antimicrobial properties of allicin from garlic. *Microbes and Infection.* 1(2):125–129.

Aydin A, et al. (2000). Garlic oil and *Helicobacter pylori* infection. *American Journal of Gastroenterology.* 95(2):563–564.

Berthold HK, et al. (1998). Effect of a garlic oil preparation on serum lipoproteins and cholesterol metabolism. A randomized controlled trial. *Journal of the American Medical Association.* 279:1900–1902.

Blumenthal M, et al. (2000). *Herbal Medicine: Expanded Commission E Monographs* (pp. 139–148). Austin, TX: American Botanical Council.

Breithaupt-Grogler K, et al. (1997). Protective effect of chronic garlic intake on elastic properties of aorta in the elderly. *Circulation.* 98(8):2649–2655.

Budoff MJ, et al. (2004). Inhibiting progression of coronary calcification using aged garlic extract in patients receiving statin therapy: A preliminary study. *Preventive Medicine.* Nov;39(5):985–991.

Dikasso D, et al. (2002). Investigation on the antibacterial properties of garlic (*Allium sativum*) on pneumonia causing bacteria. *Ethiopian Medical Journal.* Jul;40(3):241–249.

Dirsch VM, et al. (1998). Effect of allicin and ajoene, two compounds of garlic, on inducible nitric oxide synthase. *Atherosclerosis.* 139(2):333–339.

Dorant E, et al. (1993). Garlic and its significance for the prevention of cancer in humans: A critical view. *British Journal of Cancer.* 67:424–429.

Dorant E, et al. (1996). Consumption of onions and a reduced risk of stomach carcinoma. *Gastroenterology.* 110(1):12–20.

Durak I, et al. (2004). Effects of garlic extract consumption on blood lipid and oxidants/antioxidant parameters in humans with high blood cholesterol. *Journal of Nutritional Biochemistry.* Jun;15(6):373–377.

Ernst E. (1997). Can allium vegetables prevent cancer? *Phytomedicine.* 4(1):79–83.

Galeone C, et al. (2006). Onion and garlic use and human cancer. *American Journal of Clinical Nutrition.* Nov;84(5): 1027–1032.

Gallicano K, et al. (2003). Effect of short-term administration of garlic supplements on single-dose ritonavir pharmacokinetics in healthy volunteers. *British Journal of Clinical Pharmacology.* Feb;55(2):199–202.

Ide N, Lau BH. (1999). Aged garlic extract attenuates intracellular oxidative stress. *Phytomedicine.* 6(2):125–131.

Isaacsohn JL, et al. (1998). Garlic powder and plasma lipids and lipoproteins. A multicenter randomized, placebo-controlled trial. *Journal of the American Medical Association.* 158:1189–1194.

Jonkers D, et al. (1999). Antibacterial effect of garlic and omeprazole on *Helicobacter pylori. Journal of Antimicrobial Chemotherapy.* 43(6):837–839.

Koch HP, Lawson LD. (1996). *The Science and Therapeutic Application of* Allium sativum *L. and Related Species*. Baltimore: Williams & Wilkins.

Koscielny J, et al. (1999). The antiatherosclerotic effect of *Allium sativum. Atherosclerosis.* 144(1):237–249.

Krest I, Keusgen M. (1999a). Quality of herbal remedies from *Allium sativum:* Differences between alliinase from garlic powder and fresh garlic. *Planta Medica.* 65(2):139–143.

Krest I, Keusgen M. (1999b). Stabilization and pharmaceutical use of alliinase. *Pharmazie.* 54(4):289–293.

Lamm DL, Riggs DR. (2000). The potential application of *Allium sativum* (garlic) for the treatment of bladder cancer. *Urologic Clinics of North America.* 27(1):157–162.

Legnani C, et al. (1993). Effects of a dried garlic preparation on fibrinolysis and platelet aggregation in healthy subjects. *Arzneimittel-Forschung.* 43:119–122.

Maldonado PD, et al. (2005). Aged garlic extract, garlic powder extract, S-allylcystein, diallyl sulfide and diallyl disulfide do not interfere with the antibiotic activity of gentamicin. *Phytotherapy Research.* Mar;19(3):252–254.

Markowitz JS, et al. (2003). Effects of garlic (*Allium sativum* L.) supplementation on cytochrome P450 2D6 and 3A4 activity in healthy volunteers. *Clinical Pharmacology and Therapeutics*. Aug;74(2):170–177.

Munday JS, et al. (1999). Daily supplementation with aged garlic extract, but not raw garlic, protects low density lipoprotein against in vitro oxidation. *Atherosclerosis*. 143(2):399–404.

Nai-lan G, et al. (1993). Demonstrations of the anti-viral activity of garlic extract against human cytomegalovirus in vitro. *Chinese Medical Journal*. 106:93–96.

Najafi Sani M, et al. (2006). Effect of oral garlic on arterial oxygen pressure in children with hepatopulmonary syndrome. *World Journal of Gastroenterology*. Apr 21;12(15): 2427–2431.

Rapp A, et al. (2006). Does garlic influence rheologic properties and blood flow in progressive systemic sclerosis? *Forsch Komplementarmed*. Jun;13(3):141–146.

Sasaki J, et al. (1999). Antibacterial activity of garlic powder against *Escherichia coli* 0-157. *Journal of Nutrition Science and Vitaminology*. 45(6):785–790.

Shoji S, et al. (1993). Allyl compounds selectively killed human immunodeficiency virus (type 1), infected cells. *Biochemisty Biophysical Research Communications*. 194:610–621.

Silagy C, Neil A. (1994a). Garlic as a lipid lowering agent: A meta-analysis. *Journal of the Royal College of Physicians of London*. 28:39–45.

Silagy C, Neil A. (1994b). A meta-analysis of the effect of garlic on blood pressure. *Journal of Hypertension*. 12:463–468.

Takasu J, et al. (2006). Aged garlic extract is a potential therapy for sickle-cell anemia. *Journal of Nutrition*. Mar;126[3 Suppl.]: 803S–805S.

Tanaka S, et al. (2006). Aged garlic extract has potential suppressive effect on colorectal adenomas in humans. *Journal of Nutrition*. Mar;126[3 Suppl.]:821S–826S.

Williams MJ, et al. (2005). Aged garlic extract improves endothelial function in men with coronary artery disease. *Phytotherapy Research*. Apr;19(4):314–319.

 NAME: Gentian Root (*Gentiana lutea*)

Common Names: Yellow gentian, European gentian

Family: *Gentianaceae*

Description of Plant

- Gentian is a long-lived perennial herb that grows in rich, well-drained mountain meadows.
- It is a protected species throughout most of Europe due to overharvesting.
- It is a difficult plant to cultivate, and small amounts of semicultivated material are now becoming available from Europe.

Medicinal Part: Dried root

Constituents and Action (if known)

- Secoiridoids
  - Gentiopicroside: cytoprotective (Ozturk et al., 2006), bitter tonic (Skenderi, 2003)
  - Gentiopicrin: bitter tonic, antimalarial, antipyretic (Skenderi, 2003)
  - Sweroside: cytoprotective, enhances collagen production (Ozturk et al., 2006)
  - Swertiamarine: cytoprotective, enhances collagen production (Ozturk et al., 2006), choleretic, hepatoprotective (Duke, 2006), bitter tonic (O'Neil et al., 2001)
- Gentianine
- Gentianine: analgesic, anti-inflammatory (Duke, 2006)

Other Actions: Antibacterial, especially for *Helicobactor pylori* (Mahady et al., 2005), antiviral, anti-inflammatory (Skenderi, 2003)

Nutritional Ingredients: Gentian root is the main ingredient in Angostura bitters and the French liquor Suze. It is also an ingredient in the old-fashioned soft drink Moxie.

Traditional Use

- Anti-inflammatory, analgesic (mild), aperient, anthelmintic, bitter tonic, cholagogue, febrifuge
- Gentian has been used for millennia as a digestive bitter for indigestion, gas, nausea, and abdominal bloating.
- This bitter root has also been used to increase uric acid excretion for treating gout (Mitchell, 2003) and to kill pinworms.

- The Eclectic physicians recommended gentian for anorexia, morning sickness, catarrhal diarrhea (mucous colitis), and dyspepsia of the aged (Ellingwood, 1919).
- The noted Physiomedicalist physician William H. Cook recommended this herb to promote appetite; slowly enhance circulation; to tonify the stomach, gallbladder, intestines, and uterus; and for treating agues (intermittent fevers) (Cook, 1869). Interestingly, he also mentions that it is effective topically for poorly healing sores. This is not a common use for this plant, but a recent in vivo study suggests that constituents of gentian enhance wound healing (Mahady et al., 2005).
- A Chinese species of gentian (*G. macrophylla*) is used as an anti-inflammatory for arthritic pain and to relieve rebellious *qi* (hiccoughs, GERD).

Current Use

- Gentian is one of the finest bitter tonics in the entire materia medica (Mitchell, 2003). Bitters are a very effective method of enhancing digestion, absorption, and elimination. Taking bitters 5 to 10 minutes before a meal stimulates gastric HCL, small intestine, and pancreatic juices, bile secretion, and bile excretion (Mills & Bone, 2000). This herb is very effective when combined with warming bitters (angelica, turmeric, fenugreek) and other cooling bitters (dandelion root, chicory root) to promote digestion, relieve achlorhydria, flatulence, borborygmus, and poor fat digestion (Winston, 2006). In a European study, 205 patients with various digestive problems such as nausea, vomiting, poor appetite, constipation, heartburn, and gas were given a dry extract of this root for 15 days. Sixty-eight percent of the patients reported significant improvement or total relief of symptoms (Wegener, 1998).
- It also enhances hepatic bile production and stimulates the gallbladder to secrete bile as well. Bile acts as a natural aperient or mild laxative. Regular use of bitters enhances normal bowel function (ESCOP, 2003) and helps to lower cholesterol and triglyceride levels (Winston, 2006).

Available Forms, Dosage, and Administration Guidelines
Preparations: Tea, capsules, tincture
Typical Dosage
- *Tea:* 1/2 tsp dried root to 8 oz water, decoct 10 minutes, let steep 15 to 20 minutes; take 2 oz before meals
- *Capsules:* Two 500-mg capsules before meals. Capsules are the least effective way to take bitters.
- *Tincture* (1:5, 30% alcohol): 10 to 20 gtt (0.5–1.0 mL) three times a day before meals

Pharmacokinetics—If Available (form or route when known): Not known

Toxicity: None known

Contraindications: Hyperchlorhydria; use cautiously with gastric ulcers or gastritis (Mills & Bone, 2005)

Side Effects: Large doses can cause nausea, GI irritation, and headaches (ESCOP, 2003).

Long-Term Safety: Safe when used in normal therapeutic doses

Use in Pregnancy/Lactation/Children: Avoid use of large quantities during pregnancy. Small amounts are probably safe. This herb has a long history of use as a digestive bitter (usually as part of a formula), and millions of pregnant women have ingested it with no apparent negative effects. In rabbit studies, gentian had no effect on reproduction, fertility, or teratogenic effects (ESCOP, 2003).

Drug/Herb Interactions and Rationale (if known): None known

Special Notes: There are three cases in the German literature of poisonings due to adulteration of gentian with the toxic plant *Veratrum*. This emphasizes the importance of definitive botanical identification of herbs in the marketplace. Due to the increasing scarcity of wild gentian, either use the semicultivated herb grown in Germany and Switzerland or use other more common bitters such as artichoke leaf, dandelion root, or chicory root.

BIBLIOGRAPHY

Cook WM. (1869). *The Physiomedical Dispensatory* (pp. 444–446). Sandy, OR: Eclectic Medical Publications.

Duke J. Dr. Duke's phytochemical and ethnobotanical databases. Retrieved September 30 2006, from www.ars-grin.gov/ cgi-bin/duke/chemactivities.

Ellingwood F. (1919). *American Materia Medica, Therapeutics, and Pharmacognosy* (pp. 267–268). Evanston, IL: Ellingwood's Therapeutist.

European Scientific Cooperative on Phytotherapy. (2003). *ESCOP Monographs*. (2nd ed.; pp. 174–177). Stuttgart: Thieme.

Mahady GB, et al. (2005). In vitro susceptibility of *Helicobacter pylori* to botanical extracts used traditionally for the treatment of gastrointestinal disorders. *Phytotherapy Research*. Nov;19(11):988–991.

Mills S, Bone K. (2005). *The Essential Guide to Herbal Safety* (pp. 418–419). St. Louis, MO: Elsevier.

Mills S, Bone K. (2000). *Principles and Practice of Phytotherapy* (pp. 38–41). Edinburgh: Churchill Livingstone.

Mitchell W. (2003). *Plant Medicine in Practice* (pp. 374–375). Edinburgh: Churchill Livingstone.

O'Neil M, et al. [Eds.]. (2001). The Merck Index. 13th ed. Hoboken, NJ: John Wiley & Sons.

Ozturk N, et al. (2006). Effects of gentiopicroside, sweroside and swertiamarine, secoiridoids from gentian (*Gentiana lutea* ssp. symphyandra), on cultured chicken embryonic fibroblasts. *Planta Medica*. Mar;72(4):289–294.

Plants For a Future. *Gentiana lutea* L., yellow gentian. Retrieved September 30 2006, from www.pfaf.org/database/plants.php .

Skenderi G. (2003). *Herbal Vade Mecum* (pp. 167–168). Rutherford, NJ: Herbacy Press.

Wegener T. (1998). Anwendung eines trockenextrakes aus gentiana lutea radix bei dyspeptischem symptomcomplex. *Zeit Phytotherapie*. 19:163–164.

Winston D. (2006). *Winston's Botanic Materia Medica*. Washington, NJ: DWCHS.

 NAME: Ginger (*Zingiber officinale*)

Common Names: Jamaica ginger, ginger root

Family: *Zingiberaceae*

Description of Plant
- An erect perennial herb with thick tuberous rhizomes underground and stems that grow to 2' to 4' tall. Linear-lanceolate leaves are 6" to 12" long.
- Grows in the tropics; major producers are Jamaica, India, China, Thailand, Mexico, and Australia

Medicinal Part: Rhizome

Constituents and Action (if known)
- EOs (1%–3%): give ginger its characteristic aroma; may inhibit bacteria (Mills & Bone, 2000)
  - Monoterpenes (geranial, neral)
  - Sesquiterpenes (zingiberene, sesquiphellandrene, beta-bisabolene)
- Antiemetic activity (Bone & Wilkinson, 1990; Fischer-Rasmussen et al., 1991; Phillips et al., 1993; Stewart et al., 1991)
- Pungent principals (1.0%–2.5%)
  - Gingerols (gradually decompose into shogaols during storage) inhibit prostaglandins and leukotrienes; may reduce inflammation and pain of arthritis (Srivastava & Mustafa, 1992); account for pungent effects and flavor; cardiotonic effects and inotropic effect (Shoji et al., 1982); decrease thromboxanes and platelet activity (Srivastava, 1989); inhibits nonsteroidal anti-inflammatory agent injury to stomach (Yoshikawa et al., 1992)
  - Shogaols: cardiotonic, antipyretic, antitussive activity; enhances GI motility (Yamahura et al., 1990)
- Diarylheptanoids: may reduce inflammation and pain of arthritis, inhibit inflammatory prostaglandins

Other Actions: Improves production and secretion of bile from liver (Yamahura et al., 1985)

Nutritional Ingredients: As a spice, used to flavor food and drinks. Frequently used in Chinese, Thai, and Indian cuisine. Roots can also be candied.

Traditional Use

- Antiemetic, carminative, expectorant, emmenagogue, anti-inflammatory, diaphoretic, circulatory stimulant
- Commonly used in TCM for thousands of years. Fresh ginger (shen jiang) and dry ginger (gan jiang) are used slightly differently. The fresh rhizome is used for damp coughs, colds, influenza, diarrhea, and nausea. The dry root is used for deficient (cold) bleeding, arthralgias, and cold hands and feet and is considered more effective for digestive upsets, such as nausea, gas, and vomiting.
- In China, ginger root and stem are used as pesticides against aphids and fungal spores.

Current Use

- Anti-inflammatory for arthralgias: studies have shown that patients with osteoarthritis and rheumatoid arthritis and chronic muscular pain experienced relief from pain and swelling with no adverse effects (Altman & Marcussen, 2001).
- Lowers fevers and decreases the severity of colds: diaphoretic, antipyretic (lowered fevers by 38% in rats), antirhinoviral activity (in vitro)
- Decreases motion sickness, vomiting, and morning sickness: numerous studies have confirmed ginger's ability to reduce seasickness, motion sickness, postsurgical nausea, chemotherapy-induced nausea, vomiting, and hyperemesis gravidarum. The herb compared very favorably with conventional medications without the side effects associated with metoclopramide (Chaiyakunapruk et al., 2006; Manusirivithaya et al., 2004; Smith et al., 2004).
- May protect against ulcers from stress, alcohol, and aspirin, and combined with clarithromycin, it potentiates the pharmaceutical's ability to inhibit *H. pylori* infections (Nostro et al., 2006)
- Relieves dizziness and vestibular disorders

Available Forms, Dosage, and Administration Guidelines
Preparations: Fresh or dried root; capsules, tablets, tinctures

Typical Dosage
- *Capsules:* Up to eight 500- to 600-mg capsules a day
- *Fresh root:* 3–5 g three times a day as a tea
- *Dried ground root:* 0.5 to 2 tsp a day
- *Fresh tincture* (1:2, 60% alcohol): 20 to 40 gtt (1–2 mL) in water three times a day
- *Dry tincture* (1:5, 60% alcohol): 15 to 30 gtt (0.8–1.5 mL) in water three times a day
- *For migraine headache:* Two capsules at beginning of migraine to decrease nausea
- *Motion sickness:* Take 0.5 g powdered ginger or 0.5 tsp fresh ginger every 15 minutes for 1 hour before traveling; continue this dosage during the trip if any signs of illness occur.
- *Nausea from chemotherapy or surgery:* A week before chemotherapy, take 2 g powdered ginger daily. Persons who are already receiving chemotherapy have a sensitive digestive tract and should start with 250-mg powdered ginger daily, gradually increasing to a level that is comfortable and effective.
- *As a digestive tonic:* 1 g powdered ginger before or after a meal. Digestive tea can be made by simmering about 1 tsp freshing grated ginger in a cup of water for 15 minutes, then straining.
- *Colds and flu:* Take 0.5 to 1 g powdered ginger in capsules per hour for 2 to 3 days.

Pharmacokinetics—If Available (form or route when known): Onset, 25 minutes; duration, 4 hours

Toxicity: Nontoxic at normal levels. Long history of use as food, beverage, and spice.

Contraindications: None known

Side Effects: Topical applications may produce irritation in some patients. GI discomfort may occur if taken on an empty stomach or in large doses.

Long-Term Safety: Very safe

Use in Pregnancy/Lactation/Children: No adverse effects expected. Clinical trials using ginger for morning sickness have produced no adverse effects.

Drug/Herb Interactions and Rationale (if known): If given with anticoagulants, may enhance bleeding. Use together with caution. Obtain PT and INR to rule out any herb/drug interactions. In a human study, ginger in normal therapeutic doses did not significantly affect warfarin metabolism (Jiang et al., 2005). It did decrease oral bioavailability of cyclosporine in rats (Chiang et al., 2006). Avoid concurrent use.

Special Notes: There has been concern that taking ginger before surgery might increase the risk of bleeding because constituents have shown antiplatelet activity. Numerous studies have been performed in which ginger was given just before surgery to reduce postsurgical nausea. In none of these studies was increased bleeding noted (Visalyaputra et al., 1998).

BIBLIOGRAPHY

Altman RD, Marcussen KC. (2001). Effects of a ginger extract on knee pain in patients with osteoarthritis. *Arthritis and Rheumatism.* Nov;44(11):2531–2538.

Bensky D, et al. (2004). *Chinese Herbal Medicine: Materia Medica* (3rd ed.; pp. 681–684). Seattle: Eastland Press.

Bliddal H, et al. (2000). A randomized, placebo-controlled, cross-over study of ginger extracts and ibuprofen in osteoarthritis. *Osteoarthritis and Cartilage.* 8(1):9–12.

Blumenthal M, et al. (2000). *Herbal Medicine: Expanded Commission E Monographs* (pp. 153–159). Austin, TX: American Botanical Council.

Bone ME, Wilkinson DJ. (1990). Ginger root: A new antiemetic. *Anaesthesia.* 45:669–671.

Chaiyakunapruk N, et al. (2006). The efficacy of ginger for the prevention of postoperative nausea and vomiting: A meta-analysis. *American Journal of Obstetrics and Gynecology.* Jan;194(1):95–99.

Chiang HM, et al. (2006). Ginger significantly decreased the oral bioavailability of cyclosporine in rats. *American Journal of Chinese Medicine.* 34(4):845–855.

Fischer-Rasmussen W, et al. (1991). Ginger treatment of hyperemesis gravidarum. *European Journal of Obstetrics and Gynecology.* 38(1):19.

Fulder S. (1996). Ginger as an anti-nausea remedy in pregnancy. The issue of safety. *HerbalGram.* Fall;38:47–50.

Jiang X, et al. (2005). Effect of gingko and ginger on the pharmocokinetics and pharmacodynamics of warfarin in healthy subjects. *British Journal of Clinical Pharmacology.* Apr;59(4):425–432.

Manusirivithaya S, et al. (2004). Antiemetic effect of ginger in gynecologic oncology patients receiving cisplatin. *International Journal of Gynecological Cancer.* Nov-Dec;14(6): 1063–1069.

Mills S, Bone K. (2000). *Principles and Practice of Phytotherapy* (pp. 394–403). Edinburgh: Churchill Livingstone.

Nostro A, et al. (2006). Effects of combining extracts (from propolis or *Zingiber officinale*) with clarithromycin on *Helicobacter pylori. Phytotherapy Research.* May;20(3):187–190.

Phillips S, et al. (1993). *Zingiber officinale* (ginger): An antiemetic for day case surgery. *Anaesthesia.* 48:715–717.

Sharma SS, Gupta YK. (1998). Reversal of cisplatin-induced delay in gastric emptying in rats by ginger (*Zingiber officinale*). *Journal of Ethnopharmacology.* 62(1):49–55.

Smith C, et al. (2004). A randomized controlled trial of ginger to treat nausea and vomiting in pregnancy. *Obstetrics and Gynecology.* Apr;103(4):639–645.

Srivastava KC. (1989). Effect of onion and ginger consumption on platelet thromboxane production in humans. *Prostaglandins Leukotrienes and Essential Fatty Acids.* 35:183–185.

Srivastava KC, Mustafa T. (1992). Ginger (*Zingiber officinale*) in rheumatism and musculoskeletal disorders. *Medical Hypotheses.* 39:342–348.

Stewart JJ, et al. (1991). Effects of ginger on motion sickness susceptibility and gastric function. *Pharmacology.* 42:111–120.

Surh YJ, et al. (1998). Chemoprotective properties of some pungent ingredients present in red pepper and ginger. *Mutation Research.* 402(1–2):259–267.

Visalyaputra S, et al. (1998). The efficacy of ginger root in the prevention of postoperative nausea and vomiting after outpatient gynaecological laparoscopy. *Anaesthesia.* 53(5):506–510.

Yamahura J, et al. (1985). Cholagagic effect of ginger and its active constituents. *Journal of Ethnopharmacology.* 13:217–225.

Yamahura J, et al. (1990). Gastrointestinal mobility enhancing effect of ginger and its active constituents. *Chemical and Pharmaceutical Bulletin.* 38:430–431.

Yoshikawa M, et al. (1992). 6-Gingesulfonic acid, a new anti-ulcer principle, and ginger glycolipids A, B, and C, three new monoacyldigalactosylglycerols, from *Zingiberis rhizoma* originating in Taiwan. *Chemical and Pharmaceutical Bulletin.* 40:2239–2241.

NAME: Ginkgo (*Ginkgo biloba*)

Common Names: Maidenhair tree

Family: *Ginkgoaceae*

Description of Plant

- Slow-growing, deciduous tree that can grow to 125' tall, 3' to 4' in diameter, and live up to 1,000 years
- Male and female trees look slightly different and bear different flowers.
  - Male: upright flowers develop on leaf axis
  - Female: wider shape, wider crown, flowers have two terminal "naked" ovules on a stalk
- Female trees produce a small, yellow-to-orange fruit with thick fleshy layers that gives off a foul odor when mature. The fruit "hides" the highly prized inner seed.

Medicinal Part: Leaf. Highest concentration of active compounds may be present in autumn before the leaves drop from the trees. It is thought that as the chlorophyll starts to fade, flavonoids are more available, but this is not proven.

Constituents and Action (if known)

- Terpene lactones (ginkgolide B and bilobalide): inhibit platelet-activating factor, which is elevated in inflammatory and allergic reactions, improve oxygen and glucose uptake at the cellular level, improve memory, enhance mental accuracy, increase circulation to extremities, reduce infarct size in brain, and may increase neuronal growth factors
  - Ginkgolides A, B, C, J (20 carbon-diterpene): reduce the percentage of damaged neurons after ischemia, neuroprotective; reduce cholesterol transport, resulting in decreased corticosteroid synthesis; increase circulation; control mast cell degranulation (Krieglstein, 1994)
  - Bilobalide (15 carbon sesquiterpene): protects neurons from injury from ischemic damage, may stimulate regeneration of damaged nerve cells (Bruno et al., 1993)
- Flavonoids (bilobetin, ginkgetin, and about 40 others): neutralize free radicals and antagonize lipid peroxidation

- Flavonols (quercetin, kaensysferol, isorhamnetin): inhibit platelet activity, antioxidant activity
- Organic acids (vanillic acid, ascorbic acid, p-coumaric)

Other Actions: Vasoregulating effects, relaxes blood vessels and strengthens vessel walls, therefore effective in persons who bruise easily; inhibits lipid peroxidation of membranes; moderates cerebral energy metabolism; increases activity of brain waves

Nutritional Ingredients: Processed seeds have been used in Chinese medicine and for food for centuries

Traditional Use: The tree was first cultivated in the Orient, then introduced into Europe in the early 1700s and brought to the United States in the 1780s. Little traditional use of the leaves. The processed nuts have been used as a food (congee) and as a medicine for coughs, asthma, frequent urination, and damp heat leukorrhea.

Current Use
- Cerebral insufficiency (difficulty in concentration and memory, absent-mindedness, confusion, lack of energy, dizziness): improves cerebral blood flow. A gingko extract enhanced mood and ability to perform daily tasks in healthy older people (Trick et al., 2004)
- Possible reduction of muscle damage in patients with chronic disease (Parkinson's, MS) by improving blood flow
- Relieves tinnitus (ringing of ears) and may improve hearing (Holgers et al., 1994)
- Slows macular degeneration and protects retina, particularly in diabetic retinopathy (Huang et al., 2004). It also improved pre-existing visual field damage in patients with normal tension glaucoma (Ouranta et al., 2003).
- Improves peripheral vascular insufficiency (Raynaud's disease, intermittent claudication): increases walking distance and decreases leg pain (Peters et al., 1998)
- Stabilizes symptoms of Alzheimer's disease/dementia for 6 to 8 months (Maurer et al., 1997, 1998); was as effective as donepezil for treating mild to moderate Alzheimer's dementia (Mazza et al., 2006). Dog owners will be pleased

to know that this herb was also effective for reducing age-related behavior disturbances in elderly canines (Reichling et al., 2006).
- Reduces asthma symptoms through reduction of platelet-activating factor. Studies show significant clinical improvement in adults.
- Relieves vertigo associated with vestibular dysfunction
- Helps improve penile blood flow for patients with impotence caused by atherosclerosis, diabetes, and selective serotonin reuptake inhibitor use. Also reduced anorgasmia in women taking SSRIs (Kang et al., 2002).
- One controlled double-blind study showed substantial improvement in premenstrual symptoms, including breast tenderness, anxiety, and depression. A second study found that ginkgo reduced symptoms in men and women of generalized anxiety disorder or adjustment disorder with anxious mood (Woelk et al., 2007).
- It promoted substantial to complete repigmentation of skin in people with slowly spreading vitiligo (Parsad et al., 2003).

Available Forms, Dosage, and Administration Guidelines
Preparations: A highly concentrated leaf extract (50:1), standardized to 24% flavonoid glycosides (ginkgo flavone glycosides), 6% terpenoids (ginkgolides and bilobalide), with the controversial ginkgolic acid removed. Ginkgo must be used for 6 to 8 weeks before results are evident.
Typical Dosage
- *Capsules:* Standardized extract of 24% glycosides, 6% terpene lactones, and at least 0.8% ginkgolide B: 40 to 80 mg three times a day
- *For dementia:* 120 to 240 mg a day, divided into two or three doses
- *For peripheral vascular disease, vertigo, tinnitus:* 120 to 160 mg a day, divided into two or three doses
- Should be taken for at least 8 weeks before efficacy is evaluated
- *Tincture* (1:2, 70% alcohol): 40 to 60 gtt (2–3 mL) three times a day; (1:5, 70% alcohol): 60 to 100 gtt (3–5 mL) three times a day. The tincture is significantly less effective

than the standardized preparations and a tea has little or no activity.

Pharmacokinetics—If Available (form or route when known)

- Onset: readily
- Peak: 2 to 3 hours
- Duration: unknown
- Half-life: 5 hours
- Excretion: exhaled air, urine, feces

Toxicity: Very safe; seizures when unprocessed seeds and fruit are ingested

Contraindications: Vasodilative headaches

Side Effects: Minimal and transient GI upset, headache, dizziness, allergic reactions. The fruit pulp and raw seeds are toxic and are not used in medicinal preparation. Fruit can cause an allergic reaction (like poison ivy) when touched.

Long-Term Safety: Safe

Use in Pregnancy/Lactation/Children: No trials available. Regular use in Europe has shown no adverse reactions.

Drug/Herb Interactions and Rationale (if known): Use cautiously with aspirin or coumadin; may increase bleeding tendencies, although several studies indicate that it has no significant effect on bleeding (Halil et al., 2005). Obtain PT and INR to rule out possible potentiation. Ginkgo did not affect metabolism of metformin, flurbiprofen, donepezil, digoxin. It did not potentiate the bleeding time caused by cilostazol (Aruna & Naidu, 2006). Ginkgo did not affect CYP2C9, CYP1A2, CYP2D6, CYP2E1, or CYP3A4 activity (Gurley et al., 2005).

Special Notes: Standardized ginkgo extracts are regulated as drugs in Germany. In China, ginkgo is available in tablet and injectable forms. The seeds, often sold in Oriental grocery stores, should be boiled before consumption to remove toxic compounds. Ginkgo is one of the most researched herbs in the world: more than 400 research papers have been published. Several studies have shown effectiveness in treating dementia, peripheral vascular disease, and tinnitus but did not compare ginkgo with traditional drug therapy.

BIBLIOGRAPHY

Aruna D, Naidu MU. (2006). Pharmacodynamic interaction studies of *Ginkgo biloba* with cilostazol and clopidogrel in healthy human subjects. *British Journal of Clinical Pharmacology.* 63(3):333–338. Epub 2006 Sep 29.

Bruno C, et al. (1993). Regeneration of motor nerves in bilobalide-treated rats. *Planta Medica.* 59:302–307.

DeSmet P, et al. (1997). *Ginkgo Biloba.* Berlin: Springer-Verlag.

Gurley BJ, et al. (2005). Clinical assessment of effects of botanical supplementation on cytochrome P450 phenotypes in the elderly: St John's wort, garlic oil, *Panax ginseng,* and *Ginkgo biloba. Drugs and Aging.* 22(6):525–539.

Halil M, et al. (2005). No alteration in the PFA-100 in vitro bleeding time induced by the *Ginkgo biloba* special extract, Egb 761, in elderly patients with mild cognitive impairment. *Blood Coagulation and Fibrinolysis.* Jul;16(5):349–353.

Holgers KM, et al. (1994). Ginkgo biloba extract for the treatment of tinnitus. *Audiology.* 33:85–92.

Huang SY, et al. (2004). Improve haemorrheological properties by *Ginkgo biloba* extract (Egb 761) in type 2 diabetes mellitus complicated by retinopathy. *Clinical Nutrition.* Aug;23(4): 615–621.

Huguet F. (1994). Decreased cerebral 5-HTIA receptors during aging: Reversal by ginkgo biloba extract (EGb 761). *Journal of Pharmacy and Pharmacology.* 46:316–318.

Itil T. (1995). Natural substances in psychiatry (ginkgo biloba in dementia). *Psychopharmacology Bulletin.* 31:147–158.

Itil TM, et al. (1996). Central nervous system effects of ginkgo biloba, a plant extract. *American Journal of Therapeutics.* 3(1): 63–73.

Kang BJ, et al. (2002). A placebo-controlled, double-blind trial of *Ginkgo biloba* for antidepressant-induced sexual dysfunction. *Human Psychopharmacology.* Aug;17(6):L279–L284.

Kanowski S. (1996). Proof of efficacy of the ginkgo biloba special extract EGb 761 in outpatients suffering from mild to moderate primary degenerative dementia. *Pharmacopsychiatry.* 29(2): 47–56.

Kanowski S, et al. (1997). Proof of efficacy of the ginkgo biloba special extract EGb 761 in outpatients suffering from mild to moderate primary degenerative dementia of the Alzheimer type or multi-infarct dementia. *Phytomedicine.* 4(1):3–13.

Kim YS, et al. (1998). Antiplatelet and antithrombotic effects of a combination of ticlopidine and *Ginkgo biloba* ext. *Thrombosis Research.* 91(1):33–38.

Kobuchi H, et al. (1997). Ginkgo biloba extract (EGb 761): Inhibitory effect of nitric oxide production in the macrophage cell line RAW 264.7. *Biochemistry and Pharmacology.* 53: 897–903.

Krieglstein J. (1994). Neuroprotective properties of ginkgo biloba constituents. *Zeitschrift Phytotherapie.* 15:92–96.

LeBars PL, et al. (1997). A placebo-controlled, double-blind randomized trial of an extract of *Ginkgo biloba* for dementia. *Journal of the American Medical Association.* 278(16): 1327–1332.

Li CL, Wong YY. (1997). The bioavailability of ginkgolides in *Ginkgo biloba* extracts. *Planta Medica.* 63(6):563–565.

Mancini M, et al. (1993). Clinical and therapeutic effects of *Ginkgo biloba* extract versus placebo in the treatment of psychorganic senile dementia of arteriosclerotic origin. *Gazetta Medicale Italiana.* 152:69–80.

Maurer K, et al. (1997). Clinical efficacy of *Ginkgo biloba* special extract EGb 761 in dementia of the Alzheimer type. *Journal of Psychiatric Research.* 31(6):645–655.

Maurer K, et al. (1998). Clinical efficacy of *Ginkgo biloba* special extract EGb 761 in dementia of the Alzheimer type. *Phytomedicine.* 5(6):417–424.

Mazza M, et al. (2006). *Ginkgo biloba* and donepezil: A comparison in the treatment of Alzheimer's dementia in a randomized placebo-controlled double-blind study. *European Journal of Neurology.* Sep;13(9):981–985.

Ouranta L, et al. (2003). Effect of *Ginkgo biloba* extract on preexisting visual field damage in normal tension glaucoma. *Ophthalmology.* Feb;110(2):359–362.

Oyama Y, et al. (1996). *Ginkgo biloba* extract protects brain neurons against oxidative stress. *Brain Research.* 712(2):349–352.

Parsad D, et al. (2003). Effectiveness of oral *Ginkgo biloba* in treating limited, slowly spreading vitiligo. *Clinical and Experimental Dermatology.* May;28(3):285–287.

Perry N, et al. (1996). European herbs with cholinergic activities: Potential in dementia therapy. *International Journal of Geriatric Psychiatry.* 11(12):1063–1069.

Peters H, et al. (1998). Demonstration of the efficacy of ginkgo biloba special extract EGb 761 on intermittent claudication-A placebo-controlled, double-blind multicenter trial. *Vasa.* 27(2): 106–110.

Reichling J, et al. (2006). Reduction of behavioral disturbances in elderly dogs supplemented with a standardised ginkgo leaf extract. *Schweizer Archiv fur Tierheilkunde*. May;148(5): 257–263.

Sastre J, et al. (1998). A *Ginkgo biloba* extract (EGb 761) prevents mitochondrial aging by protecting against oxidative stress. *Free Radicals Biology Medicine*. 24(2):298–304.

Schatzberg AM. (1998). Ginkgo biloba for dementia. *Journal of Family Practice*. 46(1):20.

Trick L, et al. (2004). The effects of *Ginkgo biloba* extract (LI 1370) supplementation and discontinuation on activites of daily living and mood in free living older volunteers. *Phytotherapy Research*. Jul;18(7):531–537.

Wesnes KA, et al. (1997). The cognitive, subjective, and physical effects of a *Ginkgo biloba/Panax ginseng* combination in healthy volunteers with neurasthenic complaints. *Psychopharmacology Bulletin*. 33(4):677–683.

Woelk H, et al. (2007). *Ginkgo biloba* special extract EGb 761 in generalized anxiety disorder and adjustment disorder with anxious mood: A randomized, double-blind, placebo-controlled trial. *Journal of Psychiatric Research*. Sep;41(6):472–480. Epub 2006 Jun 30.

NAME: Goldenseal (*Hydrastis canadensis*)

Common Names: Ground raspberry, Indian dye, yellow Indian paint, yellow root paint, yellow puccoon, jaundice root

Family: *Ranunculaceae*

Description of Plant
- Small perennial (10"–12") found in rich woods from Vermont to Arkansas
- Dark-red berries in Autumn
- Rhizomes are gold-yellow and knotted in appearance
- Plant has been harvested almost to the point of extinction in the wild. Since the early 1990s, increased commercial farming has been started to reduce reliance on the wild plants.

Medicinal Part: Root, rhizome

Constituents and Action (if known)

- Isoquinoline alkaloids: hydrastine (3.2%–4.0%), berberine (2.0%–4.5%), hydrastinine, and canadine (0.5%–1.0%)
  - Hydrastine: antibacterial (Scazzocchio et al., 2001), constricts blood vessels, may elevate blood pressure, stimulates bile secretion, may reduce gastric inflammation
  - Berberine: stimulates bile and bilirubin secretion; antibacterial (Scazzocchio et al., 2001) and antifungal activity and some antineoplastic activity (in mice, it shrinks tumors) (Kuo et al., 1995) and enhances apoptosis.
  - Effective against many bacteria that cause diarrhea (Kuo et al., 1995), inhibit enterotoxins (Mills & Bone, 2000)
  - May lower blood pressure
  - Antitubercular activity (Gentry et al., 1998)

Nutritional Ingredients: None known

Traditional Use

- Antibacterial, cholagogue, antihemorrhagic, mucous membrane tonic, bitter tonic, anti-inflammatory, oxytocic
- To treat inflammation of mucous membranes: boggy atonic mucosa with excess secretions and a tendency toward infection, such as gingivitis, gastric and duodenal ulcers, ulceration of the cervix, postpartum hemorrhage, and menorrhagia due to a boggy uterus
- As a bitter tonic to improve appetite and treat dyspepsia
- As a cholagogue for liver disorders with inadequate bile secretion
- Antibacterial and antifungal agent for strep throat, conjunctivitis, vaginal candidiasis, tonsillitis, and otitis media and topically for cuts, ringworm, and athlete's foot

Current Use

- Effective as a mouthwash for treating periodontal disease, thrush, and aphthous stomatitis (Hwang et al., 2003)

- As a topical or local antibacterial, antifungal, and mucous membrane amphoteric: erosion of the cervix (vaginal pack), conjunctivitis, fungal or bacterial sinus infections, bacterial diarrhea, bacterial vaginosis, vaginal candidiasis, strep throat, rectal fissures (suppository). In vitro studies indicate *Hydrastis* is very effective for inhibiting *Helicobacter pylori* (Mahady et al., 2003).

Available Forms, Dosage, and Administration Guidelines

Preparations: Dried root, whole or powdered; leaf, capsules, extracts, ointments, salves, tablets, tinctures

Typical Dosage

- *Capsules:* Up to six 500- to 600-mg capsules a day
- *Tincture* (1:5, 60% alcohol): 20 to 40 gtt (1–2 mL) three or four times a day
- *Dried rhizome:* 0.5 to 1 g three times a day
- Or follow manufacturer or practitioner recommendations

Pharmacokinetics—If Available (form or route when known): None known

Toxicity: Excessive doses can cause jaundice and mild elevation of liver enzymes. The oral LD50 for goldenseal extract in mice is 1,620 mg/kg. Isolated berberine sulfate at doses of more than 0.5 g can cause GI irritation, nose bleeds, dizziness, renal irritation, and dyspnea.

Contraindications: Hypertension (theoretical concern); liver damage

Long-Term Safety: Unknown

Use in Pregnancy/Lactation/Children: Do not use in pregnancy due to possible uterine-stimulating effects (Hoffmann, 2003) or in lactation. Animal studies indicate that despite apparent cytotoxic effects in vitro, goldenseal at the dose levels used by humans is unlikely to be absorbed to the extent to be unsafe during pregnancy (Yao et al., 2005).

Drug/Herb Interactions and Rationale (if known)

- There were no significant interactions caused by taking goldenseal with digoxin (Gurley et al., 2006) or indinavir.

- May interfere or enhance hypotensive effects of antihypertensive agents; use cautiously

Special Notes

- Much of the goldenseal used in the United States is used inappropriately. If this herb were used only for truly useful therapies, the demand for this endangered plant would diminish dramatically. It is used to mask the appearance of illicit drugs on urine drug screens in humans and in racehorses; however, this belief that it is effective for this use is false and originates from a fictional literary work that depicts the plant to be useful for hiding opiate ingestion.
- It is also used as an "herbal antibiotic," which it is not. Goldenseal's antibacterial activity affects only tissues with which it comes into contact: mucous membranes, gastric mucosa, and the urinary tract. It has no profound systemic antibiotic activity.
- Many other herbs can be used as substitutes
  - Mucous membrane tonics: yerba manza, yellow root, Chinese coptis, myrrh, calendula
  - Cholagogues and bitter tonics: barberry, Oregon grape root, artichoke leaf, gentian
  - Antibacterials: garlic, thyme, Chinese coptis, usnea

BIBLIOGRAPHY

Gentry EJ, et al. (1998). Antitubercular natural products: Berberine from the roots of commercial *Hydrastis canadensis* powder. Isolation of inactive 8-oxotetrahydrothalifendine, canadine, beta-hydrastine, and two new quinic acid esters, hycandinic acid esters-1 and -2. *Journal of Natural Products*. 61(10):1187–1193.

Gurley BJ, et al. (2006). Effect of goldenseal (*Hydrastis canadensis*) and kava kava (*Piper methysticum*) supplementation on digoxin pharmacokinetics in humans. *Drug Metabolism and Disposition*. Jan;34(1):69–74.

Hoffmann D. (2003). *Medical Herbalism* (p. 448). Rochester, VT: Healing Arts Press.

Hwang BY, et al. (2003). Antimicrobial constituents from goldenseal (the rhizomes of *Hydrastis canadensis*) against selected oral pathogens. *Planta Medica*. Jul;69(7):623–627.

Kuo CL, et al. (1995). Berberine complexes with DNA in the berberine-induced apoptosis in human leukemic HL-60 cells. *Cancer Letters*. 93:193–200.

Mahady GB, et al. (2003). In vitro susceptibility of *Helicobacter pylori* to isoquinolone alkaloids from *Sanguinara canadensis* and *Hydrastis canadensis*. *Phytotherapy Research.* May;17(3):217–221.

Mills S, Bone K. (2000). *Principles and Practice of Phytotherapy* (pp. 286–296). Edinburgh: Churchill Livingstone.

Rehman J, et al. (1999). Increased production of antigen-specific immunoglobulins G and M following in vivo treatment with the medicinal plants *Echinacea angustifolia* and *Hydrastis canadensis*. *Immunology Letters.* 68(2–3):391–395.

Scazzocchio F, et al. (2001). Antibacaterial activity of *Hydrastatis canadensis* extract and its major isolated alkaloids. *Planta Medica.* Aug;67(6):561–564.

Snow JM. (1997). *Hydrastis canadensis* L. (Ranunculaceae). *Protocol Journal of Botanical Medicine.* 2(2):25–27.

Yao M, et al. (2005). A reproductive screening test of goldenseal. *Birth Defects Research. Part B, Developmental and Reproductive Toxicology.* Oct;74(5):399–404.

NAME: Gotu Kola (*Centella asiatica*)

Common Names: Indian pennywort, Brahmi, gotu cola

Family: *Apiaceae*

Description of Plant
- Weedy, creeping, low-growing herb native to tropical areas of India, Sri Lanka, and southeast Asia
- Member of the parsley family. Has round-lobed leaves and tiny pink flowers.

Medicinal Part: Fresh and dried aerial parts

Constituents and Action (if known)
- Triterpenoids: responsible for wound healing and anti-inflammatory properties, strengthen varicose veins (Babu et al., 1995). A total triterpenic fraction (TTFCA) from the herb has been used successfully to reduce diabetic and hypertensive microangiopathy and edema (Çesarone et al., 2001; Incandela et al., 2001a), inhibit deposition of femoral plaques (Incandela et al., 2001b), and relieve chronic venous insufficiency (Incandela et al., 2001c).
  ○ Asiatic acid, madecassic acid, brahmic acid (triterpene acids)

○ Asiaticoside A + B: randomized double-blind study versus placebo with topical application in 94 patients with chronic venous insufficiency showed subjective (reduction of edema, leg pain, heaviness of legs) and objective (plethysmographic measurements of vein tone) improvements (Gruenwald et al., 2004)

○ Oxyasiaticoside: inhibited tuberculosis bacilli in vivo (Emboden, 1985)

○ Madecassoside, isothankuniside, brahmiside, brahminoside

- Volatile oils: camphor, cineole
- Flavonoids (quercetin, astragalin, keampferol): anti-inflammatory
- Polyacetylenes

Nutritional Ingredients: Used in making a soft drink in Thailand, and the leaves are eaten raw and cooked as a green vegetable.

Traditional Use

- Anxiolytic, memory and brain tonic, nervine, antispasmodic, vulnerary, sedative, antibacterial, anti-inflammatory
- In India's traditional Ayurveda medicine, it was used as a calming and rejuvenating herb, especially for strengthening the nerves and the brain cells. It is used to increase intelligence, longevity, and memory, retarding aging and senility. Also used to reduce anxiety, treat petit mal epilepsy, for rheumatic pain, as a diuretic, and for varicose veins. Often used as a wash topically for skin infections, leprosy, and burns.
- In Chinese medicine, it was often used interchangeably with several other species of low-growing, round-leaved plants under the name of *Zhi xue cao*. Used for treating dermatitis, wounds, sores, dysentery, tuberculosis, jaundice, hematuria, and hemoptysis and as a nerve tonic.

Current Use

- Oral: reduces stress and fatigue, improves memory, improves learning ability, reduces anxiety and depression (DeLucia & Sertie, 1997)
- Topical: relieves inflammation, rebuilds damaged skin, promotes wound and burn healing, shows promise in

treating psoriasis, decutitus ulcers, scarring, and varicose veins (Caldecott, 2006; Gruenwald et al., 2004)
- Reduced formation of ulcers in animal studies
- Clinical herbalists and naturopathic physicians use it orally for skin and connective tissue conditions where the tissue is red, hot, and inflamed. Often used with sarsaparilla for psoriatic arthritis, rheumatoid arthritis, scleroderma, psoriasis, and eczema (Winston, 2006). It can be used for periodontal disease (Sastravaha et al., 2005), venous insufficiency, and phlebitis.

Available Forms, Dosage, and Administration Guidelines

Preparations: Dried herb, cut and sifted or powdered; capsules, tablets, tinctures, teas. Some products are standardized to asiaticoside.

Typical Dosage
- *Capsules:* Up to eight 400- to 500-mg capsules a day
- *Tea:* Steep 1 tsp dried herb in 1 cup of hot water for 10 to 15 minutes; take 4 oz three times a day
- *Tincture* (1:2, 30% alcohol): 30 to 60 gtt (1.5–3 mL) up to three times a day
- Or follow manufacturer or practitioner recommendations

Pharmacokinetics—If Available (form or route when known): None known

Toxicity: Topical applications can cause contact dermatitis in rare cases.

Contraindications: None known

Side Effects: None known

Long-Term Safety: Long-term use as a beverage and medicine in India, China, and other East Asian countries suggests reasonable safety. There is a report of three patients in Argentina developing hepatotoxicity, supposedly induced by gotu kola (Jorge & Jorge, 2005), but several things about this report are problematic. First, this herb has been used for thousands of years and is frequently used in India and Europe with no previous history of liver damage. The report does not mention if the physicians had the herb analyzed to be sure that it actually was gotu kola (there is a possibility of adulteration), and it is odd that two physicians in Argentina would uncover the only three cases of gotu kola–induced liver damage in the literature.

Use in Pregnancy/Lactation/Children: Not known; best avoided in pregnant and breast-feeding women

Drug/Herb Interactions and Rationale (if known): Can potentiate action of anxiolytic medications

Special Notes
- Gotu kola is also known as Brahmi, as is another herb, *Bacopa monnieri*. There is much confusion and debate in Ayurvedic medicine as to which herb is the true Brahmi of ancient Indian medical literature.
- Gotu kola is not related to *Cola nitida* (kola nuts, kola, cola), and it does not contain caffeine.

BIBLIOGRAPHY
Babu TD, et al. (1995). Cytotoxic and anti-tumor properties of certain Taxa of *Umbelliferae* with special reference to *Centella asiatica* (L.) Urban. *Journal of Ethnopharmacology*. 48:53.

Caldecott T. (2006). *Ayurveda. The Divine Essence of Life* (pp. 240–243). Edinburgh: Mosby/Elsevier.

Çesarone MR, et al. (2001). Effects of the total triterpene fraction of *Centella asiatica* in venous hypertensive microangiopathy: A prospective, placebo-controlled, randomized trial. *Angiology*. Oct;52[Suppl. 2]:S15–S18.

Chakraborty T, et al. (1996). Preliminary evidence of antifilarial effect of *Centella asiatica* on canine dirofilariasis. *Fitoterapia*. 67(2):110–112.

DeLucia R, Sertie JAA. (1997). Pharmacological and toxicological studies on *Centella asiatica* extract. *Fitoterapia*. 68(5):413–416.

Emboden W. (1985). The ethnopharmacology of *Centella asiatica* (L.) Urban (Apiaceae). *Journal of Ethnobiology*. 5(2):101–107.

Gruenwald J, et al. [Eds.]. (2004). *PDR for Herbal Medicines* (3rd ed.; pp. 395–399). Montvale, NJ: Medical Economics.

Incandela L, et al. (2001a). Treatment of diabetic microangiopathy and edema with total triterpenic fraction of *Centella asiatica*: A prospective, placebo-controlled study. *Angiology*. Oct;52[Suppl. 2]: S27–S31.

Incandela L, et al. (2001b). Modification of the echogenicity of femoral plaques after treatment with total triterpenic fraction of

Centella asiatica: A prospective, placebo-controlled study. *Angiology.* Oct;52[Suppl. 2]:S69–S73.

Incandela L, et al. (2001c). Total triterpenic fraction of *Centella asiatica* in chronic venous insufficiency and in high-perfusion microangiopathy. *Angiology.* Oct;52[Suppl. 2]:S69–S73.

Jorge OA, Jorge AD. (2005). Hepatotoxicity associated with the ingestion of *Centella asiatica. Revista Espanola de Enfermedades Digestivas.*Feb;97(2):115–124.

Nalini K, et al. (1992). Effect of *Centella asiatica* fresh leaf aqueous extract on learning and memory and biogenic amine turnover in albino rats. *Fitoterapia.* 63(3):232–236.

Sastravaha G, et al. (2005). Adjunctive periodontal treatment with *Centella asiatica* and *Punica granatum* extracts in supportive periodontal therapy. *Journal of the International Academy of Periodontology.* Jul;7(3):70–79.

Shukla A, et al. (1999). In vitro and in vivo wound healing activity of asiaticoside isolated from *Centella asiatica. Journal of Ethnopharmacology.* 65(1):1–12.

Srivastava R, et al. (1997). Antibacterial activity of *Centella asiatica. Fitoterapia.* 68(5):466–467.

Winston D. (2006). *Winston's Botanic Materia Medica.* Washington, NJ: DWCHS.

 NAME: Grape Seed Extract

Common Names: Red grape seed extract

Family: *Vitaceae*

Description of Plant: The common grape is cultivated throughout the world. The leaves and fruits are used as a food and to make wine and the seeds as a source of procyanidolic oligomers (PCOs). Another source of PCOs (also known as OPCs) is a product called *pycnogenol®*, which is made from the bark of maritime pine trees.

Medicinal Part: Seed or skin extract

Constituents and Action (if known)

- Flavonoids called proanthocyanidins (Maffei-Facino et al., 1994)
  - Strong antioxidant (Busserolles et al., 2006)

- ○ Improve circulation (Clifton, 2004)
- ○ Reduce inflammation
- ○ Protect collagen from natural degradation
- ○ In animal studies, grape seed PCOs helped to prevent renal ischemia, lowered blood pressure, enhanced doxorubicin's antitumor activity, was neuroprotective, and inhibited several types of cancers.
- ○ Inhibit xanthine oxidase activity (the enzyme that triggers the oxyradical cascade) (Maffei-Facino et al., 1994) and aromatase (which converts androgens to estrogens) and is found in high levels in breast cancer (Kijima et al., 2006)
- ○ Improve capillary permeability and decrease fragility (Maffei-Facino et al., 1994)
- ○ Inhibit platelet activity without increasing bleeding time (Vitseva et al., 2005)
- Essential fatty acids and tocopherols: protect liver (Oshima et al., 1995), protect vitamin E from oxidation
- Tannins: enhance cell renewal in intestinal tract (Vallet et al., 1994)

Traditional Use: None

Current Use
- Reduces inflammation in joints, prevents changes in synovial fluid and collagen (McCaleb et al., 2000)
- Inhibits tumor promotion (Kijima et al., 2006), angiogenesis and promotes insulin-like growth factor binding protein-3 (Singh et al., 2004).
- Improves circulation (particularly in peripheral vascular disease), reduces capillary fragility associated with hypertension, diabetes, and obesity (Vitseva et al., 2005)
- Slows macular degeneration, diabetic retinopathy, and retinitis pigmentosa; improves nearsightedness (McCaleb et al., 2000)
- Possibly protects against cancer and heart disease (Kijima et al., 2006; Sharma et al., 2004)
- Possibly equal to aspirin in its effect on platelet activity but unlike aspirin does not affect clotting
- Reduces postsurgical swelling and edema

- Protects the gastric mucosa from inflammation and irritation associated with disease (ulcers, gastritis) and pharmaceuticals (acetaminophen)
- Improved chloasma: an acquired hypermelanosis (Yamakoshi et al., 2004)
- In a human study, a combination of grape seed proanthocyandins and niacin-bound chromium reduced LDL cholesterol levels (Preuss et al., 2000).

Available Forms, Dosage, and Administration Guidelines: Products are usually standardized to contain 92% to 95% PCOs. Recommended dosage is 50 to 100 mg PCOs a day for the healthy patient, 150 to 300 mg PCOs a day to treat illness. Follow manufacturer or practitioner recommendations.

Pharmacokinetics—If Available (form or route when known): Not known

Toxicity: None known

Contraindications: None known

Side Effects: Gastric upset, rash (rare)

Long-Term Safety: Safe

Use in Pregnancy/Lactation/Children: Unknown

Drug/Herb Interactions and Rationale (if known): None known

BIBLIOGRAPHY

Bagchi M, et al. (1997a). Protective effects of vitamins C and E, and a grape seed proanthocyanidin extract (GSPE) on smokeless tobacco-induced oxidative stress and apoptopic cell death in human oral keratinocytes. Paper presented at the Fourth Annual Meeting of the Oxygen Society, San Francisco, Nov. 22, 1997.

Bagchi D, et al. (1997b). Comparative in vitro and in vivo free radical scavenging abilities of grape seed proanthocyanidins and selected antioxidants. *FASEB Journal.* 11(3):4.

Bagchi D, et al. (1998). Protective effects of grape seed proanthocyanidins and selected antioxidants against TPA-induced hepatic and brain lipid peroxidation and DNA fragmentation, and peritoneal macrophage activation in mice. *General Pharmacology.* 30(5):771–776.

Brooker S, et al. (2006). Double-blind, placebo-controlled, randomised phase II trial of IH636 grape seed proanthocyanidin extract (GSPE) in patients with radiation-induced breast induration. *Radiotherapy and Oncology.* Apr;79(1):45–51.

Busserolles J, et al. (2006). In vivo antioxidant activity of procyanidin-rich extracts from grape seed and pine (*Pinus maritima*) bark in rats. *International Journal for Vitamin and Nutrition Research.* Jan;76(1):22–27.

Clifton PM. (2004). Effect of grape seed extract and quercetin on cardiovascular and endothelial parameters in high-risk subjects. *Journal of Biomedicine and Biotechnology.* 2004(5):272–278.

Der Marderosian A, Beutler J. [Eds.]. (2004). *The Review of Natural Products.* St. Louis, MO: Facts and Comparisons.

Facino R, et al. (1998). Photoprotective action of procyanidins from *Vitis vinifera* seeds on UV-induced damage: In vitro and in vivo studies. *Fitoterapia.* 69(5):39–50.

Kijima I, et al. (2006). Grape seed extract is an aromatase inhibitor and a suppressor of aromatase expression. *Cancer Research.* Jun 1;66(11):5960–5967.

Maffei-Facino R, et al. (1994). Free radicals scavenging action and anti-enzyme activities of procyanidins from *Vitis vinifera.* A mechanism for their capillary protective action. *Arzneimittel-Forschung.* 44(5):592.

McCaleb RS, et al. (2000). *Encyclopedia of Popular Herbs* (pp. 229–237). Roseville, CA: Prima Publishers.

Oshima Y, et al. (1995). Powerful hepatoprotective and hepatotoxic plant oligostilbenes, isolated from the Oriental medicinal plant *Vitis coigetiae* (Vitaceae). *Experientia.* 51(1):63.

Preuss HG, et al. (2000). Effects of niacin-bound chromium and grape seed proanthocyanidin extract on the lipid profile of hypercholesterolemic subjects: A pilot study. *Journal of Medicine.* 31(5–6):227–246.

Sharma G, et al. (2004). Synergistic anti-cancer effects of grape seed extract and conventional cytotoxic agent doxorubicin against human breast carcinoma cells. *Breast Cancer Research and Treatment.* May;85(1):1–12.

Singh RP, et al. (2004). Grape seed extract inhibits advanced human protstate tumor growth and angiogenesis and upregulates insulin-like growth factor binding protein-3. *International Journal of Cancer.* Feb 20;108(5):733–740.

Vallet J, et al. (1994). Dietary grape seed tannins: Effects of nutritional balance and on some enzymic activities along the crypt-villus axis of rat small intestine. *Annals of Nutrition and Metabolism.* 38(2):75.

Vitseva O, et al. (2005). Grape seed and skin extracts inhibit platelet function and release of reactive oxygen intermediates. *Journal of Cardiovascular Pharmacology.* Oct;46(4):445–451.

Yamakoshi J, et al. (2004). Oral intake of proanthocyanidin-rich extract from grape seeds improves chloasma. *Phytotherapy Research.* Nov;18(11):895–899.

NAME: Green Tea (*Camellia sinensis*)

Common Names: Ceylon tea, Assam tea, white tea

Family: *Theaceae*

Description of Plant

- Tea plants are cultivated in India, Sri Lanka, and China.
- An evergreen shrub with white flowers, usually kept pruned to 2' to 4' tall
- Green tea is prepared from the dried tea leaves. For black tea, the leaves are withered, rolled, enzymatically fermented, and then dried. Oolong tea is semifermented, about halfway between green and black. White tea is made from the new growth buds and immature leaves, which are steamed and dried.

Medicinal Part: Leaves

Constituents and Action (if known)

- Polyphenols (35% of dry weight of tea leaves)
  - Free radical scavengers (Prior & Cao, 1999; Yang et al., 1998)
  - Anticancer activity (Kuroda & Hara, 1999; Yang et al., 1998): inhibit cytochrome P-450 activation of carcinogens, reduce oxidative DNA damage in patients with liver cancer (Luo et al., 2006)
  - Decreased cardiovascular disease: delay lipid peroxidation (Yokozawa et al., 1997); increase high-density lipoproteins, decrease low-density lipoproteins (Watanabe et al., 1998;

Yang et al., 1997); however, Tsubono et al. (1997) did not confirm this finding

- ○ Antioxidant: green, white and black tea both have antioxidant activity, but black tea has a lower level of polyphenols and is only 20% as active. Milk totally inactivates the antioxidant value of both teas but not the catechin content (Vanhet Hof et al., 1998)
- ○ Inhibit the growth of *Streptococcus* in mouth to prevent plaque formation (Rasheed & Haider, 1998)
- ○ Enhance activity of B and T lymphocytes and natural killer cells
- Epigallocatechin gallate (EGCG)
  - ○ Antioxidant 100 times more effective than vitamin C and 25 times more effective than vitamin E (Katiyar et al., 1999; Pietta et al., 1998)
  - ○ Applied topically, protects skin from ultraviolet light by up to 61%, so may prevent skin cancer
- Catechins: cancer-preventing activity; apoptosis-increasing activity (Hibasami et al., 1998)
  - ○ Inhibit MRSA (Hamilton-Miller & Shah, 1999; Yam et al., 1997)
  - ○ Tea and curcumin (turmeric) and the anticancer drug doxorubicin are additive in their antitumor effect (Sadzuka et al., 1998).
  - ○ May support P53 gene, which suppresses cancer development
- Flavonols: lower gastrointestinal cancer risk (Constable et al., 1996)
- Catechols: reduce carcinogenic activity (Ji et al., 1997)
- Tannins: lower risk of dental caries; lower risk of chromosomal mutations so lowers cancer risk; astringent for wounds, skin disorders, and eye problems (use as a poultice for baggy or tired eyes)
- Theophylline, theobromine, and other methylxanthines (caffeine): may cause nervousness, anxiety, tachycardia, and heartburn but may also help various headaches and enhance water excretion. Caffeine increases sex hormone–binding globulin, which can lower estradiol levels, thus lowering the risk of breast cancer (Nagata et al., 1998).

- Lignans and isoflavonoids: anticancer, antimutagenic, antiatherosclerosic effects
- Volatile oils (hexenal, henenol, aldehydes, phenols, geraniol)

Nutritional Ingredients: B vitamins, ascorbic acid (in green tea only)

History: The word *tea* can be traced back to 1655, when the Dutch introduced the word and beverage to England.

Traditional Use
- Used for more than 4,000 years as a beverage
- Chinese believe that green tea helps to prevent cancer and is a longevity tonic.
- Used to increase concentration and mental clarity
- Used as a diuretic
- Topically, a cold wash is used for minor burns.

Current Use
- The world's second most widely consumed beverage; only water is consumed more frequently
- It is an active diuretic
- Green tea has many proposed anticancer mechanisms: antioxidative reactions, enzyme activities, inhibition of lipid peroxidation, irradiation, inhibition of cellular proliferation, and anti-inflammatory activity (Fujiki et al., 1999; Katiyar et al., 1999; Tanaka et al., 1998). This suggests that green tea may be useful as an unconventional therapy for breast cancer—cancer onset in tea drinkers is delayed by years; may inhibit metastasis. Green tea tablets and capsules do not appear to have a cancer protection effect (Yang et al., 1998).
- Consumption of green tea lowers the risk of prostate cancer (Gupta & Ahmad, 1999; Gupta et al., 1999).
- Green tea may enhance the P450 cytochrome system in the liver and protect against the heterocyclic amino mutagens found in cooked meat (Dashwood et al., 1999).
- Protects the liver against oxidative damage
- Improves cardiovascular health: lowers low-density lipoproteins and increases high-density lipoproteins, decreases clotting tendencies and reduces atherosclerotic markers in the blood (Sung et al., 2005)

- Promotes healthy teeth by inhibiting growth of streptococci and other bacteria that cause plaque; is a source of natural fluoride (Rasheed & Haider, 1998)
- Boosts immune function
- Antioxidant: green tea can lower the oxidative stress in the body related to cigarette smoking (Klaunig et al., 1999), and it enhances flow-mediated endothelium dependent vasodilation in smokers (Kim et al., 2006)
- Green tea inhibits calcium oxalate kidney stone formation and enhances urinary oxalate excretion (Jeong et al., 2006).

Available Forms, Dosage, and Administration Guidelines: One cup or more a day; steep tea in hot water for 1 to 2 minutes. It is unknown whether green tea extract (pill form) confers the same degree of protection; if you do use tablets, purchase brands that are standardized for polyphenol content.

Pharmacokinetics—If Available (form or route when known): Peak antioxidant effect occurs 30 to 50 minutes after ingestion.

Toxicity
- May be associated with tea-induced asthma
- Extremely large intake of tea daily may be linked with increased risk of esophageal cancer

Contraindications: Daily consumption of an average of 250 mL of tea by infants has been shown to impair iron metabolism.

Side Effects: Hyperactivity in children; may deplete calcium from the bones; increased urination

Long-Term Safety: Safe

Use in Pregnancy/Lactation/Children: Caffeine is best avoided during pregnancy, but recent studies show no effect on the fetus. Thousands of years of human use suggest reasonable safety. Do not give to infants.

Drug/Herb Interactions and Rationale (if known): None known

Special Notes

- Separate milk from tea by at least 1 hour: milk complexes with polyphenols and renders them resistant to gastric breakdown and absorption, possibly by increasing the gastric pH.
- Tea contains caffeine (green tea, 10 mg a cup; black tea, 40 mg a cup).
- Never drink tea too hot because it may change the DNA structure in the esophagus and predispose it to esophageal cancer.
- Antimicrobial activity of tea decreases with the amount of oxidation. Thus, green tea is the highest in microbial activity, and black tea is the lowest (Chou et al., 1999).
- Tea made from instant powders probably offers few benefits because active ingredients are lost in the processing (Constable et al., 1996).

BIBLIOGRAPHY

Chou CC, et al. (1999). Antimicrobial activity of tea as affected by the degree of fermentation and manufacturing season. *International Journal of Food Microbiology*. 48(2):125–130.

Constable A, et al. (1996). Antimutagenicity and catechin content of soluble instant teas. *Mutagenesis*. 11(2):189–194.

Dashwood RH, et al. (1999). Cancer chemopreventive mechanisms of tea against heterocyclic amine mutagens from cooked meat. *Proceedings of the Society for Experimental Biology and Medicine*. 220(4):239–243.

Fujiki H, et al. (1999). Mechanistic findings of green tea as cancer preventive for humans. *Proceedings of the Society for Experimental Biology and Medicine*. 220(4):225–228.

Gupta S, Ahmad N. (1999). Prostate cancer chemoprevention by green tea. *Seminars in Urology and Oncology*. 17(2): 70–76.

Gupta S, et al. (1999). Prostate cancer chemoprevention by green tea: In vitro and in vivo inhibition of testosterone-mediated induction of ornithine decarboxylase. *Cancer Research*. 59(9): 2115–2120.

Hamilton-Miller JM, Shah S. (1999). Disorganization of cell division of methicillin-resistant *Staphylococcus aureus* by a component of tea (*Camellia sinensis*): A study by electron microscopy. *FEMS Microbiology Letters*. 176(2):463–469.

Green Tea (*Camellia sinensis*)

Hibasami H, et al. (1998). Induction of apoptosis in human stomach cancer cells by green tea catechins. *Oncology Reports.* 5(2):527–529.

Jeong BC, et al. (2006). Effects of green tea on urinary stone formation: An in vivo and in vitro study. *Journal of Endourology.* May;20(5):356–361.

Ji B, et al. (1997). Green tea consumption and the risk of pancreatic and colorectal cancers. *International Journal of Cancer.* 70(3):255–258.

Katiyar S, et al. (1999). Polyphenolic antioxidant (-)-epigallocatechin-3-gallate from green tea reduces UVB-induced inflammatory responses and infiltration of leukocytes in human skin. *Photochemistry and Photobiology.* 69(2):148–153.

Kim W, et al. (2006). Effect of green tea consumption on endothelial function and circulating endothelial progenitor cells in chronic smokers. *Circulation Journal.* Aug;70(8):1052–1057.

Klaunig JE, et al. (1999). The effect of tea consumption on oxidative stress in smokers and nonsmokers. *Proceedings of the Society for Experimental Biology and Medicine.* 220(4):249–254.

Kuroda Y, Hara Y. (1999). Antimutagenic and anticarcinogenic activity of tea polyphenols. *Mutation Research.* 436(1):69–97.

Luo H, et al. (2006). Phase IIa chemoprevention trial of green tea polyphenols in high-risk individuals of liver cancer: Modulation of urinary excretion of green tea polyphenols and 8-hydroxydeoxyguanosine. *Carcinogenesis.* Feb;27(2):262–268.

Nagata C, et al. (1998). Association of coffee, green tea, and caffeine intakes with serum concentrations of estradiol and sex hormone-binding globulin in premenopausal Japanese women. *Nutrition and Cancer.* 30(1):21–24.

Pietta P, et al. (1998). Relationship between rate and extent of catechin absorption and plasma antioxidant status. *Biochemisty and Molecular Biology International.* 46(5):895–903.

Prior RL, Cao G. (1999). Antioxidant capacity and polyphenolic components of teas: Implications for altering in vivo antioxidant status. *Proceedings of the Society for Experimental Biology and Medicine.* 220(4):255–261.

Rasheed A, Haider M. (1998). Antibacterial activity of *Camellia sinensis* extracts against dental caries. *Archives of Pharmaceutical Research.* 21(3):348–352.

Sadzuka Y, et al. (1998). Modulation of cancer chemotherapy by green tea. *Clinical Cancer Research.* 4(1):153–156.

Sung H, et al. (2005). The effects of green tea ingestion over four weeks on atherosclerotic markers. *Annals of Clinical Biochemistry.* Jul;42[Pt. 4]:292–297.

Tanaka K, et al. (1998). Inhibition of N-nitrosation of secondary amines in vitro by tea extracts and catechins. *Mutation Research.* 412(1):91–98.

Tsubono Y, et al. (1997). Green tea intake in relation to serum lipid levels in middle-aged Japanese men and women. *Annals of Epidemiology.* 7(4):280–284.

Vanhet Hof KH, et al. (1998). Bioavailability of catechins from tea: The effect of milk. *European Journal of Clinical Nutrition.* 52(5):356–359.

Watanabe J, et al. (1998). Isolation and identification of acetyl-CoA carboxylase inhibitors from green tea. *Bioscience, Biotechnology, and Biochemistry.* 62(3):532–534.

Weisburger JH. (1999). Tea and health: The underlying mechanisms. *Proceedings of the Society for Experimental Biology and Medicine.* 220(4):271–275.

Yam T, et al. (1997). Microbiological activity of whole and fractionated crude extracts of tea and of tea components. *FEMS Microbiology Letters.* 152(1):169–174.

Yang CS, et al. (1998). Tea and tea polyphenols inhibit cell hyperproliferation, lung tumorigenesis, and tumor progression. *Experimental Lung Research.* 24(4):629–639.

Yang T, et al. (1997). Hypocholesterolemic effects of Chinese tea. *Pharmacologic Research.* 35(6):505–512.

Yokozawa T, et al. (1997). Influence of green tea and its 3 major components upon low-density lipoprotein oxidation. *Experimental Toxicology and Pathology.* 49(5):329–335.

 NAME: Guarana (*Paullinia cupana*)

Common Names: Brazilian cocoa

Family: *Sapindaceae*

Description of Plant

- Fast-growing, woody evergreen liana
- Native to the Amazonian region of Brazil and Venezuela
- Bears orange-yellow fruit containing up to three seeds each

Medicinal Part: Dried paste made from crushed seeds

Constituents and Action (if known)

- Methylxanthine alkaloids: caffeine (2.6%–5.0%) (coffee beans contain 1%–2% and dried tea leaves 1%–4%)

(Bempong & Houghton, 1992; Willard & McCormick, 1992). Guaranine, the methylxanthine found in guarana, is absorbed more slowly than caffeine from coffee or tea.

- Alkaloids (theophylline, theobromine): found only in bark, flowers, and leaves, not in seeds
- Tannins (12%; catachutannic acid, catechol): impart astringent taste, antioxidant properties, control diarrhea (Straten, 1994)
- Saponins (timbonise): antioxidant activity (Mattei et al., 1998), reduce absorption of guaranine (Straten, 1994)

Other Actions: Inhibits platelet aggregation (Bydlowski et al., 1988, 1991)

Nutritional Ingredients: Classified as a food additive and dietary supplement; syrups, extracts used as flavoring and source of caffeine by soft drink industry

Traditional Use: In South America, guarana is used as a stimulant, diuretic, and an aphrodisiac; used to treat migraines, diarrhea, reduce fatigue, and poor concentration.

Current Use

- Diet aid (Breum et al., 1994); included in many thermogenic weight-loss formulas. Studies have shown the combination of ephedrine and caffeine has a synergistic effect of increasing the metabolic rate and reducing body weight. The widespread and unsupervised use of such products, especially in overdose, has caused adverse effects ranging from nervousness and increased blood pressure to death. Diet products with ephedrine were banned in 2004; products containing caffeine are still available in the marketplace.
- Found in smoking cessation products to curb appetite and improve mood and energy
- May be beneficial for migraine headaches
- In a clinical study, guarana, ginseng, and a combination of the two herbs enhanced memory, attention span, and task performance in human volunteers. The guarana and combination product (guarana and ginseng) had the most significant effects. The researchers believe that the low level of caffeine in the product meant that the effects are not attributable to that compound (Kennedy et al., 2004). A second study also showed enhanced cognitive function from

guarana and lower doses (37.5 mg and 75 mg) produced more significant improvement in mood, memory, and alertness than higher doses (150 mg, 300 mg) (Haskell et al., 2007).

Available Forms, Dosage, and Administration Guidelines
Preparations: Capsules and tablets
Typical Dosage
- *Capsules:* Two 500-mg capsules a day; daily dose should not exceed 3 g

Pharmacokinetics—If Available (form or route when known): Onset is more gradual than caffeine in coffee or tea; duration, 1 to 3 hours

Toxicity: None reported, but persons sensitive to caffeine should use with caution

Contraindications: Cardiovascular disease such as hypertension, angina, congestive heart failure; psychological disorders, especially mania

Side Effects: Increased diuresis, insomnia, nervousness, stomach upset; with excessive intake, diarrhea, headache, irritability, nausea, vomiting, hypertension, seizures, tremors, tachycardia, arrhythmias

Long-Term Safety: Unknown; tannin content may be carcinogenic with long-term use in humans (not proven by research)

Use in Pregnancy/Lactation/Children: Contraindicated

Drug/Herb Interactions and Rationale (if known)
- Do not use with respiratory drugs because of increased likelihood of side effects.
- Do not use with oral contraceptives, cimetidine, quinolone antibiotics, and verapamil, as they lower caffeine clearance by 30% to 50%.
- Do not use with benzodiazepines: may be less effective.
- Do not use with monoamine oxidase inhibitors: increased blood pressure.

- Monitor patient carefully if used with beta-adrenergic agonists: may potentiate activity.
- Do not use with adenosine: may lower response.
- Do not use with lithium: may inhibit lithium clearance.

Special Notes: The stimulating effect of guarana is associated with its caffeine content, but some studies question this premise (Kennedy et al., 2004).

BIBLIOGRAPHY

Bempong DK, Houghton PJ. (1992). Dissolution and absorption of caffeine from guarana. *Journal of Pharmacy and Pharmacology.* 44(9):769–771.

Breum L, et al. (1994). Comparison of an ephedrine/caffeine combination and dexfenfluramine in the treatment of obesity. A double-blind multi-centre trial in general practice. *International Journal of Obesity and Related Metabolic Disorders.* 18:99–103.

Bydlowski SP, et al. (1991). An aqueous extract of guarana (*Paullinia cupana*) decreases platelet thromboxane synthesis. *Brazilian Journal of Medical Research.* 24(4):421–424.

Der Marderosian A, Beutler J. [Eds.]. (2004). *The Review of Natural Products.* St. Louis, MO: Facts and Comparisons.

Galduroz JC, Carlini EA. (1996). The effects of long-term administration of guarana on the cognition of normal, elderly volunteers. *Revista Paulista de Medicina.* 114(1): 1073–1078.

Haskell CF, et al. (2007). A double-blind, placebo-controlled, multi-dose evaluation of the acute behavioral effects of guarana in humans. *Journal of Psychopharmacology.* 21(1): 65–70.

Kennedy DO, et al. (2004). Improved cognitive performance in human volunteers following administration of guarana (*Paullinia cupana*) extract: Comparison and interaction with *Panax ginseng. Pharmacology, Biochemistry and Behavior.* Nov;79(3):401–411.

Mattei R, et al. (1998). Guarana (*Paullinia cupana*): Toxic behavioral effects in laboratory animals and anti-oxidant activity in vitro. *Journal of Ethnopharmacology.* 60:111–116.

Straten M. (1994). *Guarana.* Saffron Walden, UK: CW Daniel Co.

Willard T, McCormick J. (1992). *Textbook of Advanced Herbology* (p. 171). Calgary: Wild Rose College of Natural Healing, Ltd.

NAME: Guggul (*Commiphora mukul*)

Common Names: Gum guggulu, gum guggul, guggulipid (brand name), Indian bdellium

Family: *Burseraceae*

Description of Plant
- Small thorny shrub widely distributed in India
- Same genus as *Commiphora myrrha*, the myrrh of the Bible

Medicinal Part: Gum resin

Constituents and Action (if known)
- Lipid steroids (Z-guggulsterone and E-guggulsterone): with lignans and diterpenoids, show lipid-lowering activity by increasing clearance and uptake and breakdown of low-density lipoprotein cholesterol by the liver and also reducing triglycerides (Das Gupta, 1990; Nityanand et al., 1989); demonstrate thyroid-stimulating activity (Panda & Kar, 2005); protective effect on cardiac enzymes and on the cytochrome P-450 system against drug-induced necrosis (Singh et al., 1990)

Additional Actions
- Mild effect on inhibiting platelet aggregation and promoting fibrinolysis
- Prevents formation of atherosclerosis and may cause regression of pre-existing atherosclerotic plaques
- Anti-inflammatory activity (Duwiejua et al., 1993; Singh et al., 2003)
- Antibacterial (Saeed & Sabir, 2004)

Nutritional Ingredients: None known

Traditional Use: Used in traditional Ayurvedic medicine to treat arthritis, psoriasis, diabetes, gout, and obesity; currently used in Ayurvedic medicine to lower cholesterol

Current Use
- Protects against atherosclerosis, inhibits platelet aggregation, and may reduce risk of stroke and pulmonary embolism
- Earlier studies indicate that guggul reduces both cholesterol (24%) and triglycerides (23%) (Nityanand et al., 1989) and

increases high-density lipoprotein cholesterol (16%); activity begins in 2 to 4 weeks. Especially effective for type 2b and type IV hyperlipidemia (Agarwal et al., 1986). A more recent study of a standardized guggul product over 8 weeks found that it failed to improve levels of serum cholesterol, and it may have slightly raised levels of LDL cholesterol (Szapary et al., 2003).

- Reduces inflammation of nodulocystic acne (Thappa & Dogra, 1994)
- Anti-inflammatory for osteoarthritis (Singh et al., 2003)
- Mildly stimulates thyroid activity, making this herb useful for mild hypothyroid conditions with obesity and hyperlipidemia (Panda & Kar, 2005)

Available Forms, Dosage, and Administration Guidelines: Always use processed gum guggal. Commercial guggul extracts are standardized to 2.5% guggulsterones. Normal dosage is 1,000 mg three times a day.

Pharmacokinetics—If Available (form or route when known): Not known

Toxicity: There is a case report of a patient taking guggul who also developed rhabdomyolysis. At this time, there are no other reports of this, and the authors of the study seem to assume that if statin drugs can cause this problem, guggul, which is believed to help lower cholesterol, can as well. Since no other cases have come to light and the mechanisms of action of these two products are so different, it seems unlikely that this report is accurate in assigning cause (Bianchi et al., 2004).

Contraindications: Avoid using in women trying to get pregnant; hyperthyroidism.

Side Effects: Minor GI disturbance, mild headache, nausea, hiccups, skin rashes

Long-Term Safety: Appears to be safe; no adverse effects expected

Use in Pregnancy/Lactation/Children: Avoid using during pregnancy, in breast-feeding women, and with children.

Drug/Herb Interactions and Rationale (if known): Do not use with beta-blockers and calcium channel blockers such as diltiazem and propranolol: diminished efficacy and responsiveness (Dalvi et al., 1994).

Special Notes: Inhibition of platelet aggregation is reversible, so patients need only discontinue medication 1 to 2 days before surgery.

BIBLIOGRAPHY

Bianchi A, et al. (2004). Rhabdomyolysis caused by *Commiphora mukul*, a natural lipid-lowering agent. *Annals of Pharmacotherapy*. Jul-Aug;38(7–8):1222–1225.

Dalvi SS, et al. (1994). Effect of gugulipid on bioavailability of diltiazem and propranolol. *Journal of the Association of Physicians of India*. 42(6):454–455.

Das Gupta R. (1990). A new hypolipidaemic agent. *Journal of the Association of Physicians of India*. 38(2):186.

Duwiejua M, et al. (1993). Antiinflammatory activity of resins from some species of the plant family Burseraceae. *Planta Medica*. 59:12.

Nityanand S, et al. (1989). Clinical trials with gugulipid. A new hypolipidaemic agent. *Journal of the Association of Physicians of India*. 37(5):323–328.

Panda S, Kar A (2005). Guggulu (*Commiphora mukul*) potentially ameliorates hypothyroidism in female mice. *Phytotherapy Research*. Jan;19(1):78–80.

Saeed MA, Sabir AW. (2004). Antibacterial activities of some constituents from oleo-gum resin of *Commiphora mukul*. *Fitoterapia*. Mar;85(2):204–208.

Singh BB, et al. (2003). The effectiveness of *Commiphora mukul* for osteoarthritis of the knee: An outcomes study. *Alternative Therapies in Health and Medicine*. May-Jun;9(3):74–79.

Singh V, et al. (1990). Stimulation of low-density lipoprotein receptor activity in liver membrane of guggulsterone-treated rats. *Pharmacologic Research*. 22:37.

Szapary PO, et al. (2003). Guggulipid for the treatment of hypercholesterolemia: A randomized controlled trial. *Journal of the American Medical Association*. Aug 13;290(6):765–772.

Thappa DM, Dogra J. (1994). Nodulocystic acne: Oral gugulipid versus tetracycline. *Journal of Dermatology*. Oct;21(10): 729–731.

NAME: Gymnema (*Gymnema sylvestre*)

Common Names: Gurmar (Hindi), meshasingi (Sanskrit)

Family: *Asclepiadaceae*

Description of Plant: Native climbing vine of India and Australia

Medicinal Part: Leaves

Constituents and Action (if known)

- Saponins (gymnemic acids [gymnenin])
  - Lower blood sugar similar to the way sulfonylureas act by stimulating release of endogenous insulin stores
  - May block glucose receptors (Bone, 1996)
  - May act by increasing cell permeability for insulin (done in rats) (Persaud et al., 1999)
  - Diminish the ability to taste sweet substances and decrease appetite for up to 90 minutes
  - May lower glycogen content of tissue (done in rats) (Chattopadhyay, 1998)
  - Lowers cholesterol in hypertensive rats (Preuss et al., 1998)
  - May promote pancreatic function in persons with diabetes
- Polypeptide (gurmarin): reduces sweet taste on tongue
- The herb regulated blood sugar levels in alloxan diabetic rabbits and increased the activity of enzymes that stimulate the use of glucose by insulin-dependent pathways. Uptake of glucose into glycogen and protein was increased in the kidney, liver, and muscle (Bone, 1996).
- Liquid extract or tea inhibits the ability to taste bitter or sweet but does not interfere with the ability to taste sour, astringent, or pungent substances.

Nutritional Ingredients: None known

Traditional Use: Traditional treatment in Ayurvedic medicine for diabetes, obesity, coughs, dyspnea, and fevers, as a diuretic, and as an oral and topical remedy for snake bites

Current Use

- May be useful in reducing cravings for sweets for weight control
- Used in management of blood sugar disorders. Two long-term human studies yielded interesting results. In the first study, use of gymnema in patients with insulin-dependent diabetes mellitus reduced insulin requirements and fasting blood glucose, glycosylated hemoglobin, and glycosylated plasma protein levels. This study also showed what may be the enhancement of endogenous insulin production and perhaps pancreatic beta-cell regeneration (Shanmugasundaram et al., 1990). In the second study, conducted with patients with noninsulin-dependent diabetes, the results were very similar: both fasting and postprandial serum insulin levels increased compared with the control group taking conventional medication (Baskaran et al., 1990).

Available Forms, Dosage, and Administration Guidelines

Preparations: Dried herb, tea, capsules, tablets, tincture. Some patients may respond quickly, but it is best if taken for 6 to 12 months to maximize effects.

Typical Dosage

- *Leaf powder:* 2 to 4 g a day

To lower blood sugar levels

- *Capsules:* Two 500-mg capsules twice a day
- *Tincture* (1:5, 30% alcohol): 60 to 100 gtt (3–5 mL) twice a day

To reduce cravings for sweets and as an appetite suppressant

- *Tincture* (1:5, 30% alcohol): 20 to 40 gtt (1–2 mL) in a small amount of water; swish in the mouth for 30 seconds. Repeat every 2 to 3 hours as needed.

Pharmacokinetics—If Available (form or route when known): None known

Toxicity: Long-term (1 year) rat studies found no detectable abnormalities in blood chemistry, weight, or organ histology (Ogawa et al., 2004).

Contraindications: None known

Side Effects: Occasional gastric upset

Long-Term Safety: Not known

Use in Pregnancy/Lactation/Children: No studies available

Drug/Herb Interactions and Rationale (if known): In patients taking hyperglycemic drugs and insulin, monitor blood sugar levels carefully so that dosage of drugs can be adjusted.

Special Notes: Most research has been done in rats and indicates a significant variation in the herb's ability to lower blood sugar. It appears to have no effects in the normal glycemic person (Chattopadhyay, 1999). More research needs to be done, but the herb looks very promising.

BIBLIOGRAPHY

Alschuler L. (1998). *Gymnema sylvestre*'s impact on blood sugar levels. *American Journal of Natural Medicine.* 5(9):26–30.

Baskaran K, et al. (1990). Antidiabetic effect of a leaf extract from *Gymnema sylvestre* in non-insulin dependent diabetes mellitus patients. *Journal of Ethnopharmacology.* 30:295–300.

Bone K. (1996). *Clinical Applications of Ayurvedic and Chinese Herbs* (pp. 115–117). Warwick: Phytotherapy Press.

Chattopadhyay RR. (1998). Possible mechanism of antihyperglycemic effect of *Gymnema sylvestre* leaf extract, part I. *General Pharmacology.* 31(3):495–496.

Chattopadhyay RR. (1999). A comparative evaluation of some blood sugar-lowering agents of plant origin. *Journal of Ethnopharmacology.* 67(3):367–372.

Der Marderosian A, Beutler J. [Eds.]. (2004). *The Review of Natural Products.* St. Louis, MO: Facts and Comparisons.

Ogawa Y, et al. (2004). *Gymnema sylvestre* leaf extract: A 52-week dietary toxicity study in Wistar rats. *Shokuhin Eiseigaku Zasshi.* Feb;45(1):8–18.

Persaud SJ, et al. (1999). *Gymnema sylvestre* stimulates insulin release in vitro by increased membrane permeability. *Journal of Endocrinology.* 163(2):207–212.

Preuss HG, et al. (1998). Comparative effects of chromium, vanadium and *Gymnema sylvestre* on sugar-induced blood pressure elevations

in SHR. *Journal of the American College of Nutrition.*
17(2):116–123.

Shanmugasundaram ER, et al. (1990). Use of *Gymnema sylvestre* leaf
extract in the control of blood glucose in insulin-dependent
diabetes mellitus. *Journal of Ethnopharmacology.*
Oct;30(3):281–294.

Williamson E. (2002). *Major Herbs of Ayurveda* (pp. 167–171).
Edinburgh: Elsevier.

H

 NAME: Hawthorn (*Crataegus monogyna, C. laevigata*)

Common Names: Maybush, Whitethorn

Family: *Rosaceae*

Description of Plant
- Small, spiny tree, native to Europe
- May be grown as a hedge but can grow to 15' to 18'
- Produces white flowers with pink anthers from April to
  June
- Spherical bright-red fruit contains one to three nuts

Medicinal Part: Blossoms, fruit, leaves. Many traditional
preparations use only the ripe fruit.

Constituents and Action (if known)
- Flavonoids (0.044%–0.150% berries, 1.78%–2.1% leaves
  and flowers)
  - Increase contractility of the heart and have a mild positive
    inotropic effect; reduce peripheral vascular resistance,
    reduce afterload (similar to captopril), thus increasing
    cardiac output and cardiac performance (Nasa et al.,
    1993), antioxidants (Upton, 1999)
  - Slightly inhibit Na^+/K^+ ATPase, might also be responsible
    for positive inotropic action (Loew, 1994)
  - Inhibit angiotensin-converting enzyme, thus reducing
    blood pressure
  - Hyperoside
  - Vitexin 2-0-rhamnoside; positive inotropic (Upton,
    1999)

- Procyanidins (0.1%–6.9%): epicatechin: cardiotonic, positive inotropic, mild hypotensive, sedative (Upton, 1999)
- Oligomeric procyanidins (1.9%–3.26%): antioxidants, circulation enhancers (Upton, 1999)
- Triterpenid acids (0.3%–1.4%)
  - Ursolic acid: increased coronary blood flow (Mills & Bone, 2000)
  - Crateagolic acid: positive inotropic
  - Isovitexin
- Flavonal aglycones (quercetin, rutin): positive inotropic (Upton, 1999)
- Chlorogenic acid

Nutritional Ingredients: Flavonoids, vitamin C; fruits are made into jam; flowers have been used to make May wines

Traditional Use
- Nutritive, heart tonic, mild diuretic, nervine
- Use dates back to Dioscorides for stomach ailments and dropsy
- Used since the 1600s for heart problems, as a diuretic, and for urinary calculi
- The eclectic physicians used hawthorn for the aging or senile heart. Indications included angina, valvular deficiency, cardiac edema, palpitations, irregular and intermittent pulse, and dyspnea. They often recommended giving it with stronger cardiac medications such as cactus (*Selenicereus grandiflorus*) and lily of the valley.

Current Use
- Reduces congestive heart failure (Gildor, 1998). Best in New York Heart Association (NYHA) stage I and II cardiac insufficiency (Degenring et al., 2003; Pittler et al., 2003; Schmidt et al., 1994; Tauchert et al., 1994; Zapfe jun, 2001).
- Stabilizes angina, improves myocardial and coronary circulation and myocardial tolerance of oxygen deficiency (ESCOP, 2003)
- Reduces abnormal cardiac rhythms (premature ventricular contractions)

- Mild hypertension: mildly lowers blood pressure (Walker et al., 2002; Walker et al., 2006)
- Reduction of blood lipids: increased bile acid excretion, increased the binding of low-density lipoproteins to liver plasma membranes (Mills & Bone, 2000)
- Beneficial for attention deficit hyperactive disorder as a solid extract (Winston, 2006)
- Stabilizes collagen and arteries, antioxidant for inflammatory connective tissue disorders and atherosclerosis (Winston, 2006)
- A study of a product containing hawthorn, California poppy, and magnesium was effective for treating mild to moderate anxiety disorders (Hanus et al., 2004).

Available Forms, Dosage, and Administration Guidelines

Preparations: Dried berries, leaves, flowers. Most research has been done on flowers and leaves. In Germany, only flowers and leaves are approved, not berries. Standardized in Europe to oligomeric procyanidins and flavonoids. To be effective, hawthorn may need to be administered for 2 weeks or more. Occasional dosing is of little value. Take regularly.

Typical Dosage

- *Capsules:* Up to nine 500- to 600-mg nonstandardized capsules a day. If standardized to either oligomeric procyanidins (18.75%) or total flavonoid content, usually calculated as vitexin (2.2%): 160 to 900 mg a day, for at least 4 to 8 weeks.
- *Tea from berries:* Decoct 1–2 tsp dried berries in 8 oz of water for 10 to 15 minutes, steep an additional half-hour; take 8 oz three times a day.
- *Tea from blossoms:* 1 to 2 tsp in 8 oz hot water, infuse for 10 to 15 minutes; take two or three cups a day
- *Tincture* (1:5, 40% alcohol): 60 to 90 gtt (3–5 mL) up to three times a day, or follow manufacturer or practitioner recommendations
- *Fluid extract* (1:1): 1 to 2 mL three times a day
- *Freeze-dried berries:* 160-mg capsules, two to four a day
- *Solid extract* (native extract): 0.25 tsp twice a day

Pharmacokinetics—If Available (form or route when known): Oligomeric procyanidins: rapid absorption. Plasma half-life is 5 hours, indicating a prolonged presence in the blood (Mills & Bone, 2000).

Toxicity: None

Contraindications: Diastolic congestive heart failure

Side Effects: Products made with more than 50% leaf occasionally cause gastric upset; other reported side effects include dizziness, headache, and nausea.

Long-Term Safety: Safe for a lifetime of use

Use in Pregnancy/Lactation/Children: Safe

Drug/Herb Interactions and Rationale (if known)

- Use cautiously and under a physician's supervision with digitalis products: several texts have stated concerns about taking hawthorn with digitalis-based medications. In a study designed to look at this issue, no changes in pharmacokinetic parameters were seen, and the authors state that the two products can be co-administered safely (Tankanow et al., 2003).
- Monitor blood pressure if used with antihypertensives, nitrates: increased risk of hypotension.
- Use cautiously with beta-blockers: may potentiate action.

Special Notes: Hawthorn is a cardiovascular trophorestorative and is appropriate for most adult patients as a nontoxic preventive therapy as well as a mild but useful treatment for cardiovascular disease.

BIBLIOGRAPHY

Daniele C, et al. (2006). Adverse-event profile of *Crataegus* spp.: A systematic review. *Drug Safety.* 29(6):523–535.

Degenring FH, et al. (2003). A randomised double-blind placebo controlled clinical trial of a standardised extract of fresh *Crataegus* berries (Crataegisan) in the treatment of patients with congestive heart failure NYHA II. *Phytomedicine.* 10(5): 363–369.

European Scientific Cooperative on Phytotherapy. (2003). *ESCOP Monographs* (pp. 98–106). New York: Thieme.

Gildor A. (1998). *Crataegus oxycantha* and heart failure. *Circulation.* 98(19):2098.

Hanus M, et al. (2004). Double-blind, randomised, placebo-controlled study to evaluate the efficacy and safety of a fixed combination containing two plant extracts (*Crataegus oxyacantha* and *Eschscholtzia californica*) and magnesium in mild-to-moderate anxiety disorders. *Current Medical Research and Opinion.* Jan;20(1):63–71.

Loew D. (1994). Pharmacological and clinical results with *Crataegus* special extracts in cardiac insufficiency. *ESCOP Phytotelegram.* 6:20–26.

Mills S, Bone K. (2000). *Principles and Practice of Phytotherapy* (pp. 438–447). Edinburgh: Churchill Livingstone.

Nasa Y, et al. (1993). Protective effect of *Crataegus* extract on the cardiac mechanical dysfunction in isolated perfused working heart. *Arzneimittelforschung.* 43(9):945–949.

Pittler MH, et al. (2003). Hawthorn extract for treating chronic heart failure: meta-analysis of randomized trials. *American Journal of Medicine.* Jun 1;114(8):665–674.

Schmidt U, et al. (1994). Efficacy of hawthorn (*Crataegus*) preparation of LI 132 in 78 patients with chronic congestive heart failure. *Phytomedicine.* 1:17–24.

Tankanow R, et al. (2003). Interaction study between digoxin and a preparation of hawthorn (*Crataegus oxyacantha*). *Journal of Clinical Pharmacology.* Jun;43(6):637–642.

Tauchert M, et al. (1994). Effectiveness of hawthorn extract LI 132 compared with the ACE inhibitor captopril. *Munchener Medizinische Wochenschrift.* 136[Suppl.]:S27–S33.

Upton R. (Ed.). (1999). *American Herbal Pharmacopoeia and Therapeutic Compendium—Hawthorn Berry.* Santa Cruz, CA: AHP.

Walker AF, et al. (2002). Promising hypotensive effect of hawthorn extract: A randomized double-blind pilot study of mild, essential hypertension. *Phytotherapy Research.* Feb;16(1): 48–54.

Walker AF, et al. (2006). Hypotensive effects of hawthorn for patients with diabetes taking prescription drugs: A randomized controlled trial. *British Journal of General Practice.* Jun;56(527):437–443.

Winston D. (2006). *Winston's Botanic Materia Medica.* Washington, NJ: DWCHS.

Zapfe jun G. (2001). Clinical efficacy of *Crataegus* extract WS 1442 in congestive heart failure NYHA class II. *Phytomedicine.* Jul;8(4):262–266.

 NAME: Holy Basil (*Ocimum sanctum*, syn. *O. tenuiflorum*)

Common Names: Tulsi, tulasi, sacred basil

Family: *Lamiaceae*

Description of Plant

- It is a small, fragrant, herbaceous annual with green-purple leaves that grows wild and is widely cultivated in India and southeast Asia.
- The herb is easily cultivated in more temperate climates, similar to garden basil.
- There are three varieties of this plant: Rama tulsi (green leaves), Krishna tulsi (red-purple leaves), and Vana tulsi (*O. gratissimum*).

Medicinal Part: The fresh or dried herb

Constituents and Action (if known)

- Terpines
  - Oleanolic acid—antioxidant, immunomodulator, antiviral, antiallergic (Duke, 2006)
  - Ursolic acid—antibacterial, hypoglycemic, hepatoprotective (Duke, 2006)
- Flavonoids including rosmarinic acid—anti-inflammatory (Duke, 2006), radioprotective (Uma Devi et al., 1999)
- EO
  - Eugenol—antibacterial (Ben Arfa et al., 2006), antioxidant, antiulcer, carminative (Duke, 2006)
  - Carvacrol—antibacterial (Ben Arfa et al., 2006), antioxidant, antiulcer, carminative (Duke, 2006), antifungal, anthelmintic (O'Neil et al., 2001)

- ○ Linalool—antiallergic, antihistamine, antiviral (Duke, 2006), nervine (Hoferl et al., 2006), anti-inflammatory (Peana et al., 2004)
- ○ β-Caryophyllene—anti-inflammatory, antiulcer (Duke, 2006), antifungal, antioxidant, antibacterial (Jutea et al., 2002)
- ○ Other actions of the EO: antibacterial (Omoregbe et al., 1996), antifungal (Nwosu & Okafor, 1995), antioxidant (Siurin, 1997), antiviral (Yamasaki et al., 1998), antiasthmatic (Siurin, 1997), antitumor (Williamson, 2002)

Nutritional Ingredients: Holy basil is used in Indian and Thai cooking as a spice.

Traditional Use
- Adaptogen, antibacterial, antidepressant, antiviral, carminative, diaphoretic, diuretic, expectorant, galactagogue, immunomodulatory, nootropic, hypotensive
- Tulsi is a rasayana or rejuvenative herb in Ayurvedic medicine. It is used for indigestion, diarrhea, nausea, poor memory, lack of concentration (especially caused by excessive cannabis use), ulcers, bronchitis, asthma, diabetes, and for colds and influenza.

Current Use
- Holy basil is an adaptogen which re-regulates HPA axis and SAS (sympatho-adrenal system) function (Singh & Hoette, 2002). It has an antistress activity, preventing excess adrenalin and cortisol production, while enhancing dopamine and serotonin levels (Singh & Hoette, 2002).
- It is an immune amphoteric, downregulating excess immune response (allergic asthma, allergic rhinitis) while promoting immune competence and protecting against radiation-induced immune suppression (Winston & Maimes, 2007).
- This herb enhances cerebral circulation and memory, concentration, and mental acuity. It is used with ginkgo, bacopa, or rosemary for menopausal "brain fog," age-related depression, ADD, and to help speed recovery from head trauma injuries (Winston & Maimes, 2007).

- Traditional use and modern research agree that tulsi can lower blood sugar levels. In a placebo-controlled study, patients given this herb had reductions of fasting (17.6%) and postprandial (7.3%) blood glucose (Agrawal et al., 1996). Combining it with other hypoglycemic herbs such as fenugreek seed, American ginseng, or *Gymnema sylvestre* can enhance the blood sugar–lowering effects.
- In human trials, this herb reduced airway reactivity in bronchitis patients. It enhanced survival rates and reduced cognitive impairment in patients with viral encephalitis. It reduced stress-induced hypertension and helped to prevent liver damage caused by environmental toxins (Williamson, 2002).

Available Forms, Dosage, and Administration Guidelines

Preparations: Tea, capsules, tincture

Typical Dosage

- *Tea:* 1 to 2 tsp dried herb to 8 oz hot water; infuse 15 to 20 minutes. Take two to three cups a day.
- *Capsules:* One to two 500-mg capsules, twice a day
- *Tincture* (1:2 or 1:5): 40 to 80 gtt (2–4 mL) three times a day

Pharmacokinetics—If Available (form or route when known): Not known

Toxicity: None known

Contraindications: None known

Side Effects: None known

Long-Term Safety: Safe

Use in Pregnancy/Lactation/Children: Safe. Holy basil is frequently used in India for pregnant and lactating women as well as for children.

Drug/Herb Interactions and Rationale (if known): Holy basil may promote phase I liver detoxification (CYP-450) and may possibly stimulate drug metabolism.

Special Notes: Tulsi is a sacred plant to Hindu people. Having this herb planted around your home protects the family against misfortune and negative influences.

BIBLIOGRAPHY

Agrawal P, et al. (1996). Randomized placebo-controlled, single blind trial of holy basil leaves in patients with noninsulin-dependent diabetes mellitus. *International Journal of Clinical Pharmacology and Therapeutics.* Sep;34(9):406–409.

Ben Arfa A, et al. (2006). Antimicrobial activity of carvacrol related to its chemical structure. *Letters in Applied Microbiology.* Aug;43(2):149–154.

Duke J. Dr. Duke's phytochemical and ethnobotanical databases. Retrieved October 5 2006, from www.ars-grin.gov/cgi-bin/duke/chemactivities.

Gupta SK, et al. (2002). Validation of traditional claim of tulsi, *Ocimum sanctum* Lin. as a medicinal plant. *Indian Journal of Experimental Biology.* 40(7):765–773.

Hoferl M, et al. (2006). Chirality influences the effects of linalool on physiological parameters of stress. *Planta Medica.* Oct;72(13):1188–1192. Epub 2006 Sep 18.

Jutea F, et al. (2002). Antibacterial and antioxidant activities of *Artemisia annua* essential oil. *Fitoterapia.* Oct;73(6):532–535.

Lu L. (2002). Study on effect of *Cordyceps sinensis* and *Artemisinin* in preventing recurrence of lupus nephritis. *Zhongguo Zhong Xi Yi Jie He Za Zhi.* Mar;22(3):169–171.

Nwosu MO, Okafor JI. (1995). Preliminary studies of the antifungal activities of some medicinal plants against *Basidiobolus* and some other pathogenic fungi. *Mycoses.* 38(5–6):191–195.

Omoregbe RE, et al. (1996). Antimicrobial activity of some medicinal plants extracts on *Escherichia coli, Salmonella paratyphi* and *Shigella dysenteriae. African Journal of Medicine and Medical Sciences.* 25(4):373–375.

O'Neil M, et al. (2001). *The Merck Index: An Encyclopedia of Chemicals, Drugs, and Biologicals.* Rahway, NJ: Merck.

Panda S, Kar A. (1998). *Ocimum sanctum* leaf extract in the regulation of thyroid function in the male mouse. *Pharmacological Research.* 38(2):107–110.

Peana AT, et al. (2004). Effects of (-)-linalool in the acute hyperalgesia induced by carrageenan, L-glutamate and prostaglandin E2. *European Journal of Pharmacology.* Aug 30;497(3):279–284.

Singh N, Hoette Y. (2002). *Tulsi, the Mother Medicine of Nature.* Lucknow, India: International Institute of Herbal Medicine.

Siurin SA. (1997). Effects of essential oil on lipid peroxidation and lipid metabolism in patients with chronic bronchitis. *Klinischeskaia Meditsina (Moskva)*. 75(10):43–45.

Uma Devi P, et al. (1999). In vivo radioprotection by *Ocimum* flavonoids: Survival of mice. *Radiation Research*. 151(1):74–78.

Williamson E. [Ed.]. (2002). *Major Herbs of Ayurveda* (pp. 201–205). Edinburgh: Churchill Livingstone.

Winston D. (2006). *Winston's Botanic Materia Medica*. Washington, NJ: DWCHS.

Winston D, Maimes S. (2007). *Adaptogens, Herbs For Strength, Stamina, and Stress Relief* (pp. 167–171). Rochester, VT: Inner Traditions.

Yamasaki K, Nakamo M, et al (1998), Anti-HIV-1 Activity of Herbs in Labiatae. *Biol Pharm Bull*. 21(8):829–33.

 NAME: Hops (*Humulus lupulus*)

Common Names: European hops, common hops, lupulin (resin)

Family: *Cannabaceae*

Description of Plant
- Climbing perennial vine with male and female flowers on separate plants
- May attain height of 25'
- Cultivated throughout the world
- The only other member of this plant family is cannabis

Medicinal Part: Strobiles (female influorescence) and lupulin (a yellow, sticky powder found in the strobiles)

Constituents and Action (if known)
- Bitter principles (15%–25%) consisting of a soft resin and a hard resin
- Humulones (lipophilic soft resins): alpha-acids
- Lupolones (lipophilic soft resins): beta-acids
  - Have antimicrobial activity (Leung & Foster, 1996), inhibit the mouth muscles, inhibit tumor promotion in mouse skin (Yasukawa et al., 1995), inhibit arachidonic acid–induced inflammatory ear edema in mice (Yasukawa et al., 1995), inhibits colon cancer metastasis in mice (Lamy et al., 2007)

- Xanthohumols: inhibit dracylglycerol (the extramicrosomal hepatic enzyme) (Tabata et al., 1997), may have antiproliferative activity against breast and ovarian cancer (Miranda et al., 1999)
- EOs (myrcene, humulene, carophyllene): sedative and hypnotic effects
- Beta-bitter acid: estrogenic activity, but this still needs to be researched (Milligan et al., 1999)

Nutritional Ingredients: Major use as an ingredient and flavoring in beer

Traditional Use
- Diuretic and used for nervous bladder
- Digestive bitter useful for nervous stomach and to treat GI tract spasms
- Sedative/analgesic for insomnia, anxiety, nervousness, tension headaches
- Placed in small pillows next to bed to induce sleep

Current Use
- Insomnia, especially with difficulty falling asleep; restlessness, anxiety, and tension caused by stress; usually combined with other sedative botanicals such as valerian, California poppy, chamomile
- In animal and in vitro studies, hops has shown an ability to bind with estrogen receptors alpha and beta. This suggests a possible use for menopausal symptoms (Chadwick et al., 2006; Liu et al., 2001). In one human trial, a hops preparation significantly reduced hot flashes (ESCOP, 2003).

Available Forms, Dosage, and Administration Guidelines
Preparations: Tea, capsules, tincture
Typical Dosage
- *Tea:* 1 tsp dried herb to 8 oz hot water, steep 20 minutes; take 4 oz three times a day
- *Capsules:* Up to six 500-mg capsules a day
- *Tincture* (1:5, 60% alcohol): 30 to 60 gtt (1.5–3 mL) up to three times daily

Pharmacokinetics—If Available (form or route when known): None known

Toxicity: Safe in recommended doses

Contraindications: Clinical depression; hops allergies or sensitivities; estrogen-positive tumors because they may be stimulated (Zava et al., 1998)

Side Effects: Contact dermatitis to plant; sedation; bronchial irritation when ground herb dust is inhaled

Long-Term Safety: Has been consumed as a part of beer by a large percentage of the world's population for thousands of years; no adverse response expected

Use in Pregnancy/Lactation/Children: No data; use cautiously. In Ireland, Guinness (a beer rich in hops) is used as a galactogue.

Drug/Herb Interactions and Rationale (if known)

- Use cautiously with central nervous system depressants (anticholinergics, antihistamines, anxiolytics, antidepressants, antipsychotics, alcohol): may cause additive effects
- Use cautiously with drugs metabolized by the cytochrome P-450 system: may cause decreased plasma levels of these drugs (theoretical concern)
- Avoid with phenothiazine-type antipsychotics: may cause additive effects or hyperthermia

Special Notes: Long storage of hops (more than 1 year) causes the labile soft resin compounds to degrade into hard resin compounds, which are mostly inert.

BIBLIOGRAPHY

Chadwick LR, et al. (2006). The pharmacognosy of *Humulus lupulus* L. (hops) with an emphasis on estrogenic properties. *Phytomedicine.* Jan;13(1–2):119–131.

European Scientific Cooperative on Phytotherapy. (2003). *ESCOP Monographs* (pp. 306–311). New York: Thieme.

Goese M, et al. (1999). Biosynthesis of bitter acids in hops. A (13)C-NMR and (2)H-NMR study on the building blocks of humulone. *European Journal of Biochemistry.* 263(2):447–454.

Lamy V, et al. (2007). Chemopreventive effects of lupoline, a hop β-acid, on human colon cancer-derived metastatic SW620 cells and in a rat model of colon carcinogenesis. *Carcinogenesis.* 28(7):1575–1581.

Leung AY, Foster S. (1996). *Encyclopedia of Common Natural Ingredients Used in Food, Drugs, and Cosmetics* (pp. 300–302). New York: John Wiley & Sons.

Liu J, et al. (2001). Evaluation of estrogenic activity of plant extracts for the potential treatment of menopausal symptoms. *Journal of Agricultural and Food Chemistry.* May;49(5):2472–2479.

Milligan SR, et al. (1999). Identification of a potent phytoestrogen in hops (*Humulus lupulus* L.) and beer. *Journal of Clinical Endocrinology and Metabolism.* 84(6):2249–2252.

Miranda CL, et al. (1999). Antiproliferative and cytotoxic effects of prenylated flavonoids from hops (*Humulus lupulus*) in human cancer cell lines. *Food Chemistry and Toxicology.* 37(4):271–285.

Tabata N, et al. (1997). Xanthohumols, diacylglycerol acyltransferase inhibitors, from *Humulus lupulus. Phytochemistry.* 46(4):683–687.

Wichtl M, Bisset NG. [Eds.]. (1994). *Herbal Drugs and Phytopharmaceuticals* (pp. 305–308). Stuttgart: Medpharm.

Zava DT, et al. (1998). Estrogen and progestin bioactivity of foods, herbs and spices. *Proceedings of the Society for Experimental Biology and Medicine.* 217:369–378.

 NAME: Horse Chestnut (*Aesculus hippocastanum*)

Common Name: Buckeye (this name is often used for the American species that are not used for medicine)

Family: *Hippocastanaceae*

Description of Plant

- Deciduous tree with gray-brown bark; may achieve height of 75'
- Cultivated worldwide; has palmate leaves with five to seven leaflets
- Has pink and white flowers that develop into a fruit with a leathery husk containing one to three dark seeds or nuts

Medicinal Part: Seeds

Constituents and Action (if known)

- Escin (Aescin), a complex mixture of triterpene glycosides (saponins): reduces capillary wall permeability, anti-inflammatory activity, potentiates contractile response to norepinephrine, increases venous tone, stabilizes endothelium

(Bielanski & Piotrowski, 1999; Rehn et al., 1996); reduces cutaneous capillary hyperpermeability induced by histamine or serotonin, thus reducing edema
- Condensed tannins
- Flavones (quercetin, kaempherol): antioxidant, anti-inflammatory
- Fatty acids

Nutritional Ingredients: None known

Traditional Use
- To relieve venous congestion with dull, aching pain and a feeling of fullness, especially for varicose veins, rectal spasms, and hemorrhoids
- Arthritis, rheumatism, neuralgias
- Lotions and creams have been used to speed healing of blunt sports injuries.

Current Use
- Improves vascular tone, so it is beneficial in chronic venous insufficiency, varicose veins, hemorrhoids, lymphedema, leg edema, leg heaviness, and peripheral vascular disease (Siebert et al., 2002; Suter et al., 2006) (use with ginkgo, blueberry, or hawthorn)
- Reduces tissue injury in bruises, sprains, and postsurgical trauma
- Reduces nighttime leg cramps, itching, and leg edema (Siebert et al., 2002; Suter et al., 2006)
- Topical applications are beneficial for hemorrhoids, varicose veins, and trauma injuries (Mills & Bone, 2000)
- Injectable forms are available in Europe and are used to treat severe head trauma and deep vein thrombosis and to reduce swelling in surgery.

Available Forms, Dosage, and Administration Guidelines
Preparations: Capsules, tablets, tinctures, standardized products. Use products with dosage equivalent to 100-mg escin a day.
Typical Dosage
- *Tablets* (standardized to 40 mg escin): two or three 200-mg tablets a day

- *Capsules* (dried herb): two to four 500-mg capsules a day for a maximum of 1 to 2 g a day
- *Tincture* (1:5, 40% alcohol): 30 to 60 gtt (1.5–3 mL) three times a day

Pharmacokinetics—If Available (form or route when known): Saponins are large molecules with low bioavailability when taken orally. They can be hydrolyzed by the gut flora, and the sapogenins or liver metabolites may be the primary active form of escin.

Toxicity: Bark, leaves, and fruit capsules are potentially toxic. FDA classifies it as unsafe because of glycosides, saponins, and esculin. Signs of toxicity include muscle twitching, weakness, dilated pupils, vomiting, diarrhea, paralysis, stupor, and hepatic injury. The seed and its extract have a very low risk associated with oral or topical use in the recommended dosage.

Contraindications: Do not use topically on broken or ulcerated skin.

Side Effects: Rarely, nausea, stomach upset, urticaria

Long-Term Safety: Long-term use in Europe and many clinical studies show no problems associated with long-term use.

Use in Pregnancy/Lactation/Children: Horse chestnut seed extracts have been used in numerous clinical studies that included pregnant women. Some studies excluded women in their third trimester. No adverse effects have been reported, but do not use without a clinician's recommendation. Avoid use in breast-feeding women and children.

Drug/Herb Interactions and Rationale (if known): None known

Special Notes: Many European companies are including this herb or its purified extract escin in cosmetics for sensitive skin, pimples, and sunburn.

BIBLIOGRAPHY
Bielanski TE, Piotrowski ZH. (1999). Horse-chestnut seed extract for chronic venous insufficiency. *Journal of Family Practice.* 48(3):171–172.

Bombardelli E, et al. (1996). A review: *Aesculus hippocastanum* L. *Fitoterpia*. 67:483–511.

Diehm C, et al. (1996). Comparison of leg compression stocking and oral horse chestnut seed extract in patients with chronic venous insufficiency. *Lancet*. 347:292–294.

European Scientific Cooperative on Phytotherapy. (2003). *ESCOP Monographs* (pp. 248–256). New York: Thieme.

Greeske K, Pohlmann BK. (1996). Horse chestnut seed extract: An effective therapy principle in general practice. Drug therapy of chronic venous insufficiency. *Fortschritte der Medizin*. 114(15): 196–200.

Mills S, Bone K. (2000). *Principles and Practice of Phytotherapy* (pp. 448–455). Edinburgh: Churchill Livingstone.

Pittler MH, Ernst E. (1998). Horse-chestnut seed extract for chronic venous insufficiency. A criteria-based systematic review. *Archives of Dermatology*. 134(11):1356–1360.

Rehn D, et al. (1996). Comparative clinical efficacy and tolerability of oxerutins and horse chestnut extract in patients with chronic venous insufficiency. *Arzneimittelforschung*. 5:483–487.

Siebert U, et al. (2002). Efficacy, routine effectiveness, and safety of horsechestnut seed extract in the treatment of chronic venous insufficiency. A meta-analysis of randomized controlled trials and large observational studies. *International Angiology*. Dec;21(4): 305–315.

Suter A, et al. (2006). Treatment of patients with venous insufficiency with fresh plant horse chestnut seed extract: A review of 5 clinical studies. *Advances in Therapy*. Jan-Feb;23(1): 179–190.

 NAME: Huang Qin (*Scutellaria baicalensis*)

Common Names: Scute root, baical scullcap

Family: *Lamiaceae*

Description of Plant
- A small perennial member of the mint family with blue-violet flowers
- Grows in dry, sandy soils in the mountains of northeast and southwest China

Medicinal Part: Root

Constituents and Action (if known)

- Flavones and flavone glycosides
  - Baicalein: antiallergic effect, inhibits histamine release from mast cells (Bensky et al., 2003), choleretic, antioxidant, anti-inflammatory, antileukemic, renal protective (Bone, 1996), inhibits androgen receptor and prostate cancer in lab and animal studies (Bonham et al., 2005)
  - Baicalin (6.4%–17%): central nervous system sedative, antitumor
  - Wogonin: inhibited platelet aggregation
  - Wogonoside
  - Norwogonin
  - Scullcap flavone I, II
  - Scutellarein, skullcap flavone
- The extract inhibits phosphodiesterase, which increases cAMP and causes antiplatelet activity and hypotensive (vasodilation) effects (Bone, 1996).
- The herb has broad-spectrum antibacterial activity against *Staphylococcus aureus, Corynebacterium diphtheriae, Pseudomonas aeruginosa, Streptococcus pneumoniae*, and *Neisseria meningitidis*.
- Significant in vitro and in vivo (animal studies) antitumor activity. Inhibited lymphoma and myeloma cell lines by inducing apoptosis and cell cycle arrest at clinically achievable concentrations (Kumagai et al., 2007).

Nutritional Ingredients: None

Traditional Use: Antibacterial, antiallergic, diuretic, anti-inflammatory, antipyretic, hypotensive, choleretic. In TCM, scute root clears damp heat conditions (diarrhea; dysentery; bronchitis with profuse yellow, green, or bloody sputum; urinary tract infections with painful urination; and hematuria). The root is also used as an adjunct for treating damp heat jaundice (hepatitis), to prevent miscarriage, and for liver fire symptoms (headache; red, painful eyes; red head or ears; and a persistent bitter taste in the mouth), and it can also be used topically for boils.

Current Use

- Hyperimmune response: useful for reducing histamine release from mast cells (allergic hives, allergic asthma, allergic rhinitis). Also can be useful with immune amphoterics such as reishi, grifola, or licorice for autoimmune conditions (rheumatoid arthritis, scleroderma, lupus) (Bone, 1996; Winston, 2006).
- Chronic hepatitis: may be used with milk thistle, turmeric, schisandra to prevent and treat liver disease (Bone, 1996)
- Useful with other antibacterial agents (coptis, gardenia fruit) for acute respiratory, urinary tract, and bowel infections (You-ping, 1998), including bacterial diarrhea, dysentery, bronchitis, pneumonia, and prostatitis
- Mild cases of hypertension have been effectively treated using this herb (Bensky et al., 2003).

Available Forms, Dosage, and Administration Guidelines

Preparations: Dried herb, tea, tincture

Typical Dosage

- *Dried herb:* 2 to 6 g a day
- *Tea:* 1 tsp dried root in 8 oz hot water, decoct 15 minutes, steep 40 minutes; take two or three cups a day
- *Tincture* (1:5, 45% alcohol): 30 to 80 gtt (1.5–4 mL) three times a day

Pharmacokinetics—If Available (form or route when known): Not known

Toxicity: Low potential for toxicity

Contraindications: Chronic low-grade (cold) diarrhea

Side Effects: Rarely, GI disturbance and diarrhea

Long-Term Safety: Safe when used in normal therapeutic doses

Use in Pregnancy/Lactation/Children: Traditionally used to prevent miscarriage. Use under professional supervision only.

Drug/Herb Interactions and Rationale (if known)

- Theoretical interaction with blood thinners; use cautiously together

- In rats, concurrent use of huang qin and oral cyclosporine dramatically increased blood levels of the medication (Lai et al., 2004). Do not use together.

Special Notes: Like most Chinese herbs, it is rarely if ever used alone. It is combined with other herbs based on classic formulas.

BIBLIOGRAPHY

Bensky D, et al. (2003). *Chinese Herbal Medicine: Materia Medica* (pp. 131–134). Seattle: Eastland Press.

Bone K. (1996). *Clinical Applications of Ayurvedic and Chinese Herbs* (pp. 75–79). Queensland, Australia: Phytotherapy Press.

Bonham M, et al. (2005). Characterization of chemical constituents in *Scutelleria baicalensis* with antiandrogenic and growth-inhibitory activities toward prostate carcinoma. *Clinical Cancer Research*. May 15;11(10):3905–3914.

Chung CP, et al. (1995). Pharmacological effects of methanolic extract from the root of *Scutellaria baicalensis* and its flavonoids on human gingival fibroblast. *Planta Medica*. 61(2):150–153.

Gao Z, et al. (1999). Free radical scavenging and antioxidant activities of flavonoids extracted from the radix of *Scutellaria baicalensis* Georgi. *Biochimica et Biophysica Acta*. 1472(3):643–650.

Hui KM, et al. (2000). Interaction of flavones from the roots of *Scutellaria baicalensis* with the benzodiazepine site. *Planta Medica*. 66(1):91–93.

Kumagai T, et al. (2007). *Scutellaria baicalensis*, a herbal medicine: Anti-proliferative and apoptotic activity against acute lymphocytic leukemia, lymphoma, and myeloma cell lines. *Leukemia Research*. Apr;31(4):523–530. Epub 2006 Sept 25.

Lai MY, et al. (2004). Significant decrease of cyclosporine bioavailability in rats caused by a decoction of the roots of *Scutellaria baicalensis*. *Planta Medica*. Feb;70(2):132–137.

Smolianinov ES, et al. (1997). Effect of *Scutellaria baicalensis* extract on the immunologic status of patients with lung cancer receiving antineoplastic chemotherapy. *Eksperimentalna Klinika Farmakologiia*. 60(6):49–51.

Winston D. (2006). *Winston's Botanic Materia Medica*. Washington, NJ: DWCHS.

You-ping Z. (1998). *Chinese Materia Medica: Chemistry Pharmacology and Applications* (pp. 127–135). Amsterdam: Harwood.

NAME: Hyssop (*Hyssopus officinalis*)

Common Name: Hysope (French)

Family: *Lamiaceae*

Description of Plant

- Aromatic perennial member of the mint family, originally from Mediterranean, now cultivated throughout the United States, Britain, and Canada
- Tubular blue-purple flowers bloom July to October, grows 2' tall, similar to many other members of the mint family in appearance

Medicinal Part: Dried flowering herb

Constituents and Action (if known)

- Tannins: antiviral activity against herpes simplex when applied topically (Gollapudi et al., 1995)
- Volatile oils (pinocamphone, isopinocamphone, alpha- and beta-pinene, camphene, alpha-terpenene): make up 70% of the EO
- Glucosides (hyssopin)
- Rosmarinic acid: antioxidant, antiherpetic, antiviral, antibacterial (Duke, 2006)
- Marubin: bitter principle
- Flavonoids (diosmin and hesperidin): antihistamine, antioxidant, anti-inflammatory, antiviral (Duke, 2006)
- Polysaccharides (MR-10) have anti-HIV activity.

Nutritional Ingredients: Used as a flavoring for liqueurs (Chartreuse, Benedictine), puddings, and candies

Traditional Use

- Antibacterial, antiviral, carminative, diaphoretic, expectorant, emmenagogue, antispasmodic
- Antibacterial/antiviral for colds, influenza, sore throats, bronchitis, and pneumonia
- Expectorant for damp coughs
- Emmenagogue for delayed menses
- Antispasmodic for petit mal seizures
- Carminative for digestive upset, gas, and intestinal viruses
- EO used as an insect repellent, insecticide, and pediculicide; also used in perfumery

Current Use
- Gargle for sore throats; mix with thyme, sage, or Chinese coptis (Winston, 2006)
- Expectorant and antiviral for bronchitis, viral pneumonia, bronchial catarrh, colds and flu (Bartram, 1995)
- Demonstrates antiviral activity (extracts of dried leaves); use topically for herpes infections (oral or genital), mix with lemon balm
- Promotes menstrual flow: for delayed menses (due to stress, travel) or menses with a scanty, clotty flow

Available Forms, Dosage, and Administration Guidelines

Preparations: Dried herb, capsules, tinctures

Typical Dosage
- *Capsules:* Up to six 400- to 500-mg capsules a day
- *Tea:* Steep 1 tsp dried herb in 1 cup hot water (covered) for 10 to 15 minutes; take three times a day for cough, colds.
- *Tincture* (1:5, 40% alcohol): 40 to 60 gtt (2–3 mL) up to four times a day; or follow manufacturer or practitioner recommendations

Pharmacokinetics—If Available (form or route when known): Unknown

Toxicity: Safe for short-term use at recommended doses

Contraindications: None known

Side Effects: Stomach upset, nausea, diarrhea

Long-Term Safety: Generally recognized as safe (GRAS) by the FDA

Use in Pregnancy/Lactation/Children: Emmenagogue: do not use

Drug/Herb Interactions and Rationale (if known): None known

Special Notes: The EO, like all EOs, is highly concentrated and can be toxic if used internally in excess dosage. Topically, it is nonirritating and nonsensitizing to human skin.

BIBLIOGRAPHY

Bartram T. (1995). *Encyclopedia of Herbal Medicine* (p. 244). Dorset: Grace Publishers.

Der Marderosian A, Beutler J. [Eds.]. (2004). *The Review of Natural Products*. St. Louis, MO: Facts and Comparisons.

Duke J. Dr. Duke's phytochemical and ethnobotanical databases. Retrieved October 15 2006, from www.ars-grin.gov/cgi-bin/duke/chemactivities.

Gollapudi S, et al. (1995). Isolation of a previously unidentified polysaccharide (MAR-10) from *Hyssop officinalis* that exhibits strong activity against human immunodeficiency virus type 1. *Biochemistry and Biophysics Research Communications*. 210(1):145.

Gruenwald J, et al. [Eds.]. (2004). *PDR for Herbal Medicine* (pp. 454–455). Montvale, NJ: Medical Economics.

Kreis W, et al. (1990). Inhibition of HIV replication by *Hyssop officinalis* extracts. *Antiviral Research*. 14(6):323–338.

Winston D. (2006). *Winston's Botanic Materia Medica*. Washington, NJ: DWCHS.

K

 NAME: Kava Kava (*Piper methysticum*)

Common Names: Ava, awa, kawa, kava, yagana

Family: *Piperaceae*

Description of Plant
- Sprawling shrub in the black pepper family
- Cultivated throughout the South Pacific; it no longer grows in the wild
- More than 20 varieties have been identified

Medicinal Part: Four- to 6-year-old dried root

Constituents and Action (if known)
- Resins: kava lactones (kava pyrones; 5%–9%)—sedative activity (Lehmann, 1996; Singh et al., 1998) induces sleep; local anesthetic activity through nonopiate pathways
  - Methysticin: local anesthetic activity, skeletal muscle relaxant (Munte, 1993)
  - Kavain: mild sedative, analgesic, and muscle-relaxing effects, similar to lidocaine

- Flavonoids (flavokavains)
- Kava modifies GABA receptors in brain, reduces anxiety (Lehmann, 1996; Singh et al., 1998; Voltz & Kieser, 1997)
- May act directly on the limbic system
- Suppresses emotional excitability (Munte, 1993) and enhances mood, possibly by binding with GABA receptors; blocks norepinephrine uptake; fungistatic activity

Nutritional Ingredients: None known

Traditional Use
- Antispasmodic, anxiolytic, diuretic, topical and urinary analgesic, sedative
- Used for hundreds of years by natives of the South Pacific islands as a ceremonial and celebratory nonalcoholic, calming drink
- Also used by South Pacific islanders to treat gonorrhea, urinary conditions, bronchitis, rheumatism, headaches, colds, and sore throats and to enhance wound healing
- Eclectic physicians used kava for urinary tract pain, renal colic, chronic urethritis, neuralgias (optic, trigeminal), mouth and throat pain, and dyspepsia.

Current Use
- Relieves anxiety, nervousness, and tension without affecting alertness. German studies have shown that kava is as effective a treatment for anxiety disorders as tricyclic antidepressants (opripramol) and benzodiazepines, without the side effects and tolerance issues (Boerner et al., 2003; Geier & Konstantinowicz, 2004; Pittler & Ernst, 2003).
- Relieves tension headaches and muscle spasms: restless legs syndrome, back pain, torticollis, temporomandibular joint pain
- Relieves insomnia, enhances REM sleep without morning grogginess; also benefits anxiety-induced insomnia (Lehrl, 2004)
- Relieves menopausal anxiety and sleep disorders; may also help other menopausal symptoms, including hot flashes
- May be used for pain control (analgesia through nonopiate pathways): urinary tract pain, muscle pain, mouth and throat pain, fibromyalgia (with ashwagandha) (Winston, 2006)

- In Europe, combined with pumpkin seeds to treat irritable bladder syndrome
- May have some antiseizure activity through the GABA receptors

Available Forms, Dosage, and Administration Guidelines

Preparations: Dried root, capsules, tablets, tinctures

Typical Dosage: Absorption may be enhanced if taken with food. Do not use more than 3 to 4 months continuously for self-diagnosed anxiety and sleep disorders.

- *Dried root:* 1.5 to 3 g a day
- *Capsules:* Up to six 400- to 500-mg capsules a day (100–200 mg kava lactones a day)
- *Tea:* 1 to 2 tsp of the dried, cut, sifted root to 8 oz boiling water, decoct 10 to 15 minutes, steep 30 minutes; take 4 oz two or three times a day
- *Tincture* (1:3, 60% alcohol): 30 to 60 gtt (1.5–3 mL) in water up to three times a day
- Or follow manufacturer or practitioner recommendations

Pharmacokinetics—If Available (form or route when known): Metabolism of kava lactones is more rapid and three to five times higher when ingesting whole root extracts rather than isolated lactone extracts.

Toxicity

- Skin discoloration (yellowing of skin, hair, nails), or "kava dermopathy," occurs with abuse only. It may be caused by disruption of cholesterol metabolism (Norton & Ruze, 1994).
- Chronic ingestion in large excessive doses may lead to kawaism: dry, flaking, discolored skin, blood count abnormalities (increased red blood cells, decreased platelets, decreased lymphocytes), some pulmonary hypertension, and reddened eyes (also possibly related to interference with cholesterol metabolism). All symptoms are reversible when kava intake is stopped.
- Some authors believe that alcohol may increase toxicity, but Herberg's 1993 study showed no synergistic effects or increased toxicity when combining kava with moderate levels of alcohol.

- There have been a number of reports of kava-induced hepatotoxicity. Kava as a tea and tincture have not been implicated in liver damage. An animal study found no signs of toxicity in rats ingesting kava tincture for 3 to 6 months (Sorrentino et al., 2006). The products associated with this problem are all standardized extracts. Several reports suggest that one problem may be poor manufacturing with some companies using cheap stem peelings rather than the traditional part, the root. An alkaloid, pipermethystine, found mostly in the stem, has been shown to negatively affect the liver (Nerurkar et al., 2004). This may explain the rare cases of kava-induced liver damage and why there are no reported cases when used as a traditional preparation.

Contraindications: Parkinson's disease: tremors may increase

Side Effects: Changes in motor reflexes and judgment (Spillane et al., 1997), visual disturbances. With chronic, heavy use, low platelet and white blood cell counts; dry, flaky, yellow skin; increased patellar reflexes; shortness of breath; pulmonary hypertension; reduced plasma proteins.

Long-Term Safety: Safe in moderate doses and short-term. Kava abuse is a possibility. Withdrawal symptoms have occurred on discontinuation. Twenty-five cases of hepatitis have been associated with long-term use of standardized kava products. Do not use more than 4 to 6 weeks. Do not use in patients with a history of liver diseases or with known hepatotoxic drugs.

Use in Pregnancy/Lactation/Children: Do not use if pregnant or breast-feeding; safety is unknown in children.

Drug/Herb Interactions and Rationale (if known)
- Do not use with antiparkinsonian drugs: may increase tremors and make medications less effective.
- May potentiate action of alcohol (Herberg, 1993), tranquilizers (barbiturates), and antidepressants. In one case, a patient taking kava and alprazolam was admitted to the hospital in a lethargic and disoriented state; may have been a drug/herb interaction (Almeida et al., 1996).
- Kava did not affect digoxin metabolism in a human study (Gurley et al., 2006).

Special Notes: Research demonstrates that kava can be an alternative to benzodiazepines and tricyclic antidepressants in anxiety disorders. Take care when operating machinery or driving a vehicle. Do not take kava for depression.

BIBLIOGRAPHY

Almeida J, et al. (1996). Coma from health food store: interaction between kava and alprazolam. *Annals of Internal Medicine.* 125:940.

Boerner RJ, et al. (2003). Kava-kava extract LI 150 is as effective as opipramol and busipirone in generalised anxiety disorder—An 8-week randomized, double-blind multi-centre clinical trial in 129 out-patients. *Phytomedicine.* 10[Suppl. 4]:38–49.

Cantor C. (1997). Kava and alcohol. *Medical Journal of Australia.* 167:560.

Geier FP, Konstantinowicz T. (2004). Kava treatment in patients with anxiety. *Phytotherapy Research.* Apr;18(4):297–300.

Gurley BJ, et al. (2006). Effect of goldenseal (*Hydrastatis candadensis*) and kava kava (*Piper methysticum*) supplementation on digoxin pharmacokinetics in humans. *Drug Metabolism and Disposition.* Feb;35(2):240–245.

Herberg KW. (1993). Effect of kava special extract WS 1490 combined with ethyl alcohol on safety relevant performance parameters. *Blutalkohol.* 30:96–105.

Jussogie A, et al. (1994). Kavapyrone extract enriched from *Piper methysticum* as modulator of the GABA binding site in different regions of the rat brain. *Psychopharmacology (Berlin).* 116:469–474.

Lehmann E. (1996). Efficacy of a special kava extract (*Piper methysticum*) in patients with states of anxiety, tension and excitedness of non-mental origin: A double-blind placebo-controlled study of four weeks of treatment. *Phytomedicine.* 3:113–119.

Lehrl S. (2004). Clinical efficacy of kava extract WS 1490 in sleep disturbances associated with anxiety disorders. Results of a multicenter, randomized, placebo-controlled, double-blind clinical trial. *Journal of Affective Disorders.* Feb;78(2):101–110.

Munte TF. (1993). Effects of oxazepam and an extract of kava roots on event-related potentials in a word recognition task. *Neuropsychobiology.* 27:46–53.

Nerurkar PV, et al. (2004). In vitro toxicity of kava alkaloid, pipermethystine, in hepg2 cells compared to kavalactones. *Toxicological Sciences.* May;79(1):106–111.

Norton S, Ruze P. (1994). Kava dermopathy. *Journal of the American Academy of Dermatology.* 31(1):89–97.

Pittler MH, Ernst E. (2003). Kava extract for treating anxiety. *Cochrane Database of Systematic Reviews.* (1):CD003383.

Singh NN, et al. (1998). A double-blind, placebo controlled study of the effects of kava (Kavatrol) on daily stress and anxiety in adults. *Alternative Therapies.* 4(2):97–98.

Sorrentino L, et al. (2006). Safety of ethanolic kava extract: Results of a study of chronic toxicity in rats. *Phytomedicine.* Sep;13(8):542–549.

Spillane PK, et al. (1997). Neurological manifestations of kava intoxication. *Medical Journal of Australia.* 167:172–173.

Voltz HP, Kieser M. (1997). Kava-kava extract WS 1490 versus placebo in anxiety disorders: A randomized placebo-controlled 25-week outpatient trial. *Pharmacopsychiatry.* 30(1):1–5.

Winston D. (2006). *Winston's Botanic Materia Medica.* Washington, NJ: DWCHS.

NAME: Kudzu *(Pueraria montana* var. *lobata, P. thunbergiana)*

Common Names: Kuzu, ge gen (Chinese), *Pueraria montana* (synonym)

Family: *Fabaceae*

Description of Plant
- A fast-growing perennial vine native to China, Korea, Japan, Burma, and Thailand
- Introduced into the southeastern United States to control erosion, it has now become an aggressive and invasive weed.

Medicinal Part: Dried root (usually with the outer bark removed)

Constituents and Action (if known)
- Isoflavones and isoflavone glycosides (average 7.6%)
  - Puerarin: inhibits platelet aggregation and is a beta-adrenergic blocking agent in vitro
  - Daidzein: immunostimulant

- ○ Daidzein-4, 7-diglucoside, formononetin, genistin: antioxidant, anticancer, hepatoprotective, spasmolytic
- Coumestan derivative (puerarol)
- Aromatic glycosides (puerosides A and B)
- Sapogenins (kudzusapogenols A, B, C, sophoradiol): anti-inflammatory
- Starch (up to 27%): demulcent
- Root extracts (20 g) for 14 days modestly reduced elevated blood pressure in renal hypertensive dogs. The root is a vasodilator, reducing peripheral vascular resistance (You-ping, 1998).

Nutritional Ingredients: Used in Japanese cooking, the root starch is used as a thickening agent and to make noodles. The leaves are eaten raw and cooked as a green.

Traditional Use
- Antipyretic, antispasmodic, decongestant, demulcent, cardiotonic, hypotensive, vasodilator
- Flowers (ge hua) are used to treat alcohol poisoning (hangovers).
- In TCM, kudzu root is used to reduce fevers and associated headaches, stiff neck, and muscle pain. It is also indicated to treat diarrhea, dysentery, constant thirst, and to promote the eruption of measles.

Current Use
- Useful for treating irritable bowel syndrome, diarrhea, dysentery, and mucous colitis. Combine with sarsaparilla, yarrow, wild yam, and chamomile (Winston, 2006).
- One hundred ten patients were given an extract (6:1) of pueraria and hawthorn for angina pain. Ninety percent experienced pain relief, and 43% had improved electrocardiograms. This combination can also be used for mild congestive heart failure.
- It is very useful for treating stiff neck (torticollis) caused by fevers and hypertension. In hypertensive patients, it also improves other symptoms, including headaches, tinnitus, vertigo, and numbness of the extremities (You-ping, 1998).

- In laboratory studies, alcoholic Syrian golden hamsters voluntarily and significantly reduced their alcohol consumption when given a water extract of kudzu. A human study showed similar results with reduced alcohol consumption by heavy drinkers (Lukas et al., 2005).
- A mild decongestant, pueraria can be effective for allergic rhinitis, sinus headaches, and painful otitis media.
- Women given a pueraria isoflavone extract experienced no benefits for menopausal symptoms but had enhanced cognitive function (Woo et al., 2003). A related species, *Pueraria mirifica*, was useful for alleviating perimenopausal hot flashes and night sweats (Lamiertkittikul & Chandeving, 2004).

Available Forms, Dosage, and Administration Guidelines
Preparations: Dried root, tea, capsules, tincture
Typical Dosage
- *Dried root:* 9 to 15 g
- *Tea:* 1 to 2 tsp dried root in 8 oz water, decoct 20 minutes, steep 30 minutes; take two or three cups a day
- *Capsules* (4:1 extract): two 500-mg capsules three times a day
- *Tincture* (1:5, 40% alcohol): 40 to 80 gtt (2–4 mL) four times a day

Pharmacokinetics—If Available (form or route when known): Peurarin is quickly but only partially absorbed: 37% was recovered from rat feces in 24 hours. In humans, it is also rapidly absorbed and reaches peak absorption in 2 hours. The half-life was 4.3 hours (Penetar et al., 2006).

Toxicity: Safe: long history of use as a food and medicine. Large doses in animals produced no toxic effects.

Contraindications: Do not use kudzu tincture (alcohol extract) to reduce alcohol cravings.

Side Effects: None known

Long-Term Safety: Safe

Use in Pregnancy/Lactation/Children: Safe

Drug/Herb Interactions and Rationale (if known): In rats, concurrent use of pueraria and methotrexate caused dramatic increases in methotrexate levels and increased mortality in the animals (Chiang et al., 2005). Avoid concurrent use.

Special Notes: Kudzu is an amazing plant. It has taken over the southeastern United States and is considered a noxious and invasive weed. At the same time, the plant can provide medicine (root, flower), food (root starch, root, and young leaves), animal fodder (leaves), and basketry materials (vines) and can provide a source of pulp for paper.

BIBLIOGRAPHY

Chiang HM, et al. (2005). Life-threatening interaction between the root extract of *Pueraria lobata* and methotrexate in rats. *Toxicology and Applied Pharmacology*. Dec 15;209(3):263–268.

de Padua LS, et al. (1999). *Plant Resources of Southeast Asia— Medicinal and Poisonous Plants* (pp. 417–420). Leiden, Germany: Backhuys Publishing.

Kueng W, et al. (1998). Kudzu root: An ancient Chinese source of modern antidipsotropic agents. *Phytochemistry*. 47(4):499–506.

Lamiertkittikul S, Chandeving V. (2004). Efficacy and safety of *Pueraria mirifica* (Kwao Kruea Khao) for the treatment of vasomotor symptoms in perimenopausal women: Phase II study. *Journal of the Medical Association of Thailand*. Jan;87(1):33–40.

Leung A, Foster S. (1996). *Encyclopedia of Common Natural Ingredients* (pp. 333–336). New York: John Wiley & Sons.

Lukas SE, et al. (2005). An extract of the Chinese herbal root kudzu reduced alcohol drinking by heavy drinkers in a naturalistic setting. *Alcoholism Clinical and Experimental Research*. May;29(5): 756–762.

Penetar DV, et al. (2006). Pharmacokinetic profile of the isoflavone puerarin after acute and repeated administration of a novel kudzu extract to human volunteers. *Journal of Alternative and Complementary Medicine*. 12(6):543–548.

Wagner H, et al. (2003). *Chinese Drug Monographs and Analysis— Radix puerariae—Ge Gen, Kolzting/Bayer*. Wald, Germany: Verlag Fur Ganzheitliche Medizin.

Winston D. (2006). *Winston's Botanic Materia Medica*. Washington, NJ: DWCHS.

Woo J, et al. (2003). Comparison of *Pueraria lobata* with hormone replacement therapy in treating the adverse health consequences of menopause. *Menopause*. Jul-Aug;10(4):352–361.

Xie C, et al. (1994). Daidzein, an antioxidant isoflavonoid, decreases blood alcohol levels and shortens sleep time induced by ethanol intoxication. *Alcoholism Clinical and Experimental Research*. 18(6):1443–1447.

You-ping Z. (1998). *Chinese Materia Medica, Chemistry, Pharmacology, and Applications* (pp. 92–97). Amsterdam: Harwood.

L

NAME: Lavender (*Lavandula angustifolia*)

Common Names: English lavender, True lavender

Family: *Lamiaceae*

Description of Plant
- A strongly aromatic, shrubby member of the mint family with blue flowers
- Native to the low mountains of the Mediterranean

Medicinal Part: Dried flowers and EO

Constituents and Action (if known)
- Volatile oils (1%–5%): linalool (25%–38%), linalyl acetate (25%–45%), antispasmodic, inhibited caffeine stimulation by 50%, relaxant, camphor, B-ocimene, and cineole
- Hydroxycoumarins (umbelliferone, herniarin, coumarin)
- Caffeic acid derivatives (rosmarinic acid): antioxidant, anti-inflammatory, antiallergic
- Flavonoids (luteolin): antimutagenic
- Tannins (up to 12%)

Nutritional Ingredients: Flowers are occasionally used in baking cookies and tea cakes. The EO is used in tooth powders.

Traditional Use
- Antibacterial, antidepressant, carminative, cholagogue, diuretic, nervine, rubefacient

- Used for digestive disturbances including gas, nausea, vomiting, biliousness, poor fat digestion, intestinal colic, and nervous stomach
- Used with St. John's wort and lemon balm for "stagnant" depression (Winston, 2006)
- The tea has a long history of use for irritability, insomnia, headaches, and seizures.
- The EO has been used topically (diluted) for muscle pain, arthralgias, neuralgia, and Bell's palsy.

Current Use

- Effective treatment for flatulence, borborygmus, nervous stomach, and abdominal bloating. Mix with fennel or chamomile (Winston, 2006).
- EO (1–2 gtt) in a sitz bath is antibacterial and anti-inflammatory; promotes healing for episiotomy incisions. EOs can also be used topically for first-degree and small second-degree burns, athlete's foot, cuts, and muscle pain. Studies show that the EO is active orally against *Giardia duodenalis*, *Trichomonas vaginalis*, and *Candida albicans* (D'Auria et al., 2005; Moon et al., 2006). The EO, used as aromatherapy, has been effective for depression, anxiety, restlessness, irritability, and insomnia of old age and menopause (Holmes et al., 2002; Lee & Lee, 2006). The EO also reduced travel-induced excitement in dogs (Wells, 2006).
- Lavender baths are calming and mildly sedating for occasional insomnia, irritability, premenstrual anger, and stress-induced headaches.
- Lavender tea has also been shown to have diuretic activity (Elhajili et al., 2001), and the tincture, given along with the antidepressant imipramine, was more effective than the pharmaceutical alone (Aknondzadeh et al., 2003).

Available Forms, Dosage, and Administration Guidelines

Preparations: Tea, tincture, EO

Typical Dosage

- *Tea:* 1 tsp dried flowers in 8 oz hot water, steep covered for 20 to 30 minutes; take 4 oz three times a day

- *Tincture* (1:5, 70% alcohol): 30–40 gtt (1.5–2 mL) three to four times a day
- *EO:* 1 to 2 gtt two or three times a day

Pharmacokinetics—If Available (form or route when known): Not known

Toxicity: Herb: none known; EO in overdose can be toxic

Contraindications: None known

Side Effects: Herb: none known; EO rarely causes skin irritation

Long-Term Safety: Safe

Use in Pregnancy/Lactation/Children: No adverse effects expected from the herb. Avoid using the EO internally during pregnancy.

Drug/Herb Interactions and Rationale (if known): None known

Special Notes: Lavender's enduring popularity as a medicine and its use in cosmetics and perfumes has a great deal to do with its odor's ability to alter mood via the olfactory receptors.

BIBLIOGRAPHY

Akhondzadeh S, et al. (2003). Comparison of *Lavandula angustifolia* Mill. tincture and imipramine in the treatment of mild to moderate depression: A double blind, randomized trial. *Progress in Neuro-Psychopharmacology and Biological Psychiatry.* Feb;27(1):123–127.

Bruneton J. (1999). *Pharmacognosy, Phytochemistry, Medicinal Plants* (2nd ed.; pp. 528–530). Paris: Lavoisier.

Cornwall S, Dale A. (1995). Lavender oil and perineal repair. *Modern Midwife.* 5(3):31–33.

D'Auria FD, et al. (2005). Antifungal activity of *Lavandula angustifolia* essential oil against *Candida albicans* yeast and mycelial form. *Medical Mycology.* Aug;43(5):391–396.

Elhajili M, et al. (2001). Diuretic activity of the infusion of flowers from *Lavandula officinalis. Reproduction Nutrition Development.* Sep-Oct;41(5):393–394.

Holmes C, et al. (2002). Lavender oil as a treatment for agitated behaviour in severe dementia: A placebo controlled study. *International Journal of Geriatric Psychiatry.* Apr;17(4):305–308.

Lee IS, Lee GJ. (2006). Effects of lavender aromatherapy on insomnia and depression in women college students. *Taehan Kanho Hakhoe Chi.* Feb;36(1):136–143.

Moon T, et al. (2006). Antiparasitic activity of two lavandula essential oils against *Giardia duodenalis, Trichomonas vaginalis,* and *Hexamita inflata. Parasitology Research.* Nov;99(6):722–728.

Morris N. (2002). The effects of lavender (*Lavendula angustifolium*) baths on psychological well-being: Two exploratory randomised control trials. *Complementary Therapies in Medicine.* Dec;10(4):223–228.

Tisserand R, Balics T. (1995). *EO Safety* (pp. 144–145). Edinburgh: Churchill Livingstone.

Weiss RF. (1988). *Herbal Medicine* (pp. 96, 302). Beaconsfield, England: Beaconsfield Publishing.

Wells DL. (2006). Aromatherapy for travel-induced excitement in dogs. *Journal of the American Veterinary Medical Association.* Sep 15;229(6):964–967.

Wichtl M, Bisset NG. [Eds.]. (1994). *Herbal Drugs and Phytopharmaceuticals* (pp. 292–294). Stuttgart: Medpharm.

Winston D. (2006). *Winston's Botanic Materia Medica.* Washington, NJ: DWCHS.

NAME: Lemon Balm (*Melissa officinalis*)

Common Names: Balm, melissa, sweet balm

Family: *Lamiaceae*

Description of Plant
- Small perennial herb in the mint family with ovate or heart-shaped leaves
- Has a lemon odor when leaves are rubbed
- Indigenous to Mediterranean but is cultured worldwide

Medicinal Part: Fresh or dried leaves harvested before flowers bloom

Constituents and Action (if known)
- EO (0.2%–0.5%), monoterpenoids, citronellal: sedative and antispasmodic properties (Hener et al., 1995), geranial, neral
  - Sesqueterpenes (beta-caryophyllene, germacrene D)
  - EO is antibacterial, antiviral, and antifungal (Bruneton, 1999).

- Flavonoids (quercitrin, rhamnocitrin, the 7-glucosides of apigenin, and luteolin)
- Phenolic acids (rosmarinic acid, caffeic acid—up to 4.0%): antioxidant effects (may have an effect 10 times greater than vitamin C and E); antiviral activity against herpes simplex cold sores (Nolkemper et al., 2006)
- Freeze-dried extracts bind thyroid-stimulating immunoglobulin and may reduce circulating thyroid hormone.
- Inhibits C3 and C5 in complement cascade, thus reducing inflammation (Peake et al., 1991)

Nutritional Ingredients: Used as a beverage tea

Traditional Use
- Antiviral, antidepressant, carminative, diaphoretic
- Carminative for gas, nausea, and digestive disturbances of children and adults
- Diaphoretic: useful for children's fevers, mixes well with elder flower and peppermint
- In Ancient Greece, lemon balm was thought to strengthen the mind, and students wore sprigs of lemon balm in their hair as they studied. Steeped in wine, it was also used as a surgical dressing for wounds and to treat venomous bites and stings.

Current Use
- Relieves nervousness, stress-induced headaches, has a mild sedative effect, improves sleep, reduces restlessness and overexcitability (children with attention deficient disorder) (Kennedy et al., 2004; Muller & Klement, 2006)
- Antiviral: relieves symptoms and improves healing of herpes simplex cold sores (topically) (Nolkemper et al., 2006)
- Shown to interfere with cholinesterase, which breaks down acetylcholine; thus, may be helpful in lowering the incidence or slowing the progression of Alzheimer's disease (Perry et al., 1996)
- Mild antidepressant: can be useful for seasonal affective disorder when mixed with St. John's wort (Winston, 2006)
- Thyroxin antagonist: used for hyperthyroidism and Graves' disease (Aufmkolk et al., 1985a, 1985b); use with buglewood and motherwort
- GI disturbances: epigastric bloating, flatulence, eructations

Available Forms, Dosage, and Administration Guidelines

Preparations: Cream, capsules, tea, tincture

Typical Dosage

- *Cream:* Apply as directed at early stages of cold sores and genital herpes
- *Capsules:* 300- to 400-mg capsules up to nine times a day
- *Tea:* steep 1 to 2 tsp dried herb in 1 cup hot water for 10 to 15 minutes; take two to four cups a day
- *Tincture* (1:5, 30% alcohol): 60 to 90 gtt (3–5 mL) three to four times a day

Pharmacokinetics—If Available (form or route when known): None known

Toxicity: None known

Contraindications: None known

Side Effects: None known

Long-Term Safety: Safe

Use in Pregnancy/Lactation/Children: Safe

Drug/Herb Interactions and Rationale (if known): Large doses may act as a thyroxin antagonist and affect the action of medications such as levothyroxine.

Special Notes: The EO, used in aromatherapy, may be beneficial for mild depression.

BIBLIOGRAPHY

Akhondzadeh S, et al. (2003). *Melissa officinalis* extract in the treatment of patients with mild to moderate Alzheimer's disease: A double-blind, randomised, placebo controlled trial. *Journal of Neurology Neurosurgery and Psychiatry.* Jul;74(7):863–866.

Aufmkolk M, et al. (1985a). Extracts and auto-oxidized constituents of certain plants inhibit the receptor-binding and biological activity of Graves' immunoglobulins. *Endocrinology.* 116(5):1687.

Aufmkolk M, et al. (1985b). The active principles of plant extracts with antithyrotropic activity: Oxidation products of derivatives of 3,4-dihydroxycinnamic acid. *Endocrinology.* 116(5):1677.

Bruneton J. (1999). *Pharmacognosy, Phytochemistry, Medicinal Plants* (2nd ed.; pp. 530–532). Paris: Lavoisier.

Hener U, et al. (1995). Evaluation of authenticity of balm oil (*Melissa officinalis* L.). *Pharmazie*. 50(1):60.

Kennedy DO, et al. (2002). Modulation of mood and cognitive performance following acute administration of *Melissa officinalis* (lemon balm). *Pharmacology Biochemistry and Behavior*. Jul;72(4):953–964.

Kennedy DO, et al. (2004). Attenuation of laboratory-induced stress in humans after acute administration of *Melissa officinalis* (lemon balm). *Psychosomatic Medicine*. Jul-Aug;66(4):607–613.

Muller SF, Klement S. (2006). A combination of valerian and lemon balm is effective in the treatment of restlessness and dyssomnia in children. *Phytomedicine*. Jun;13(6):383–387.

Nolkemper S, et al. (2006). Antiviral effect of aqueous extracts from species of the *Lamiaceae* family against herpes simplex virus type I and type 2 in vitro. *Planta Medica*. 72:e366–e367.

Peake PW, et al. (1991). The inhibitory effect of rosmarinic acid on complement involves the C5 convertase. *International Journal of Immunopharmacology*. 13(7):853.

Perry N, et al. (1996). European herbs with cholinergic activities: Potential in dementia therapy. *International Journal of Geriatric Psychiatry*. 11(12):1063–1069.

Wichtl M, Bisset NG. [Eds.]. (1994). *Herbal Drugs and Phytopharmaceuticals* (pp. 329–332). Stuttgart: Medpharm.

Winston D. (2006). *Winston's Botanic Materia Medica*. Washington, NJ: DWCHS.

NAME: Licorice (*Glycyrrhiza glabra*)

Common Names: Sweet root, Persian licorice, Spanish licorice, Chinese licorice (*G. uralensis*)

Family: *Fabiaceae*

Description of Plant

- Shrub 4' to 5' tall, cultivated in Turkey, Spain, Pakistan, and China
- *Glycyrrhiza* means "sweet root;" the yellow rhizome is intensely sweet.
- Spanish licorice has pea-like blue flowers; Chinese licorice has pale yellow flowers.

Medicinal Part: Rhizome

Constituents and Action (if known)

- Triterpenoid: glycyrrhizin (glycyrrhizic acid)—content varies (2%–6%) depending on growing season and soil
  - Pseudoaldosterone effects (sodium retention, hypertension, and edema) may be seen with doses of 700 to 1,400 mg licorice a day (Bernardi et al., 1994).
  - Suppresses scalp sebum secretion (10% glycyrrhizin shampoo) for an additional 24 hours compared with citric acid shampoo (Snow, 1996)
  - Binds to mineralocorticoid and glucocorticoid receptors in vitro (Farese et al., 1991; MacKenzie et al., 1990)
  - Reduces mucosal injury associated with aspirin administration; may increase gastric mucosal blood flow (Snow, 1996) Stimulates gastric mucosa repair (Mills & Bone, 2000).
  - Inhibits production of oxygen free radicals by neutrophils (Akamatsu et al., 1991)
  - Mild anti-inflammatory and antiarthritic activity
  - May enhance clearance of immune complexes, so may benefit autoimmune disease (Matsumoto, 1996)
- Flavonoids (1%–1.5%; liquiritin, isoliquiritin, glabrol)
- Isoflavones (formononetin, glabrone)
- Coumarins

Nutritional Ingredients: Used as a sweetening and flavoring agent. Licorice is 50 times sweeter than sugar and is used in candies and liqueurs. Contains starches and sugars (glucose, mannose, sucrose).

Traditional Use

- Adaptogen, carminative, expectorant, antispasmodic, anti-inflammatory, immune amphoteric, antiviral, hepatoprotective, gastroprotective
- Used by ancient Greek and Roman physicians such as Hippocrates and Pliny the Elder (AD 23) as an expectorant and antitussive for asthma and dry coughs and as a carminative
- In China, licorice is one of the most frequently prescribed herbs. It is used to treat sore throats and sticky, hard-to-expectorate mucus; to tonify the stomach, spleen, and lungs; to control abdominal spasms; and as an antidote for arsenic and pesticide poisoning.

Current Use

- Expectorant, antitussive (similar to but milder than codeine): useful for bronchial congestion, spastic coughs, pertussis, bronchitis, and allergies
- Mild systemic anti-inflammatory: similar in action to cortisone
- Soothes irritated mucous membranes (gastritis, gastric and duodenal ulcer, irritable bowel syndrome, and sore throat). It has been shown in clinical studies to be as effective as cimetidine for treating ulcers and has a superior ability to prevent recurrence.
- Heals herpetic lesions and shingles (topical use). A licorice gel was effective for treating atopic dermatitis (Saeedi et al., 2003).
- Hepatoprotective and antiviral activity (intravenous): has shown benefits in Japanese studies with patients with active hepatitis C (Arase et al., 1997)
- Used to support adrenal exhaustion and mild cases of Addison's disease with Asian ginseng (Winston, 2006)
- Immune amphoteric and adaptogen: studies have shown that licorice is beneficial for autoimmune conditions such as lupus and immune deficiency conditions such as chronic fatigue syndrome (Baschetti, 1995) and HIV/AIDS (Mills & Bone, 2000)
- Inhibits low-density lipoprotein cholesterol peroxidation
- Polycystic ovarian disease: licorice, along with white peony, was given to eight women in an uncontrolled study. After 8 weeks, serum testosterone levels had become normal in seven patients, and six of the women were ovulating regularly (Mills & Bone, 2000).
- Improves vasovagal syncope (Blythe, 1999)
- A human study found that licorice could reduce body weight, but the safety of this as a long-term therapy is questionable (Armanini et al., 2003).

Available Forms, Dosage, and Administration Guidelines

Preparations: Dried root, capsules, extracts, tablets, tinctures, standardized products. European products are formulated to deliver 5 to 15 g (1–2 tsp) root, which contains 200- to 600-mg glycyrrhizin. Several studies have assessed the efficacy of deglycyrrhizinated licorice (DGL), in which all the glycyrrhizin is removed, with inconclusive results. DGL products show none of the serious side effects associated with licorice.

Typical Dosage

- *Capsules:* Up to six 400- to 500-mg capsules a day for no more than 4 to 6 weeks
- *Tincture* (1:5, 30% alcohol): 30 to 60 gtt (1.5–3 mL) up to three times a day
- *Powdered root:* 1 to 2 g one to three times a day
- *Solid (dry powder) extract* (4:1): 250 to 500 mg
- *DGL extract:* 380 to 760 mg three times a day
- Or follow manufacturer or practitioner recommendations

Pharmacokinetics—If Available (form or route when known): Studies have shown that glycyrrhizin is less bioavailable and has less toxicity when given in a whole extract rather than as an isolated substance (Cantelli-Forti et al., 1994).

Toxicity: A mineralocorticoid-like effect can occur that can cause lethargy, headache, hypertension, hypokalemia, sodium retention and edema, weight gain, and pulmonary hypertension.

Contraindications: Hypersensitivity to licorice; pre-existing renal, hepatic (cholestatic liver disorders), and cardiovascular (congestive heart failure) disease because of risk of side effects; essential hypertension; hypokalemia. Elderly patients and women may be more sensitive to licorice (Sigurjonsdottir et al., 2003).

Side Effects: Hyperaldosteronism, hypertension, edema, hypokalemia, sodium retention. The DGL form will not cause any of these side effects.

Long-Term Safety: Long history of human use as a food and medicine. Safe when used in small quantities or for limited periods of time.

Use in Pregnancy/Lactation/Children: Cautious use is advised. Use low doses in children. Avoid using for more than 2 weeks during pregnancy because it may increase blood pressure.

Drug/Herb Interactions and Rationale (if known)

- Do not use with diuretics: inhibits fluid loss and increases potassium loss.
- Do not use with digitalis: decreases effectiveness and increases side effects related to K^+ and Na^+.
- Use cautiously with antihypertensives: may inhibit activity.
- Use cautiously with corticosteroids: can potentiate effects. Dosage of medication may need to be adjusted.
- Use cautiously with laxatives: may increase potassium loss and cause hypokalemia.

Special Notes: Licorice preparations can be deglycyrrhizinated. This removes the side effects of pseudoaldosteronism but may reduce some of the herb's activity. Much of the licorice candy in the United States is flavored with anise oil and does not really contain licorice. Do not overconsume licorice. Eat a diet high in K^+ and low in sodium when taking licorice. Monitor patient's blood pressure regularly. Most cases of hyperaldosteronism have occurred with overconsumption of real licorice candies; there are fewer reports of adverse reactions in patients who take recommended therapeutic doses of whole licorice extracts.

BIBLIOGRAPHY

Akamatsu H, et al. (1991). Mechanism of anti-inflammatory action of glycyrrhizin: Effect on neutrophil functions including reactive oxygen species generation. *Planta Medica.* 57:119–121.

Arase Y, et al. (1997). The long-term efficacy of glycyrrhizin in chronic hepatitis C patients. *Cancer.* 79:1494–1500.

Armanini D, et al. (2003). Effect of licorice on the reduction of body fat mass in healthy subjects. *Journal of Endocrinological Investigation.* Jul;26(7):646–650.

Baschetti R. (1995). Chronic fatigue syndrome and liquorice [letter]. *New Zealand Medical Journal.* Apr 25:156–157.

Bernardi M, et al. (1994). Effects of prolonged ingestion of graded doses of licorice by healthy volunteers. *Life Sciences.* 55:863–872.

Blythe SL. (1999). Use of licorice root to treat vasovagal syncope. *HerbalGram.* 46:24.

Cantelli-Forti G, et al. (1994). Interaction of licorice on glycyrrhizin pharmacokinetics. *Environmental Health Perspectives*. 102[Suppl. 9]:65–68.

Chamberlain J, Abolnik I. (1997). Pulmonary edema following a licorice binge [letter]. *Western Journal of Medicine*. 167(3):184–185.

Farese RV, et al. (1991). Licorice-induced hypermineralocorticoidism. *New England Journal of Medicine*. 325:1223–1227.

Isbrucker RA, Burdock GA. (2006). Risk and safety assessment on the consumption of licorice root (*Glycyrrhiza* sp.). Its extract and powder as a food ingredient, with emphasis on the pharmacology and toxicology of glycyrrhizin. *Regulatory Toxicology and Pharmacology*. Dec;46(3):167–192.

MacKenzie MA, et al. (1990). The influence of glycyrrhetinic acid on plasma cortisol and cortisone in healthy young volunteers. *Journal of Clinical Endocrinology and Metabolism*. 70:1637–1643.

Matsumoto T, et al. (1996). Licorice may fight lupus. *Journal of Ethnopharmacology*. 53:1–4.

Mills S, Bone K. (2000). *Principles and Practice of Phytotherapy* (pp. 465–478). Edinburgh: Churchill Livingstone.

Saeedi, M, et al. (2003). The treatment of atopic dermatitis with licorice gel. *Journal of Dermatological Treatment*. Sep;14(3):153–157.

Sigurjonsdottir HA, et al. (2003). Subjects with essential hypertension are more sensitive to the inhibition of 11 beta-HDS by liquorice. *Journal of Human Hypertension*. Feb;17(2):125–131.

Snow JM. (1996). *Glycyrrhiza glabra* L. (*Leguminaceae*). Protocol *Journal of Botanical Medicine*. Winter:9–14.

Winston D. (2006). *Winston's Materia Medica*. Washington, NJ: DWCHS.

 NAME: Lobelia (*Lobelia inflata*)

Common Names: Asthma weed, pukeweed, Indian tobacco

Family: *Campanulaceae*

Description of Plant

- Small, hardy annual or biennial herb with pale blue flowers and inflated calyxes
- Native to eastern North America

Medicinal Part: Dried leaves and tops, seeds

Constituents and Action (if known)
- Lobeline (0.26%–0.40%): primary alkaloid, but at least 14 different piperidine alkaloids have been identified, including lobelanine and lobelanidine
  - Acts on nicotine receptors in body, crosses blood and placental barriers but is less potent than nicotine; because it binds to nicotine receptors, it decreases cravings for nicotine
  - Paradoxical effect: in low doses, stimulation; in high doses, depression by inhibiting respiratory center in brainstem (Damaj et al., 1997)
- Beta-amyrin palmitate: may possess sedative activity (Subarnas et al., 1993)

Nutritional Ingredients: None known

Traditional Use
- Antispasmodic, antiasthmatic, analgesic, bronchodilator, sedative, expectorant, emetic
- Important herbal medicine for the Thomsonians, physiomedicalists, and eclectic physicians (1822–1930). It was used to treat asthma, bronchitis (cough with a sense of oppression and a feeling of fullness in the chest, mucous rales), pertussis, pleurisy, angina, petit mal seizures, and muscle spasms.
- Topically, used for bruises, sprains, insect bites, and muscle spasms
- Lobelia and lobeline sulphate have been used as a smoking deterrent because of their nicotine-like effects. The FDA has banned its use as an antismoking aid not because of toxicity but because proof of efficacy is lacking. No companies were willing to spend the money to do sufficient research because the product could not be patented.

Current Use
- Spasmodic, asthma, and chronic obstructive pulmonary disease (Bradley, 1992). Lobelia, along with ma huang, thyme, and khella (*Ammi visnaga*), can be an effective treatment for mild asthma.

- Lobelia seed oil is a very effective topical treatment for muscle spasms, sore muscles, strains, and bruises (Winston, 2006).

Available Forms, Dosage, and Administration Guidelines

Preparations: Capsules, tinctures, tea; lobeline sulphate tablets or lozenges

Typical Dosage

- *Capsule* (usually no more than 10% of a formula): two or three capsules a day of a combination product
- *Tea:* 0.5 tsp dried herb in 8 oz hot water, steep half-hour; take 2 oz three times a day. Always mixed with milder, less acrid herbs.
- *Tincture* (1:2, 40% alcohol, 10% acetic acid): 2 to 10 gtt three times a day; (1:5, 40% alcohol, 10% acetic acid): 5 to 20 gtt three times a day
- *Lobeline sulphate:* 5 mg twice a day. Do not use more than 20 mg a day.

Pharmacokinetics—If Available (form or route when known): Absorbed well by mucous membranes (mouth; GI and respiratory tract); metabolized in liver, kidney, and lungs; excreted in kidneys (Westfall & Meldrum, 1986). Lobeline is rapidly metabolized, and its effects are rather transitory when taken orally (Bradley, 1992).

Toxicity: There is much confusion about the toxicity of this herb. Recent analysis of the literature suggests that the acute dangers of this herb have been exaggerated (Bergner, 1998). At high doses, respiratory depression and tachycardia. The isolated alkaloid lobeline sulphate is substantially more toxic than the herb or whole herb extract.

Contraindications: Nausea, dyspnea, hypotension

Side Effects: Nausea, vomiting, dizziness, dyspnea, changes in heart rate, hypotension, diaphoresis, palpitations

Long-Term Safety: Unknown

Use in Pregnancy/Lactation/Children: Contraindicated, except as an aid during childbirth (helps to relax and dilate the cervix) by trained midwives or obstetricians

Drug/Herb Interactions and Rationale (if known): Do not use with smoking cessation products: may potentiate side effects.

Special Notes: Because of the strong potential for adverse effects with this herb (especially nausea, dizziness, and dyspnea), do not use for self-medication; it should be prescribed by a knowledgeable clinician. Patients should be warned that safer methods of smoking cessation are FDA approved.

BIBLIOGRAPHY

Bartram T. (1995). *Encyclopedia of Herbal Medicine* (p. 276). Dorset: Grace Publishers.

Bergner P. (1998). Lobelia toxicity: A literature review. *Medical Herbalism.* 10(1–2):15–34.

Bradley PR. [Ed.]. (1992). *British Herbal Compendium* (pp. 149–150). Dorset: British Herbal Medicine Association.

Damaj MI, et al. (1997). Pharmacology of lobeline, a nicotine receptor ligand. *Journal of Pharmacology and Experimental Therapy.* 282:410–419.

Leung A, Foster S. (1996). *Encyclopedia of Common Natural Ingredients* (2nd ed.; pp. 354–355). New York: John Wiley & Sons.

Subarnas A, et al. (1993). Pharmacological properties of beta-amyrin palmitate, a novel centrally acting compound, isolated from *Lobelia inflata* leaves. *Journal of Pharmacy and Pharmacology.* 45(6):545–550.

Westfall TC, Meldrum MJ. (1986). Ganglionic blocking agents. In: Craig CR, Stizel RE. *Modern Pharmacology* (2nd ed.). Boston: Little, Brown & Co.

Winston D. (2006). *Winston's Botanic Materia Medica.* Washington, NJ: DWCHS.

NAME: Ma Huang (*Ephedra sinica, E. equisetina, E. intermedia*)

Common Names: Ephedra, Chinese ephedra

Family: *Ephedraceae*

Description of Plant: A small perennial evergreen shrub native to China, Japan, Tibet, India, Pakistan, and southern Siberia

Medicinal Part: Dried twigs (stem)

Constituents and Action (if known)

- Phenylproamine alkaloids (0.487%–2.436%)
  - Ephedrine (12%–75%): sympathomimetic agent acting on alpha- and beta-adrenergic receptors. Increases heart rate, blood pressure; bronchodilator; relaxes bronchi; anti-inflammatory; inhibits inflammatory PGE2 prostaglandins and other proinflammatory substances (histamine, serotonin, bradykinin, PGE1) (You-Ping, 1998)
  - Pseudoephedrine (12%–75%): bronchodilating effects; increases heart rate, blood pressure; diuretic; anti-inflammatory; inhibits inflammatory PGE2 prostaglandins and other proinflammatory substances (histamine, serotonin, bradykinin, PGE1) (You-Ping, 1998)
  - Methylephedrine
  - Methylpseudoephedrine
  - Norephedrine
  - Norpseudoephedrine
  - Ephedroxane: anti-inflammatory (AHPA, 1999)
  - Tannins: inhibit angiotensin II production
- Research suggests:
  - Volatile oils (tetramethylpyrazine, l-alpha-terpineol): antiasthmatic (AHPA, 1999)
  - Whole ephedra has fewer side effects than isolated ephedrine hydrochloride because of the balancing effect of its two major alkaloids.
  - Ephedra decoction has in vitro antibacterial activity against *Staphylococcus aureus, Bacillus anthracis, B. diphtheriae, B. dysenteriae, B. typhosus,* and *Pseudomonas aeruginosa.*
- Each species of ephedra has a different alkaloidal profile.

Nutritional Ingredients: None

Traditional Use

- Antiallergic, bronchodilator, decongestant, central nervous system stimulant, diaphoretic, diuretic
- In TCM, ma huang is used in formulas for treating bronchial asthma, nasal congestion, head colds, fevers without perspiration, and headache and as a diuretic for edema.

Current Use

- Decongestant for allergies and hay fever: isolated ephedrine sulfate is found in over-the-counter medicines used to treat allergic rhinitis, allergic sinusitis, and head colds. The herb, in combination with other herbs such as eyebright, osha root, and bayberry root, works very well with only minor side effects such as dry mouth and rare sinus headaches (Winston, 2006).
- Asthma: ephedrine sulfate is used as an over-the-counter medication in some inhalers. The herb ephedra can be a useful part of an herbal protocol for mild asthma. It can be combined with other herbs such as lobelia, thyme, licorice, schisandra, and khella (*Ammi visnaga*).
- Weight loss: the benefits of thermogenic formulas for weight loss in patients with a sluggish metabolism seem to outweigh the potential risks, as long as the patient has no contraindications and if used in the recommended dosage and monitored by a physician (along with healthy diet, exercise, and behavior modification) (Boozer et al., 2002; Hackman et al., 2006; Shekelle et al., 2003).
- Recent studies in China found that ma huang could be used to treat chronic bedwetting in children. Dosage was based on age; therapy lasted 1 month. In one study, 50 children were given a ma huang decoction every night before bed; 42 were cured with no recurrence after 6 months, 5 stopped bedwetting but resumed after the herb was discontinued, and 3 did not respond (AHPA, 1999).

Available Forms, Dosage, and Administration Guidelines

Preparations: Dried herb, tea, tincture, tablets, capsules, standardized extract. The American Herb Products Association (AHPA) has established upper limits for ephedra use of 25 mg ephedra alkaloids per dose and 100 mg ephedra alkaloids a day.

Typical Dosage

- *Dried herb:* 1 to 2 g per dose (approximately 13 mg total alkaloids) two or three times a day
- *Capsules* (ground whole herb): 500 to 1,000 mg two or three times a day
- *Standardized extract*: 12 to 25 mg total alkaloids two or three times a day

- *Tea:* 0.5 tsp dried herb in 8 oz hot water, decoct 15 minutes, steep 30 minutes; take 4 oz three times a day
- *Tincture* (1:5, 40% alcohol): 15 to 30 gtt (0.75–1.5 mL) up to three times a day

Pharmacokinetics—If Available (form or route when known): With oral administration of ephedrine, peak effect occurs in 1 hour and activity lasts up to 6 hours. Whole ephedra is absorbed more slowly; the effects are less dramatic but more sustained (AHPA, 1999).

Toxicity: Overdose is associated with hypertension, tachycardia, cardiac arrhythmia, myocardial infarction, and stroke (Rakovec et al., 2006).

Contraindications: Hypertension, insomnia, heart disease, glaucoma, benign prostatic hypertrophy, thyrotoxicosis, diabetes, pheochromocytoma, panic disorders, renal failure

Side Effects: Dry mouth, nervousness, anxiety, increased blood pressure, insomnia, palpitations, adrenal exhaustion, heartburn, headache, nausea, ventricular tachycardia

Long-Term Safety: Unknown; not appropriate for long-term use except as prescribed by a physician

Use in Pregnancy/Lactation/Children: Avoid use in pregnancy, lactation, or in children.

Drug/Herb Interactions and Rationale (if known)
- Caffeine and other xanthine alkaloids: increased effects and potential toxicity
- Monoamine oxidase inhibitors: increased sympathomimetic effects
- Cardiac glycosides (digoxin): can cause arrhythmia
- Guanethidine: antagonized the hypotensive effect (Brinker, 2001)
- Oxytocin: can increase hypertensive effects
- Halothane: may cause arrhythmias
- May antagonize hypotensive agents such as beta-blockers and ACE inhibitors (Brinker, 2001)

Special Notes: Ephedra was being used inappropriately as an "herbal amphetamine" and energy aid and for sports training.

It should not be used for any of these purposes. Due to significant drug abuse of ephedra and adverse effects, the FDA banned the use of ephedra in May 2004. It may be of some value for obesity due to sluggish metabolism but should be used only under a physician's supervision in otherwise relatively healthy patients.

BIBLIOGRAPHY

AHPA. (1999). Ephedra International Symposium Silver Spring: MD. American Herb Products Association.

Blumenthal M, et al. (2000). *Herbal Medicine: Expanded Commission E Monographs* (pp. 110–117). Austin, TX: American Botanical Council.

Blumenthal M, King P. (1995). Ma huang: Ancient herb, modern medicine regulatory dilemma. *HerbalGram*. 34:22.

Boozer CN, et al. (2002). Herbal ephedra/caffeine for weight loss: A 6-month randomized safety and efficacy trial. *International Journal of Obesity and Related Metabolic Disorders*. May;26(5): 593–604.

Brinker F. (2001). *Herb Contraindications & Drug Interactions* (pp. 87–90). Sandy, OR: Eclectic Medical Publications.

Hackman RM, et al. (2006). Multinutrient supplement containing ephedra and caffeine causes weight loss and improves metabolic risk factors in obese women: A randomized controlled trial. *International Journal of Obesity (London)*. Oct;30(10): 1545–1556.

Rakovec P, et al. (2006). Ventricular tachycardia induced by abuse of ephedrine in a young healthy woman. *Wiener Klinische Wochenschrift*. Sep;118(17–18):558–561.

Shekelle PG, et al. (2003). Efficacy and safety of ephedra and ephedrine for weight loss and athletic performance: A meta-analysis. *Journal of the American Medical Association*. Mar 26;289(12):1537–1545.

Winston D. (2006). *Winston's Botanic Materia Medica*. Washington, NJ: DWCHS.

You-Ping Z. (1998). *Chinese Materia Medica: Chemistry, Pharmacology and Applications* (pp. 45–51). Amsterdam: Harwood Academic Publishers.

 NAME: Maitake Mushroom (*Grifola frondosa*)

Common Names: Hen of the woods, sheep's head

Family: *Polyporaceae*

Description of Plant
- This mushroom grows on live, aging hardwood trees in the eastern United States and Asia
- It fruits in the autumn, producing a white-brown cauliflower-like mushroom that can weight up to 30 lbs.

Medicinal Part: Mushroom (fruiting body) and mycelia

Constituents and Action (if known)
- Beta-glucans
  - 1-6B glucan (grifolan): immunomodulator, antitumor (Hobbs, 1995; Kodama et al., 2004), antibacterial (Skenderi, 2003)
  - 1-4B-D glucans: immunomodulator, antitumor (Kodama et al., 2004), antibacterial (Skenderi, 2003)
  - 1-3B-D glucans: immunomodulator, antitumor (Kodama et al., 2004), antibacterial (Skenderi, 2003)
  - Acidic B glucans: immunomodulator, antitumor (Kodama et al., 2004), antibacterial (Skenderi, 2003)
  - Hetero B-glucans: immunomodulator, antitumor (Kodama et al., 2004)
- Ergosterol (vitamin D_2): cyclo-oxygenase (COX) enzyme inhibitor, antioxidant (Zhang et al., 2002)
- Ergostra-4,6,8 (14), 22-tetraen-3-one: enzyme inhibitor, antioxidant (Zhang et al., 2002)
- 1-oleoyl-2-linoleoyl-3-palmitoylglycenol: enzyme inhibitor, antioxidant (Zhang et al., 2002)
- Phospholipids
  - Phosphatydalcholine: neuroprotective (Rao et al., 2000)
  - Phosphatydalserine: neuroprotective (Rao et al., 2000)
  - Phosphatidylinositol: neuroprotective (Rao et al., 2000)

Nutritional Ingredients: Hen of the woods is a prized edible mushroom. It is cooked (fried, sautéed, grilled, etc.) and eaten in stir-fries, soups, and casseroles.

Traditional Use
- Antibacterial, hypocholesteremic, antifungal, antitumor agent, antiviral, immune amphoteric, hypoglycemic
- This mushroom has a long history of use as a food, but its medicinal effects have only recently been recognized.

- A related Chinese species, *Grifola umbellata* (*Polyporus umbellatus*) is known as Zhu Ling. It is used in TCM as a diuretic and for treating urinary tract infections, edema, jaundice, and diarrhea.

Current Use

- *Grifola* is an immune amphoteric that can be used for immune deficiency (cancer, CFIDS) or in hyperactive immune conditions (allergies, autoimmune disease) (Winston, 2006).
- There is a significant body of research on maitake, but most of it is either in vitro or animal studies, and often the studies are of specific beta-glucan compounds known as the "D fraction" or "MD fraction." These beta-glucans can increase tumor necrosis factor (TNF); T-4, T-8, K, NK cells (Hobbs, 1995; Winston, 2006) and macrophage cytokine production, and they have antitumor activity (Stamets, 2002). Two human studies give even greater creedance to the use of maitake as an adjunct for cancer treatment. In a nonrandomized trial of 165 advanced stage cancer patients, 11 of 15 breast cancer patients, 12 of 18 lung cancer patients, and 7 of 15 patients with hepatic cancer had tumor regression or significant improvements of symptoms while taking maitake-D-fraction (Nanba, 1997). In this same study, this product taken along with chemotherapy improved response rates by 12% to 28% (Nanba, 1997). Another study found that 62.5% of patients with lung cancer, 68.8% with breast cancer, and 58.3% with liver cancer had increased levels of immune-competent cells when maitake was taken concurrently with chemotherapy (Kodama et al., 2002).
- In animal studies, adding substantial amounts of maitake to diabetic rat diets reduced prandial and postprandial blood glucose levels (Horio et al., 2001).
- In another animal study, the ingestion of a large dose (20% of the daily diet) of powdered maitake lowered cholesterol and triglyceride levels as well as reduced weight and blood pressure.
- Additional animal studies also show that *Grifola* has hepatoprotective, tumor-regression, and antiviral (HIV and hepatitis B) activity (Hobbs, 1995).

- While these studies are not conclusive, adding maitake to protocols for treating patients with hyperlipedemia, insulin resistance, mild hypertension, NIDDM, and hepatitis B may offer some benefits with little or no risk. Two small unpublished studies (Christian & Schar, 1999; Christian et al., 1999) using maitake showed benefit for women with chronic vaginal candidiasis and for patients with HIV infections (increased CD4 counts, decreased or static viral loads, reduction of symptoms such as warts, gum infections, neuropathies, fatigue, weight loss, etc., and an increased feeling of well-being).

Available Forms, Dosage, and Administration Guidelines
Preparations: Fresh mushroom, dried mushroom, tea, capsule, tincture
Typical Dosage
- *Fresh mushroom*: 4 oz a day
- *Dried mushroom*: 5 to 10 g a day
- *Tea*: 2 to 3 tsp dried mushroom to 10 to 12 oz water, decoct at low heat (less than 225°F) for 1 hour. Take 2 to 4 cups a day.
- *Tincture* (1:5, 22.5% alcohol): 100 to 120 gtt (5–6 mL) three to four times a day
- *Capsule* (D-fraction): 1 to 2 capsules up to three times a day

Pharmacokinetics—If Available (form or route when known): Not known

Toxicity: None known

Contraindications: Mushroom allergies

Side Effects: Large quantities of the mushroom can cause gastric upset and flatulence.

Long-Term Safety: Safe

Use in Pregnancy/Lactation/Children: Safe

Drug/Herb Interactions and Rationale (if known):
Several studies indicate that maitake taken concurrently with chemotherapy enhances the effects of the drug regimen while reducing side effects (Kodama et al., 2003; Kodama et al., 2004; Nanba, 1997).

Special Notes: The Japanese name *maitake* means "dancing mushroom." The mushroom fruits in the autumn and is eagerly collected for food and medicinal use. Much of the maitake in the market is now cultivated, making the mushroom much more available.

BIBLIOGRAPHY

Christian R, et al. (1999). An evaluative study of the effects of a strain of *Grifola frondosa* (maitake) against persistent vaginal *Candida albicans* proliferation (thrush). The Herbalists of Colombia Road Think Tank, London.

Christian R, Schar D. (1999). An evaluative study of the effects of *Grifola frondosa* var. Yukiguni (maitake) on the maintenance of health of people suffering with HIV infection. The Herbalists of Colombia Road Think Tank, London.

Fukushima M, et al. (2001). Cholesterol-lowering effects of maitake (*Grifola frondosa*) fiber, shiitake (*Lentinus edodes*) fiber, and enokitake (*Flammulina velutipes*) fiber in rats. *Experimental Biology and Medicine (Maywood)*. Sep;226(8):758–765.

Hobbs C. (1995). *Medicinal Mushrooms* (pp. 110–115). Santa Cruz, CA: Botanica Press.

Horio H, et al. (2001). Maitake (*Grifola frondosa*) improves glucose tolerance of experimental diabetic rats. *Journal of Nutritional Science and Vitaminology (Tokyo)*. Feb;47(1):57–63.

Kodama N, et al. (2002). Can maitake MD-fraction aid cancer patients? *Alternative Medicine Review*. Jun;7(3):236–239.

Kodama N, et al. (2003). Effect of maitake (*Grifola frondosa*) D-fraction on the activation of NK cells in cancer patients. *Journal of Medicinal Food*. Winter;6(4):371–377.

Kodama N, et al. (2004). Administration of a polysaccharide from *Grifola frondosa* stimulates immune function of normal mice. *Journal of Medicinal Food*. Summer;7(2):141–145.

Kodama N, et al. (2005). Maitake D-fraction enhances antitumor effects and reduces immunosuppression by mitomycin-C in tumor-bearing mice. *Nutrition*. May;21(5):624–629.

Nanba H. (1997). Maitake D-fraction: Healing and preventative potential for cancer. *Journal of Orthomolecular Medicine*. (12):43–49.

Rao AM, et al. (2000). Lipid alterations in transient forebrain ischemia: Possible new mechanisms of CDP-choline neuroprotection. *Journal of Neurochemistry*. Dec;75(6):2528–2535.

Skenderi G. (2003). *Herbal Vade Mecum* (pp. 157–168). Rutherford, NJ: Herbacy Press.

Stamets P. (2002). *Mycomedicinals* (pp. 29–32). Olympia, WA: MycoMedia Productions.

Winston D. (2006). *Winston's Botanic Materia Medica*. Washington, NJ: DWCHS.

Zhang Y, et al. (2002). Cyclooxygenase inhibitory and antioxidant compounds from the mycelia of the edible mushroom *Grifola frondosa*. *Journal of Agricultural and Food Chemistry*. Dec 18;50(26):7581–7585.

 NAME: Meadowsweet (*Filipendula ulmaria*)

Common Names: Queen of the meadow, bridewort, lady of the meadow

Family: *Rosaceae*

Description of Plant
- Perennial herb growing up to 3' to 5' tall, with panicles of small white flowers
- Native to Europe but grows well in North America
- Prefers damp, moist soil

Medicinal Part: Dried herb and flowers

Constituents and Action (if known)
- Phenolic glycosides (spiraein, monotropitin, isosalicin): anti-inflammatory, antipyretic, analgesic activity (Mills & Bone, 2000; Wichtl & Bisset, 1994)
- Flavonoids (rutin, hyperoside, spiraeoside) (Wichtl & Bisset, 1994)
- Polyphenols (tannins) (10%–15%): rugosin-D has astringent properties and may help with diarrhea (Duke, 1989), antibacterial (Rauha et al., 2000).
- A heparin-like compound; may be responsible for anticoagulant activity (Kudriashov et al., 1990)
- Volatile oils (0.2%): mostly salicylaldehyde

Nutritional Ingredients: Used as a flavoring in alcoholic beverages in the United Kingdom

History
- It was considered a sacred herb by the Druids.
- Salicylic acid was first isolated from *Filipendula* (spirae) flowers. The pure salicylic acid caused acute GI distress, so

researchers found a related compound, acetylsalicylic acid, that had the benefits of the salicylic acid without as much of the adverse reactions. The word *aspirin* comes from A (acetyl) + spirae (old name for meadowsweet).

Traditional Use

- Antacid, astringent, antipyretic, analgesic, anti-inflammatory, astringent, diuretic, stomachic
- To settle the stomach and treat indigestion, heartburn, irritable bowel syndrome, and diarrhea
- To treat arthritis, bursitis, muscle pain, and rheumatic pain
- To treat headaches, fevers, and abdominal cramps
- Nonirritating antiseptic diuretic for cystitis, urinary calculi, and gout

Current Use

- Supportive therapy for colds because of its anti-inflammatory, analgesic, antipyretic activity (ESCOP, 2003).
- Digestive remedy for acid indigestion (dyspepsia), gastritis, and peptic ulcers. It is often combined with licorice, marshmallow, and chamomile (Winston, 2006).
- Used to treat rheumatic and arthritic pains (orally and topically) (Bradley, 1992).
- Intravaginal administration of meadowsweet ointment in 48 patients with cervical dysplasia resulted in an improvement in 32 women, with 25 of these having a complete remission (ESCOP, 2003).

Available Forms, Dosage, and Administration Guidelines

- *Dried flowers/herb*: 2 to 6 g
- *Tea*: 1 to 2 tsp dried herb/flowers in 8 oz hot water, steep 30 minutes; take two or three cups a day
- *Tincture* (1:5, 30% alcohol): 40 to 80 gtt (2–4 mL) up to three times a day

Pharmacokinetics—If Available (form or route when known): Not known

Toxicity: None known

Contraindications: Salicylate sensitivity

Side Effects: None known

Long-Term Safety: Not known

Use in Pregnancy/Lactation/Children: No research available; no restrictions known (McGuffin et al., 1997)

Drug/Herb Interactions and Rationale (if known): Possible interaction with anticoagulants. Use cautiously together, especially if using other herb or supplement products that could cause a cumulative effect (fish oils, vitamin E, ginkgo, garlic). Obtain prothrombin time and International Normalized Ratio (INR) to rule out possible interactions.

BIBLIOGRAPHY

Bradley PR. (1992). *British Herbal Compendium* (pp. 158–160). Dorset: British Herbal Medicine Association.

Duke J. (1989). *CRC Handbook of Medicinal Herbs* (pp. 196–197). Boca Raton, FL: CRC Press Inc.

European Scientific Cooperative on Phytotherapy. (2003). *ESCOP Monographs* (pp. 157–161). New York: Thieme.

Kudriashov B, et al. (1990). The content of a heparin-like anticoagulant in the flowers of the meadowsweet. *Farmakology Toksikologia.* 53(4):39–41.

Liapina LA, Kovalchuk GA. (1993). A comparative study of the action on the hemostatic system of extracts from the flowers and seeds of the meadowsweet. *Izvestiia Akademii Nauk. Seriia Biologicheskaia.* 4:625–628.

McGuffin M, et al. (1997). *American Herbal Product Association's Botanical Safety Handbook.* Boca Raton, FL: CRC Press.

Mills S, Bone K. (2000). *Principles and Practice of Phytotherapy* (pp. 479–482). Edinburgh: Churchill Livingstone.

Rauha JP, et al. (2000). Antimicrobial effects of Finnish plant extracts containing flavonoids and other phenolic compounds. *International Journal of Food Microbiology.* May 25;56(1):3–12.

Wichtl M, Bisset N. (1994). *Herbal Drugs and Phytopharmaceuticals* (pp. 280–282). Stuttgart, Germany: CRC Press.

Winston D. (2006). *Winston's Botanic Materia Medica.* Washington, NJ: DWCHS.

 NAME: Milk Thistle (*Silybum marianum*)

Common Names: Lady's thistle, Marion thistle, Mary's thistle, *Cardii marianus*

Family: *Asteraceae*

Description of Plant

- Annual/biennial weedy plant found in rocky soils in southern and western Europe and North Africa; naturalized in some parts of the United States
- Grows 2' to 4' high. Has dark shiny green leaves with white veins.
- The spiny flower heads are purple and bloom from June to August.

Medicinal Part: Seeds

Constituents and Action (if known)

- Silymarin (1.5%–3%) consists of several flavonolignans: silybin (antioxidant and hepatoprotection), silychristin, silydianin, and isosilybin (protected against cisplatin-induced renal damage and cycosplorin A–induced pancreatic exocrine inhibition) (Brinker, 2001).
  - Binds with hepatocellular membranes and protects against damaging chemicals and toxins (Albrecht, 1992; Awang, 1993), inhibits carcinogenesis (Deep & Agarwal, 2007)
  - Prevents lysoperoxidative hepatic damage from alcohol and drugs (Buzzelli et al., 1993; Flora et al., 1998)
  - Prevents hepatocyte damage (Flora et al., 1998)
  - Antioxidant: inhibits lipid peroxidation of hepatic microsomes (Kativar, 2005)
  - Increases level of glutathione in liver
  - Reduces blood cholesterol (Skottova & Kreeman, 1998)
  - Increases superoxide dismutase levels in red blood cells of chronic alcoholics (Muzes et al., 1991)
  - Increases protein synthesis in hepatocytes, thereby increasing liver cell regeneration (Grossman, 1995; Mascarella, 1993)
  - Prevents toxins from entering liver cells by preventing binding (Morazzoni & Bombardelli, 1995)
  - Prevents liver damage from alcohol, tetracycline, acetaminophen, thallium, erythromycin, amitriptyline, long-term phenothiazine use, carbon tetrachloride, lorazepam, and anesthesia (Morazzoni & Bombardelli, 1995; von Schonfeld et al., 1997)

- Flavonoids (quercitin, taxifolin, eriodyctiol, chrysoeriol)
- Fixed oil (20%–30%)

Additional Actions

- In vitro anti-inflammatory activity (Polyak et al., 2007)
- May enhance immune function (polymorphonuclear neutrophils, T lymphocytes)
- Increases motility of neutrophils and leukocytes
- Lowers biliary cholesterol and phospholipid concentrations without affecting bile flow (Morazzoni & Bombardelli, 1995)
- Increases bile secretion
- Decreases prostaglandin synthesis

Nutritional Ingredients: Once grown in Europe as a vegetable: the despined leaves were used as a spinach-like green, and the flower was eaten like an artichoke. The roasted seeds were used as a coffee substitute.

Traditional Use

- Used for more than 2,000 years as a liver herb and protectant
- Used in England to remove obstructions of the liver and spleen and to treat jaundice, constipation, hemorrhoids, and insufficient bile flow with clay-colored stools
- The eclectic physicians used the seed to treat hepatomegaly, splenomegaly, dry, scaly skin, pancreatitis (with ceanothus), and gallstones.
- The leaves have been used to stimulate milk production in lactating women, as a bitter digestive tonic, and as a mild liver tonic.

Current Use

- Milk thistle is the most widely researched hepatoprotective herb (Flora et al., 1998).
- Improves survival in patients with cirrhosis: slows liver disease and may reverse liver damage. Patients must stop drinking to maximize effectiveness.
- Improves immune function and appetite and reduces nausea in patients with cirrhosis
- Inhibits damage caused by chronic persistent hepatitis (A, B, and possibly C). It does not have antiviral activity but reduces inflammatory response to the virus (Torres et al., 2004).

- Reduces liver damage and helps to restore hepatic function in nonviral hepatitis (drug-induced or of unknown origin)
- Reduces side effects in patients undergoing chemotherapy for cancer
- May prevent or treat gallstones
- Persons exposed to hepatotoxins (farmers, chemical workers) use it to protect the liver from damage.
- Used in Europe for *Amanita* (death cap) mushroom poisoning: inhibits hepatic uptake of the phallotoxins and renal uptake of alpha-amanitine, thus preventing liver and kidney damage and death (primarily used as an injection)
- May reduce diabetic complications: studies showed less diabetic neuropathy resulting from prevention of inhibition of protein mono-adenosine diphosphate ribosylation (Huseini et al., 2006)
- In a human randomized, double-blind placebo-controlled study, milk thistle decreased levels of glycosylated hemoglobin (HbA1c), fasting blood glucose, total cholesterol, LDL cholesterol, triglycerides, SGOT, and SGPT compared with placebo (Huseini et al., 2006).

Available Forms, Dosage, and Administration Guidelines

Preparations: Whole or powdered seed, capsules, tablets, tinctures. Most capsules and tablets are standardized to 70% to 80% silymarin. Alcohol-based extracts should be used cautiously in patients with liver damage because of the need to administer relatively high amounts of alcohol to obtain an adequate dose of silymarin.

Typical Dosage

- *Capsules* (standardized to 70%–80% silymarin): 140 to 160 mg silymarin three times a day. After 6 weeks, reduce to 90 mg three times a day.
- *Tea*: Steep 2 to 3 tsp dried, powdered seed in 1 cup hot water for 10 to 15 minutes. Silymarin is poorly soluble in water, so aqueous preparations such as teas are only marginally effective, if at all.
- *Tincture* (1:5, 70% alcohol): 60 to 100 gtt (3–5 mL) up to three times a day
- Or follow manufacturer or practitioner recommendations

Pharmacokinetics—If Available (form or route when known): Absorbs readily: 20% to 50% of silymarin is absorbed by oral administration. Peak action occurs in 1 hour. Excretion: 80% of silymarin is excreted in the bile. Functional onset: 5 to 8 days. Reversal of liver damage occurs in 1 to 2 months; improvement of chronic hepatitis in 6 months to 1 year.

Toxicity: Considered completely safe

Contraindications: None known

Side Effects: Mostly devoid of side effects; mild laxative effect and GI symptoms, usually subside in 2 to 3 days; mild allergic reactions

Long-Term Safety: Safe with no reported toxicity

Use in Pregnancy/Lactation/Children: Safe

Drug/Herb Interactions and Rationale (if known): Milk thistle's constituent silybin has been shown to inhibit CYP3A4, CYP 2C9 and UDP glucuronosyltransferase 1AI in vitro. In a human study, milk thistle extract was given to cancer patients taking irinotecan. There was no short- or long-term interaction, and the authors concluded that the concentrations of silybin in milk thistle are too low to affect drug metabolism (Van Erp et al., 2005). Milk thistle and its constituents have been shown to protect the liver against damage caused by dilantin, acetaminophen, butyrophenones, phenothiazines, and halothane (Brinker, 2001).

BIBLIOGRAPHY

Albrecht M. (1992). Therapy of toxic liver pathologies with Legalon. *Zeitschrift fur Klinische Medizin.* 47(2):87–92.

Awang D. (1993). Milk thistle. *Canadian Pharmaceutical Journal.* 126:403–404.

Brinker F. (2001). *Herb Contraindications & Drug Interactions* (pp. 149–150). Sandy, OR: Eclectic Medical Publications.

Buzzelli G, et al. (1993). A pilot study on the liver protective effect of silybin-phosphatidylcholine complex (IdB1016) in chronic active hepatitis. *International Journal of Clinical Pharmacology Therapy and Toxicology.* 31:456–460.

Deep G, Agarwal R. (2007). Chemopreventive efficacy of silymarin in skin and prostate cancer. *Integrative Cancer Therapies.* 6(2):130–145.

Flora K, et al. (1998). Milk thistle (*Silybum marianum*) for the therapy of liver disease. *American Journal of Gastroenterology.* 93(2):139–143.

Grossman M. (1995). Spontaneous regression of hepatocellular carcinoma. *American Journal of Gastroenterology.* 90(9): 1500–1503.

Huseini HF, et al. (2006). The efficacy of *Silybum marianum* (L.) Gaertn. (silymarin) in the treatment of type II diabetes: A randomized, double-blind, placebo-controlled, clinical trial. *Phytotherapy Research.* 20:1036–1039.

Kativar SK. (2005). Silymarin and skin cancer prevention: Anti-inflammatory, antioxidant, and immunomodulatory effects (Review). *International Journal of Oncology.* Jan;26(1):169–176.

Mascarella S. (1993). Therapeutic and antilipoperoxidant effects of silybin-phosphatidycholine complex in chronic liver disease: Preliminary result. *Current Therapeutic Research.* 53(1):98–102.

Morazzoni P, Bombardelli E. (1995). *Silybum marianum* (*Carduus marianus*). *Fitoterapia.* 66(1):3–42.

Muzes G, et al. (1991). Effect of the bioflavonoid silymarin on the in vitro activity and expression of superoxide dismutase enzyme. *Acta Physiologica Hungarica.* 78:3–9.

Polyak SJ et al., (2007). Inhibition of T-cell inflammatory cytokines, hepatocyte NF-KappaB signaling, and HCV infection by standardized silymarin. *Gastroenterology.* May;132(5):1925–1936.

Skottova N, Kreeman V. (1998). Silymarin as a potential hypocholesterolaemic drug. *Physiology Research.* 47(1):1–7.

Torres M, et al. (2004). Does *Silybum marianum* play a role in the treatment of chronic hepatitis C? *Puerto Rico Health Sciences Journal.* Jun;23[2 Suppl.]:68–74.

Van Erp NP, et al. (2005). Effect of milk thistle (*Silybum marianum*) on the pharmacokinetics of irinotecan. *Clinical Cancer Research.* Nov 1;11(2):7800–7806.

von Schonfeld J, et al. (1997). Silibinin, a plant extract with antioxidant and membrane stabilizing properties, protects exocrine pancreas from cyclosporin A toxicity. *Cellular Molecular Life Sciences.* 53(11–12):917–920.

Wichtl M, Bisset NG. [Eds.]. (1994). *Herbal Drugs and Phytopharmaceuticals* (pp. 121–123). Medpharm: Stuttgart.

 NAME: Motherwort (*Leonurus cardiaca*)

Common Names: The Chinese species *L. heterophyllyus* (yi mu cao) has similar activity.

Family: *Lamiaceae*

Description of Plant
- A nonaromatic perennial member of the mint family.
- Naturalized in the United States and Canada, it grows 2' to 4' tall, with pink flowers and sharp, thorny calyxes.

Medicinal Part: Dried leaves

Constituents and Action (if known)
- Triterpenes
  - Ursolic acid: tumor-inhibiting for leukemia and lung, mammary, and colon cancers (Nagasawa et al., 1992)
  - Antiviral (Epstein-Barr virus) (Tokuda et al., 1986)
  - Cardioactive: stimulates alpha- and beta-adrenoreceptors and inhibits calcium chloride (Newall et al., 1996)
  - Cytotoxic
- Iridoid glycosides (leonuride)
- Alkaloids
  - Leonurine: produces transient central nervous system depression and hypotensive effects when given intravenously (Bradley, 1992); uterine stimulant (You-Ping, 1998)
  - L-stachydrine
- Lavandulifolioside (phyenylpropanoid): negatively chronotropic hypotensive (Milkowska-Leyck et al., 2002)
- Tannins (5%–9%)

Traditional Use
- Antispasmodic, anxiolytic, cardiotonic, emmenagogue, hypotensive, nervine/sedative
- Cardiovascular conditions such as palpitations and mild hypertension
- Reduces the pain of menstrual cramps and other smooth muscle, parasympathetic cramps, including vaginismus
- Increases or stimulates menstrual flow for women with amenorrhea or a clotty, scanty flow with cramps

Current Use
- Stress-induced cardiac disorders: palpitations and mild hypertension. For hypertension use with hawthorn, olive leaf, linden flower, and black haw (Winston, 2006).
- Nervine, mild sedative, antispasmodic, useful for general anxiety, including premenstrual and menopausal anxiety. Use

with blue vervain, scullcap, or fresh oat extract. Motherwort is also useful for pelvic and lumbar pain, including mild to moderate dysmenorrhea.

- Use for hyperthyroidism with bugleweed and lemon balm, especially if nervousness and palpitations are part of the patient's symptoms.

Available Forms, Dosage, and Administration Guidelines
Preparations: Infusion, dried herb, capsules, tincture
Typical Dosage

- Unless otherwise prescribed, 3 to 6 g a day of dried herb
- *Infusion*: 2 tsp dried herb in 8 oz hot water, steep 30 minutes; take two or three cups a day
- *Capsules*: Two or three 500-mg capsules three times a day
- *Tincture* (1:5, 30% alcohol): 60 to 100 gtt (3–5 mL) three times a day

Pharmacokinetics—If Available (form or route when known): Not known

Toxicity: None known

Contraindications: None known

Side Effects: May increase menstrual bleeding

Long-Term Safety: Safe when used in normal therapeutic doses

Use in Pregnancy/Lactation/Children: Not recommended in pregnancy because it is an emmenagogue; no restrictions in lactation

Drug/Herb Interactions and Rationale (if known): None known

Special Notes: The *Botanical Safety Handbook* notes, "A dose in excess of 3.0 grams of a powdered extract may cause diarrhea, uterine bleeding, and stomach irritation" (McGuffin et al., 1997, p. 69). There is no mention in the original literature of what type of extract was used or the concentration. This warning is not repeated anywhere else in the literature and does not apply to the crude herb or tincture.

BIBLIOGRAPHY

Bradley PR. [Ed.]. (1992). *British Herbal Compendium, Vol. 1* (pp. 161–162). Bournemouth: British Herbal Medicine Association.

McGuffin M, et al. (1997). *American Herbal Product Association's Botanical Safety Handbook* (pp. 68–69). Boca Raton, FL: CRC Press.

Milkowska-Leyck, et al. (2002). Pharmacological effects of lavandulifolioside from *Leonurus cardiaca*. *Journal of Ethnopharmacology.* Apr;80(1):85–90.

Moore M. (2003). *Medicinal Plants of the Mountain West* (pp. 168–169). Santa Fe: Museum of New Mexico Press.

Nagasawa H, et al. (1992). Further study on the effects of motherwort (*Leonurus sibiricus* L.) preneoplastic and neoplastic mammary gland growth in multiparous GR/A mice. *Anticancer Research.* 12(1):141–143.

Newall CA, et al. (1996). *Herbal Medicines: A Guide for Health Care Professionals* (pp. 197–198). London: Pharmaceutical Press.

Sherman JA. (1993). *Complete Botanical Prescriber* (3rd ed.; p. 134). Portland, OR: Author.

Tokuda H, et al. (1986). Inhibitory effects of ursolic and oleanolic acid on skin tumor promotion by 12-0-tetradecanoylphorbol-13-acetate. *Cancer Letters.* 33(3):279–285.

Weiss R. (2001). *Weiss' Herbal Medicine—Classic Edition* (p. 186). New York: Thieme.

Winston D. (2006). *Winston's Botanic Materia Medica.* Washington, NJ: DWCHS.

You-Ping Z. (1998). *Chinese Materia Medica-Chemistry, Pharmacology, and Applications* (pp. 466–468). Amsterdam: Harwood Academic Publishers.

Zou QZ, et al. (1989). Effect of motherwort on blood hyperviscosity. *American Journal of Chinese Medicine.* 17(1–2):65–70.

 NAME: Myrrh (*Commiphora myrrha, C. molmol, C. madagascariensis*)

Common Names: African myrrh, Somali myrrh, Yemen myrrh, Gum myrrh

Family: *Burseraceae*

Description of Plant

- A shrub or small tree that grows up to 30' high; native to Egypt, Sudan, Somalia, Yemen, and Ethiopia

- The gum resin exudes from natural fractures in the bark and from man-made incisions, then hardens into red-brown or yellowish-red tears.

Medicinal Part: Gum resin

Constituents and Action (if known)

- Volatile oils (limonene, dipentene, alpha coprene, elemene, lindestrene, boubonene)
- Resins: alpha, beta, and gamma commiphoric acids (25%–40%), alpha and beta heerabomyrrols, heeraboresene, burseracin
- Gum (30%–60%) contains proteoglycans
- Sesquiterpenes/lactones/terpenes (commiferin): smooth muscle relaxant (Andersson et al., 1997), local anesthetic, antibacterial, antifungal (Dolara et al., 2000)

Other Actions

- Antimicrobial, Stimulates WBC production (Hoffmann, 2003)
- Analgesic activity (Dolara et al., 2000)
- Cytoprotective effect: antiulcer effect against numerous necrotizing agents
- Prevents genotoxicity and hepatic oxidative damage caused by lead ingestion in mice (El-Ashmawy et al., 2006)

Nutritional Ingredients: Used as flavor for beverages, liqueurs, and foods

History: Used since ancient times as an incense, a medicine, and for embalming mummies in Egypt

Traditional Use

- Astringent, antibacterial, anti-inflammatory, antiulcer, carminative, analgesic, antispasmodic
- Used for sore throats, gum disease, and bronchial infections and topically for sores, infections, and muscle pain
- Long tradition of therapeutic use in traditional Chinese, Tibetan, and Unani medical traditions to treat mouth ulcers, poorly healing sores, boils, bruises, abdominal pains, and amenorrhea

Current Use

- Useful therapy with echinacea and sage for tonsillitis or pharyngitis (Winston, 2006)
- Astringent and antibacterial in mouthwashes for gingivitis and aphthous ulcers (ESCOP, 2003)
- Improves granulation and is used topically as a salve or as dusting powder to treat wounds, hemorrhoids, oozing skin conditions, and bedsores
- A number of slides have shown that myrrh has some benefits for treating heterophydiasis (Fathy et al., 2005), but its success in treating schistosomiasis is doubtful (Barakat et al., 2005).

Available Forms, Dosage, and Administration Guidelines

Preparations: Powdered gum resin, tincture, capsules, dental powders

Typical Dosage

- *Tincture* (1:5, 90% alcohol): For use in gargles, mouthwashes, and rinses; dilute with water or it may irritate mucous membranes
- *Mouthwash or gargle solution:* Add 30 to 60 gtt tincture to a glass of warm water
- *Capsule:* Two to three 400- to 500-mg capsules a day

Pharmacokinetics—If Available (form or route when known): Not known

Toxicity: None known

Contraindications: None known

Side Effects: Dermatitis from local contact (Gallo et al., 1999)

Long-Term Safety: Although no formal clinical studies have been reported, it is clear from ethnopharmacologic evidence that myrrh has been extensively used both internally and externally without apparent adverse effects (ESCOP, 2003).

Use in Pregnancy/Lactation/Children: Avoid internal use during pregnancy; topical use is fine. No known restrictions for breast-feeding and with children.

Drug/Herb Interactions and Rationale (if known): None known

BIBLIOGRAPHY

Al-Harbi MM, et al. (1997). Gastric antiulcer and cytoprotective effect of *Commiphora molmol* in rats. *Journal of Ethnopharmacology.* 55:141–150.

Andersson M, et al. (1997). Minor components with smooth muscle relaxing properties from scented myrrh (*Commiphora guidotti*). *Planta Medica.* 63(3):251–254.

Barakat R, et al. (2005). Efficacy of myrrh in the treatment of Human *Schistosomiasis mansoni. American Journal of Tropical Medicine and Hygiene.* Aug;73(2):365–367.

Blumenthal M, et al. (2000). *Herbal Medicine: Expanded Commission E Monographs* (pp. 273–277). Austin, TX: American Botanical Council.

Bradley P. (1992). *British Herbal Compendium, Vol. 1.* Bournemouth: British Herbal Medicine Association.

Der Marderosian A, Beutler J. [Eds.]. (2004). *The Review of Natural Products.* St. Louis, MO: Facts and Comparisons.

Dolara P, et al. (2000). Local anaesthetic, antibacterial and antifungal properties of sesquiterpenes from myrrh. *Planta Medica.* May;66(4):356–358.

El-Ashmawy IM, et al. (2006). Protection by turmeric and myrrh against liver oxidative damage and genotoxicity induced by lead acetate in mice. *Basic and Clinical Pharmacology and Toxicology.* Jan;98(1):32–37.

European Scientific Cooperative on Phytotherapy. (2003). *ESCOP Monographs* (pp. 340–344). New York: Thieme.

Fathy FM, et al. (2005). Effect of mirazid (*Commiphora molmol*) on experimental heterophyidiasis. *Journal of the Egyptian Society of Parasitology.* Dec;35(3):1037–1050.

Gallo R, et al. (1999). Allergic contact dermatitis from myrrh. *Contact Dermatitis.* 41(4):230–231.

Hoffmann D. (2003). *Medical Herbalism* (p. 541). Rochester, VT: Healing Arts Press.

Leung A, Foster S. (1996). *Encyclopedia of Common Natural Ingredients.* New York: John Wiley & Sons.

Winston D. (2006). *Winston's Botanic Materia Medica.* Washington, NJ: DWCHS.

NAME: Nettles (*Urtica dioica*)

Common Names: Common nettles, greater nettles, stinging nettles

Family: *Urticaceae*

Description of Plant

- Common weedy perennial found throughout the United States, Europe, and most temperate climates. Can grow 3' to 4' tall.
- Hairs on stem and leaves release formic acid when touched and can cause a burning rash (urticaria) that can last for hours.

Medicinal Part: Root, leaf, seed

Constituents and Action (if known)

- Roots and flowers: scopoletin (coumarin): anti-inflammatory activity (Chrubasik et al., 1997)
- Roots: steroids—inhibit membrane Na^+/K^+ ATPase activity of the prostate (Hirano et al., 1994)
  - Phenylpropanes
  - Lignans (secoisolariciresinol, enterodiol, enterolactone): reduced binding affinity of human sex hormone–binding globulin in vitro. Lignans may also inhibit the sex hormone–binding globulin and 5-dihydrotestosterone interaction (Mills & Bone, 2000).
- A single-chain lectin, UDA, inhibits the sex hormone–binding globulin to the receptor, thus decreasing the symptoms of benign prostatic hypertrophy (Gansser, 1995; Hartmann et al., 1996); suppresses prostate cell metabolism (Krzeski et al., 1993); inhibits cytomegalovirus and HIV (Balzarini et al., 1992)
- Leaf: flavonal glycosides—vitamins C, B complex, K, carotenoids; minerals—potassium, calcium, magnesium
- Water extracts of the leaf have shown antioxidant, analgesic, and antiulcer activity (Gulcin et al., 2004).
- Stinging hairs contain amines (histamine, serotonin, acetylcholine, formic acid).

Nutritional Ingredients: As a food, nettles contain 25% to 42% protein and are rich in Ca^{++}, Mg^{++}, zinc, K^+, selenium, silicon, and vitamins B, C, D, K, and carotenoids. Steamed nettles taste like spinach. Collect the plants when they are young, tender, light green, and no more than 6" to 10" tall. Use gloves when gathering nettles!

Traditional Use

- High iron content used to treat low hemoglobin/hematocrit and iron deficiency anemia
- Used to stop bleeding; hematuria, menorrhagia, hemoptysis; applied topically to stop nosebleeds, cuts
- Tea was applied to the head to increase hair growth.
- The Eclectics used the herb for skin conditions where the skin looks and feels like paper and tears easily
- Nonirritating diuretic used for low-grade kidney infections with low back pain

Current Use

- The leaf extract reduces inflammation (especially arthralgias) and may reduce the need for nonsteroidal anti-inflammatories by as much as 50%. Studies have found it of benefit for osteoarthritis of the thumb joint, hip, and back (Chrubasik et al., 1997; White, 1995).
- Freeze-dried product has a moderate ability to reduce allergic reaction and reduce symptoms of seasonal allergies (Mittman, 1990).
- Leaf has a mild diuretic effect (potassium-sparing) and therefore may benefit persons with hypertension, heart failure, and kidney disorders.
- Root improves urinary output and inhibits cellular proliferation in benign prostatic hyperplasia; use for stage 1 and 2 benign prostatic hyperplasia (Safarinejad, 2006). It is usually mixed with saw palmetto and/or pygeum bark (Lopatkin et al., 2006).
- Root weakly inhibits interaction between 5-alpha-reductase and dihydrotestosterone. Root also inhibits aromatase, which converts testosterone into estradiol (Winston, 1999).
- Seed is used as a kidney trophorestorative in experimental protocols for glomerulonephritis and chronic nephritis with degeneration. The initial results have been promising

(Treasure, 2003; Winston, 2006). A lectin found in nettle seed has shown an ability to protect nephons and kidneys (Mussette et al., 1996).

Available Forms, Dosage, and Administration Guidelines

Preparations: Dried leaf, dried root; capsules, tablets, tea, tincture. Studies conflict as to whether the aqueous or alcoholic extract of the root is more effective (Hryb et al., 1995; Mills & Bone, 2000). The freeze-dried herb in capsules is the most effective form for antihistamine activity.

Typical Dosage

- *Dried leaf:* 6 to 10 g a day
- *Capsules (root)* (5:1 extract): 600 to 1,200 mg a day
- *Tea (root):* Steep 1 to 2 tsp dried root in 8 oz of hot water for 30 to 40 minutes; take one or two cups daily.
- *Tea (leaf):* Steep 1 to 2 tsp dried herb in 8 oz of hot water for 20 to 30 minutes; take two to four cups daily.
- *Tincture (root)* (1:5, 30% alcohol): 40 to 60 gtt (2–3 mL) three times a day
- *Tincture (leaf)* (1:5, 30% alcohol): 60 to 100 gtt (3–5 mL) three times a day
- Or follow manufacturer or practitioner recommendations

Pharmacokinetics—If Available (form or route when known): The lectin UDA is primarily excreted via the intestines (30%–50%) and to a minor degree by the kidneys (less than 1%).

Toxicity: None known

Contraindications: Avoid using the leaf in people with hemochromatosis and hyperkalemia.

Side Effects: Contact dermatitis: the rash and blisters from nettles can last up to 12 hours. Nettle root can rarely cause nausea or vomiting; take with food. May raise glucose serum levels (Roman et al., 1992).

Long-Term Safety: Safe; has been eaten as a food for millennia

Use in Pregnancy/Lactation/Children: Herb is safe; long history of use as a food; no data for the root

Drug/Herb Interactions and Rationale (if known): Use cautiously with diuretics: may potentiate action

Special Notes: Alert patients not to self-diagnose benign prostatic hyperplasia. Recommend that they seek medical attention before beginning any prostate protocol to rule out a serious medical condition. For nettle rash, apply a compress of plantain leaf, chickweed, or jewelweed juice. International application of fresh nettles for arthritic pain is a well known (and painful) Folk therapy.

BIBLIOGRAPHY

Balzarini J, et al. (1992). The mannose-specific plant lectins from *Cymbidium hybrid* and *Epipactis helleborine* and the (N-acetylglucosamine) n-specific plant lectin from *Urtica dioica* are potent and selective inhibitors of human immunodeficiency virus and cytomegalovirus replication in vitro. *Antiviral Research.* 18(2):191–207.

Chrubasik S, et al. (1997). Evidence for antirheumatic effectiveness of Herba *Urtica dioica* in acute arthritis: A pilot study. *Phytomedicine.* 4(2):105–108.

Gansser D. (1995). Plant constituents interfering with human sex hormone-binding globulin. Evaluation of a test method and its application to *Urtica dioica* root extracts. *Zeitschrift fur Naturforschung [C].* 50:98–104.

Gulcin I, et al. (2004). Antioxidant, antimicrobial, antiulcer and analgesic activities of nettle (*Urtica dioica* L.). *Journal of Ethnopharmacology.* Feb;90(2–3):205–215.

Hartmann RW, et al. (1996). Inhibition of 5 a-reductase and aromatase by PHL-00801 (Prostatonin), a combination of PY 102 (*Pygeum africanum*) and UR 102 (*Urtica dioica*) extracts. *Phytomedicine.* 3(2):121–128.

Hirano T, et al. (1994). Effects of stinging nettle root extracts and their steroidal components on the Na^+, K^+ -ATPase of the benign prostatic hyperplasia. *Planta Medica.* 60(1):30–33.

Hryb D, et al. (1995). The effect of extracts of the roots of the stinging nettle (*Urtica dioica*) on the interaction of SHBG with its receptor on human prostatic membranes. *Planta Medica.* 61(1):31–32.

Krzeski T, et al. (1993). Combined extracts of *Urtica dioica* and *Pygeum africanum* in the treatment of benign prostatic hyperplasia: Double-blind comparison of two doses. *Clinical Therapeutics.* 15(6):1011–1020.

Lopatkin NA, et al. (2006). Combined extract of sabal palm and nettle in the treatment of patients with lower urinary tract symptoms in double blind, placebo-controlled trial. *Urologia.* Mar-Apr;(2):12,14–19.

Mills S, Bone K. (2000). *Principles and Practice of Phytotherapy* (pp. 490–498). Edinburgh, UK: Churchill Livingstone.

Mittman P. (1990). Randomized, double-blind study of freeze-dried *Urtica dioica* in the treatment of allergic rhinitis. *Planta Medica.* 56:44–47.

Mussette P, et al. (1996). *Urtica dioica* agglutinin, a V Beta 8.3-specific superantigen, prevents the development of the systemic lupus erythematosus-like pathology of MRL lpr/lpr mice. *European Journal of Immunology.* Aug;26(8):1707–1711.

Randall C, et al. (2000). Randomized controlled trial of nettle sting for treatment of base-of-thumb pain. *Journal of the Royal Society of Medicine.* Jun;93(6):305–309.

Safarinejad MR. (2006). *Urtica dioica* for treatment of benign prostatic hyperplasia: A prospective, randomized, double-blind, placebo-controlled, crossover study. *Journal of Herbal Pharmacotherapy.* 5(4):1–11.

Treasure J. (2003). Urtica semen reduces serum creatinine levels. *Journal of the American Herbalists Guild.* 4(2):22–25.

Wagner H, et al. (1994). Search for the antiprostatic principle of stinging nettle (*Urtica dioica*) roots. *Phytomedicine.* 1(3): 213–224.

White A. (1995). Stinging nettles for osteoarthritis pain of the hip. *British Journal of General Practice.* 45(392):162.

Wichtl M, Bisset N. [Eds.]. (1994). *Herbal Drugs and Phytopharmaceuticals* (pp. 505–509). Stuttgart: Medpharm.

Winston D. (1999). *Saw Palmetto for Men and Women* (pp. 62–78). Pownal, CT: Storey Publishing.

Winston D. (2006). *Winston's Botanic Materia Medica.* Washington, NJ: DWCHS.

NAME: Noni (*Morinda citrifolia*)

Common Names: Hog apple, Indian mulberry, nonu

Family: *Rubiaceae*

Description of Plant

- An evergreen shrub or small tree native to southeast Asia; has become naturalized in Polynesia, Australia, Mexico, the Caribbean, and Central America

- Has white flowers and yellow fruit about the size of a potato with a bumpy surface. Ripe fruit has cheese-like, offensive odor.

Medicinal Part: Fruit, leaves, bark

Constituents and Action (if known)
- Anthraquinones: laxative, antibacterial—trace amounts
- Fatty acids: linoleic, oleic, caproic, caprylic acids, octanic acid: insecticidal activity (Dixon et al., 1999)
- Neolignans: americanin A—antioxidant (Su et al., 2005)
- Alcohol extracts of leaves display anthelmintic activity against human *Ascaris lumbricoides*.
- Immunodulatory polysaccharide: noni PPT (Hirazumi & Furusawa, 1999)
- A researcher has claimed to have identified an "alkaloid/xeronine;" it is theorized to work at the molecular level to repair damaged cells to regulate their function (digestive, respiratory, bone, and skin can all benefit) (Hirazumi & Furusawa, 1999; U.S. Patent #5,288,491, 1994). No other researchers have validated this claim; in fact, they have dismissed this research as seriously flawed.
- Other actions: may have anticancer activity (studied in Lewis lung carcinoma in mice) by enhancing immune system activity (Hirazumi et al., 1994; Hirazumi & Furusawa, 1999)

Nutritional Ingredients: Contains vitamin A; edible fruit is usually layered in sugar; leaves are consumed raw or cooked

Traditional Use
- Traditional ethnobotanical use by Hawaiians and other Polynesian peoples was primarily as a topical application for boils, ringworm, rheumatic pain, neuralgia, bruises, gout, and infections.
- Seeds were used as a purgative and anthelmintic in the Philippines.
- In Hawaii, by the 1930s, noni had become a popular ingredient in many compound formulas (usually mixed with ginger, coconut milk, or sugar cane juice); it was

taken orally for tuberculosis, intestinal worms, and sexually transmitted diseases and for "purifying the blood."

Current Use

- Promoted as a panacea for a wide range of diseases, including cancer, atherosclerosis, AIDS, obesity, hypertension, and diabetes. There is currently no research on the effectiveness of this herb for these conditions. The product seems to have a low potential for toxicity, but it is unclear whether noni has any real health benefits.
- Based on a long history of use for topical complaints, noni may be useful as a local application for skin infections, abscesses, boils, carbuncles, abrasions, blemishes, wounds, bruises, and arthritic pain.

Available Forms, Dosage, and Administration Guidelines

Preparations: Noni juice (10%–97% noni mixed with fruit juices), dry extract, tincture

Typical Dosage: The juice product should be taken on an empty stomach 30 minutes before meals. Take 1 to 2 oz twice a day.

Pharmacokinetics—If Available (form or route when known): Not known

Toxicity: Three cases of possible noni-induced hepatotoxicity have been reported (Yuce et al., 2006). Researchers working for a company that produces the product state that in human and animal studies, this herb juice shows no evidence of liver toxicity (West et al., 2006).

Contraindications: Hyperkalemia: the juice products contain fruit juices that often have substantial potassium content (Mueller et al., 2000)

Side Effects: None known

Long-Term Safety: Has been used for thousands of years as a healing plant and food; would appear to be safe

Use in Pregnancy/Lactation/Children: According to one manufacturer of noni juice, it is safe in pregnant and lactating women and children 7 months and older. Lack of objective research confirming this statement warrants a more conservative approach. Avoid use in pregnancy, lactation, and in young children.

Drug/Herb Interactions and Rationale (if known): None known

Special Notes: Most research has been done by companies with commercial interests in the product.

BIBLIOGRAPHY

Dittmar A. (1993). *Morinda citrifolia* L.: Use in indigenous Samoan medicine. *Journal of Herbs, Spices and Medicinal Plants.* 1(3): 77–92.

Dixon AR, et al. (1999). Ferment this: The transformation of noni, a traditional Polynesian medicine (*Morinda citrifolia*, Rubiaceae). *Economic Botany.* 53(1):51–68.

Hirazumi A, et al. (1994). Anticancer activity of *Morinda citrifolia* (noni) on intraperitoneally implanted Lewis lung carcinoma in syngeneic mice. *Proceedings of the Western Pharmacologic Society.* 37:145–146.

Hirazumi A, et al. (1996). Immunomodulation contributes to the anticancer activity of *Morinda citrifolia* (noni) fruit juice. *Proceedings of the Western Pharmacologic Society.* 39:7–9.

Hirazumi A, Furusawa E. (1999). An immunomodulatory polysaccharide-rich substance from the fruit juice of *Morinda citrifolia* (noni) with antitumor activity. *Phytotherapy Research.* 13(5):380–387.

Mueller BA, et al. (2000). Noni juice (*Morinda citrifolia*): Hidden potential for hyperkalemia? *American Journal of Kidney Disease.* 35(2):310–312.

Su BN, et al. (2005). Chemical constituents of the fruits of *Morinda citrifolia* (noni) and their antioxidant activity. *Journal of Natural Products.* Apr;68(4):592–595.

West BJ, et al. (2006). Noni juice is not hepatotoxic. *World Journal of Gastroenterology.* Jun 14;12(22):3616–3619.

Yuce B, et al. (2006). Hepatitis induced by noni juice from *Morinda citrifolia:* A rare cause of hepatotoxicity or the tip of the iceberg? *Digestion.* 73(2–3):167–170.

O

 NAME: Olive Leaf (*Olea europaea*)

Common Names: Olive leaf

Family: *Oleaceae*

Description of Plant

- Evergreen tree, grows to 25' to 30' tall, source of olives and olive oil
- Native to Mediterranean but cultivated in California
- Leaves can be gathered throughout the year.

Medicinal Part: Leaves

Constituents and Action (if known)

- Secoiridoid glycosides
  - Oleuropein (oleouropeoside): antibacterial— *Staphylococcus*, *Bacillus cereus*, antiviral, antifungal properties, reduces blood pressure (in animal studies) through vasodilation, antiarrhythmic, mild calcium antagonist (Weiss & Fintelmann, 2000), inhibits oxidation of low-density lipoprotein (Zheng, 1999)
  - Antioxidant properties (Bruneton, 1999), antispasmodic, coronary vasodilator (Zarzuelo et al., 1991)
  - Antidiabetic activity by increasing peripheral uptake of glucose and potentiates glucose-induced insulin release (Gonzalez et al., 1992)
  - Calcium elenolate, a hydrolyzed form of oleuropein, shows antiviral activity (Zheng et al., 1999)
- Ligustroside, oleuroside, oleacein: inhibits vasoconstriction by blocking production of angiotensin II (Zheng et al., 1999)
- Flavonoids (rutin, glycosides of apigenin and leuteolin) (Bruneton, 1999)
- Phenols: caffeic acid, antioxidant; 2-(3,4 dihydroxyphenyl) ethanol, inhibits platelet aggregation and production of thromboxane A2 (Zheng et al., 1999)
- Triterpenes (oleanolic acid, maslinic acid, erythrodiol): hypotensive, reduced insulin resistance and inhibited atherosclerosis in rats (Somova et al., 2003)

Nutritional Ingredients: None known

Traditional Use
- Hypoglycemic agent, hypotensive, diuretic, astringent, antipyretic
- Used in Europe for mild hypertension
- Used to treat diabetes in Trinidad and Tobago as well as in European folk medicine
- Used to treat malaria
- Topical astringent and antiseptic for skin

Current Use
- To lower blood pressure: useful for mild hypertension (Cherif et al., 1996; Khayyal et al., 2002), usually combined with other herbs such as hawthorn, motherwort, black haw, and dandelion leaf (Winston, 2006)
- May be useful for borderline type 2 diabetes and insulin resistance (metabolic syndrome), but more research is needed (Somova et al., 2003)
- Many websites and articles recommend olive leaf as a broad-spectrum antiviral and antibacterial agent for a wide range of diseases. The research on olive leaf constituents as an antimicrobial is almost entirely in vitro and not confirmed by human or animal studies.

Available Forms, Dosage, and Administration Guidelines
Preparations: Dried leaf; extracts containing 6% to 15% oleuropein, tincture, pills, capsules. Take with meals to avoid GI upset.
Typical Dosage
- *Tea*: Steep 1 tsp dried leaves in 1 cup hot water for 20 minutes; take a half-cup two or three times a day.
- *Tincture* (1:5, 60% alcohol): 30 to 40 gtt (1.5–2 mL) three times a day
- *Capsules:* One or two capsules twice a day with meals to avoid GI upset or follow manufacturer recommendations

Pharmacokinetics—If Available (form or route when known): None known

Toxicity: None known

Contraindications: May lower blood sugar in patients with hypoglycemia (Gonzalez et al., 1992)

Side Effects: GI upset occasionally has been reported.

Long-Term Safety: Not known

Use in Pregnancy/Lactation/Children: No research; do not use

Drug/Herb Interactions and Rationale (if known): None known

Special Notes
- A current testimonial claims that this herb should be used for chronic fatigue syndrome, herpes and other viral infections, arthritis, yeast infections, and skin conditions. No real research exists to support these claims.
- Regular use of olive oil has been found to inhibit inflammation, mildly reduce blood lipids, and atherosclerotic changes. Olive fruit extract has been found to be effective in relieving pain and stiffness due to osteoarthritis (Bitler et al., 2007).

BIBLIOGRAPHY

Bitler CM et al., (2007). Olive extract supplement decreases pain and improves daily activities in adults with osteoarthritis and decreases plasma homocysteine in those with rheumatoid arthritis. *Nutrition Research.* 27:470–477.

Bruneton J. (1999). Pharmacognosy, *Phytochemistry, Medicinal Plants* (pp. 602–604). Paris: Lavoisier.

Cherif S, et al. (1996). A clinical trial of a titrated olea extract in the treatment of essential arterial hypertension. *Journal de Pharmacie de Belgique (Belgium).* Mar-Apr;51(2):69–71.

Gonzalez M, et al. (1992). Hypoglycemic activity of olive leaf. *Planta Medica.* 58(6):513–515.

Hansen K, et al. (1996). Isolation of an angiotensin-converting enzyme (ACE) inhibitor from *Olea europaea* and *Olea lancea. Phytomedicine.* 2(4):319–325.

Khayyal MT, et al. (2002). Blood pressure lowering effect of an olive leaf extract (*Olea europaea*) in L-NAME induced hypertension in rats. *Arzneimittelforschung.* 52(11):797–802.

Somova LI, et al. (2003). Antihypertensive, antiatherosclerotic, and antioxidant activity of triterpenoids isolated from *Olea europaea,* subspecies africana leaves. *Journal of Ethnopharmacology.* Feb;84(2–3):299–305.

Weiss R, Fintelmann V. (2000). *Herbal Medicine* (2nd ed.; pp. 173–174). Stuttgart: Thieme.

Winston D. (2006). *Winston's Botanic Materia Medica*. Washington, NJ: DWCHS.

Zarzuelo A, et al. (1991). Vasodilator effect of olive leaf. *Planta Medica*. 57(5):417–419.

Zheng QY, et al. (1999). *Review of Pharmacology and Chemistry of Olive Leaf (Olea europaea L.)*. [Unpublished manuscript.]

 NAME: Passion Flower (*Passiflora incarnata*)

Common Names: Apricot vine, passionfruit, maypop, passion vine

Family: *Passifloraceae*

Description of Plant

- Most plants in this family are vines. There are more than 400 different species. Some have edible fruit, and many have showy flowers.
- Different species are native to tropical and subtropical areas of the Americas; *P. incarnata* is a creeping vine native to the southeastern United States.

Medicinal Part: Dried or fresh above-ground herb and flower

Constituents and Action (if known)

- Flavonoids (2.5%) (shaftoside, isoshaftoside, isovitexin, isoorientin, lucenin-2, vicenin-2): may account for sedative activity (Bokstaller et al., 1997; Bourin et al., 1997
- Maltol (0.05%): relaxes skeletal muscle, reduces corneal reflexes, reduces spontaneous activity, induces sleep (Bourin et al., 1997)
- Cyanogenic glycosides (0.01%): gynocardin
- Indole alkaloids (trace amounts only) (harmine, harman, harmol): have sedative effects through monoamine oxidase inhibition; not enough present to have any activity

Other Actions

- In vitro, has antimicrobial activity against a hemolytic streptococci, *Staphylococcus aureus*, and *Candida*
- Antibacterial (Bokstaller et al., 1997)

- No single constituent or group of constituents has been found to be responsible for passion flower's activity. Recent research suggests that two unidentified compounds that are not alkaloids or flavonoids may have significant activity (Bruneton, 1999).

Nutritional Ingredients: Fruit used for juices and jellies

History: Folklore suggests that the flower resembles the crucifixion: the three styles are the nails, the five stamens are the five wounds, the ovary resembles a hammer, the corona resembles the crown of thorns, the petals represent the 10 true apostles, the white color symbolizes purity, and the purple color heaven.

Traditional Use
- Sedative, nervine, antispasmodic, anxiolytic
- The eclectic indications for this herb are insomnia with circular thinking: the patient cannot seem to turn off his or her mind.
- Used for insomnia, anxiety, nervous tachycardia, neuralgias, and nervous headaches

Current Use
- Minor sleeplessness associated with stress (Bradley, 1992); combine with hawthorn, valerian, lemon balm, or linden flower
- GI disturbance caused by stress; combine with catnip, valerian, or chamomile (Winston, 2006)
- Reduces menopausal anxiety and sleeplessness; use with motherwort and black cohosh
- Anxiety disorders (Dhawan et al., 2004); use it with Motherwort, Blue Vervain, Chinese Polygale and Bacopa (Winston, 2006).

Available Forms, Dosage, and Administration Guidelines
Preparations: Dried herb, fluid extract, tea, tincture, combination products with other nervine herbs

Typical Dosage
- *Dried herb:* 1 to 2 g three times a day
- *Tea:* Steep 1 tsp dried herb in 1 cup hot water for 15 to 20 minutes; take two cups a day.
- *Tincture* (1:5, 40% alcohol): 40 to 80 gtt (2–4 mL) up to four times a day
- *Fluid extracts* (1:1 in 25% alcohol): 0.5 to 2 mL three times a day
- Or follow manufacturer or practitioner recommendations

Pharmacokinetics—If Available (form or route when known): Not known

Toxicity: None known

Contraindications: Depression (Brinker, 2001)

Side Effects: Slight CNS depression

Long-Term Safety: Unknown

Use in Pregnancy/Lactation/Children: There is a theoretical possibility of a uterine-stimulating action caused by several constituents of this herb (Brinker, 2001). Use cautiously during pregnancy. No known restrictions for lactation or in children.

Drug/Herb Interactions and Rationale (if known): Possible additive effect with CNS depressants; theoretical concern (Carlini, 2003)

BIBLIOGRAPHY

Bokstaller S, et al. (1997). Comparative study on the content of passionflower flavonoids and sesquiterpenes from valerian root extracts in pharmaceutical preparations by HPLC. *Pharmazie.* 52:552–557.

Bourin M, et al. (1997). A combination of plant extracts in the treatment of outpatients with adjustment disorder with anxious mood: Controlled study vs. placebo. *Fundamentals of Clinical Pharmacology.* 11(2):127–132.

Bradley P. (1992). *British Herbal Compendium, Vol. 1* (pp. 171–173). Dorset: British Herbal Medicine Association.

Brinker F. (2001). *Herb Contraindications & Drug Interactions* (p. 158). Sandy, OR: Eclectic Medical Publications.

Bruneton J. (1999). *Pharmacognosy, Phytochemistry, Medicinal Plants* (pp. 331–335). Paris: Lavoisier.

Carlini EA. (2003). Plants and the central nervous system. *Pharmacology, Biochemistry and Behavior.* Jun;75(3):501–512.

Dhawan K, et al., (2004). Passiflora: A review update. *Journal of Ethnopharmacology*. Sept; 94(1):1–23.

Dhawan K, et al. (2003). Antiasthmatic activity of the methanol extract of leaves of *Passiflora incarnata*. *Phytotherapy Research*. Aug;17(7):821–822.

Israel D, et al. (1997). Herbal therapies for perimenopausal and menopausal complaints. *Pharmacotherapy*. 17(5):970–984.

Winston D. (2006). *Winston's Botanic Materia Medica*. Washington, NJ: DWCHS.

 NAME: Pau D'arco (*Tabebuia impetiginosa, T. ipe*)

Common Names: Ipe roxo, lapacho colorado, lapacho morado, purple lapacho, red lapacho, taheebo

Family: *Bignoniaceae*

Description of Plant
- Evergreen flowering trees with red, violet, and pink flowers. Species that have yellow flowers are considered to be inferior as a medicine.
- Native to South America, especially Brazil and Argentina

Medicinal Part: Inner bark

Constituents and Action (if known)
- Quinone compounds (naphthoquinones)
  - Lapachol and beta-lapachone: antimicrobial activity against gram-positive and gram-negative organisms and fungas (Guiraud et al., 1994) and MRSA (Pereira et al., 2006), antitumor activity, antimalarial, antischistosomal, antifungal, antiviral, anticoagulant (Mills & Bone, 2000; Park et al., 2006)
  - Xyloidone, deoxylapachol
- Anthroquinone: tabebuin-shows activity against H. Pylori (Park et al., 2006)
- Furonaphthoquinones

Nutritional Ingredients: None known

Traditional Use
- Anticancer, antibacterial, antiviral, antifungal, anti-inflammatory, diuretic

- Used for a broad spectrum of diseases, including dysentery, gastric ulcers, snake bites, fevers, and malaria
- Skin diseases: topically and orally for fungal infections, skin cancers, eczema, psoriasis, and wounds
- Used as a cancer cure for a wide range of carcinomas, including leukemia

Current Use

- In Brazil, it is used to treat cancer; effectiveness is unproven; may be useful as an adjunctive immune stimulant
- Adjunctive therapy to treat viral infections such as herpes, flu, and colds
- Used to treat fungal and bacterial infections (candidiasis, topical MRSA infections) (Pereira et al., 2006)
- The bark extract inhibits *Helicobacter pylori* and may be useful for treating gastritis and gastric ulcers (Park et al., 2006).
- Possible use for treating malaria and schistosomiasis; additional research needed

Available Forms, Dosage, and Administration Guidelines
Preparations: Dried bark, capsules, tincture, tea
Typical Dosage
- No therapeutic dosage has been established.
- *Capsules:* Up to four 500- to 600-mg capsules or nine 300-mg capsules a day
- *Tea:* Simmer 2 to 3 tsp inner bark in 2 cups water for 15 minutes; divide into two or three daily doses.
- *Tincture* (1:5, 40% alcohol): 20 to 50 gtt (1–2.5 mL) up to four times a day
- Or follow manufacturer or practitioner recommendations

Pharmacokinetics—If Available (form or route when known): None known

Toxicity: Very low

Contraindications: Blood clotting disorders

Side Effects: Nausea, vomiting, intestinal discomfort (isolated lapachol); pink urine; anticoagulant effects with high doses

Long-Term Safety: Unknown

Use in Pregnancy/Lactation/Children: The isolated phytochemical lapachol has abortive and teratogenic effects. The whole herb, which contains very small amounts of lapachol, should be used very cautiously if at all during pregnancy and only under clinical supervision.

Drug/Herb Interactions and Rationale (if known): Avoid concurrent use with anticoagulants; may potentiate effects.

Special Notes: Research has primarily been done in the laboratory and not on living organisms. National Cancer Institute researchers isolated lapachol in the 1960s and 1970s, with no significant findings. The anticancer activity might come from the whole bark rather than one isolated constituent. More research is necessary. Most products in the North American marketplace have very low levels of lapachol; Brazilian products have much higher levels of this therapeutically active phytochemical (Awang, 1988).

BIBLIOGRAPHY

De Miranda FG, et al. (2001). Antinociceptive and antiedematogenic properties and acute toxicity of *Tabebuia avellanedae Lor. ex Griseb.* inner bark aqueous extract. *BMC Pharmacology.* 1:6.

Dinnen RD, Ebisuzaki K. (1997). Search for novel anticancer agents: A differentiation-based assay and analysis of a folklore product. *Anticancer Research.* 17:1027–1034.

Guiraud P, et al. (1994). Comparison of antibacterial and antifungal activities of lapachol and beta-lapachone. *Planta Medica.* 60:373–374.

Mills S, Bone K. (2000). *Principles and Practice of Phytotherapy* (pp. 499–506). Edinburgh: Churchill Livingstone.

Park BS, et al. (2006). Antibacterial activity of *Tabebuia impetiginosa* Martius ex DC (Taheebo) against *Helicobacter pylori. Journal of Ethnopharmacology.* Apr 21;105(1–2):255–262.

Pereira EM, et al. (2006). *Tabebuia avellanedae* naphthoquinones: Activity against methicillin-resistant staphylococcal strains, cytotoxic activity and in vivo dermal irritability analysis. *Annals of Clinical Microbiology and Antimicrobials.* Mar 22;5:5.

Schutes RE, Raffauf, RF. (1990). The Healing Forest, Medicinal and
    Toxic Plants of the Northwest Amazonia (pp. 107–108). Portland,
    OR: Dioscorides Press.
Warashina T, et al. (2006). Constituents from the bark of *Tabebuia
    impetiginosa*. *Phytochemistry*. Jan;54(1):14–20.

 NAME: Pennyroyal (*Hedeoma pulegioides, Mentha
pulegium*)

Common Names: American pennyroyal (*H. pulegioides*),
European pennyroyal (*M. pulegium*)

Family: *Lamiaceae*

Description of Plant
- Both plants are small members of the mint family with a
  very strong mint odor.
- American pennyroyal is a small, upright annual herb;
  European pennyroyal is a creeping perennial.

Medicinal Part: Herb, EO (very toxic)

Constituents and Action (if known): Volatile oils
(monoterpene ketones): pulegone (hepatotoxic; Khojasteh-
Bakht et al., 1999), isomenthone, menthone, piperitenone

Nutritional Ingredients: None

Traditional Use
- Abortifacient, carminative, diaphoretic, emmenagogue
- Used to induce "herbal" abortions: this is a very dangerous
  procedure with the EO and not a very effective one with the
  herb or tea
- Used as a carminative for gas, nausea, and vomiting
- The hot tea was used as a diaphoretic to induce sweating
  and lower fevers.

Current Use
- The tea can be useful for scanty menstruation with a clotty
  flow and cramps. Use mixed with ginger, chamomile, and
  motherwort. Short-term use only.

- The EO has been found to kill *Pediculus capitis* (head lice) diluted in a carrier oil and applied topically and as a fumigant (Yang et al., 2004). How safe the EO is on the skin or inhaled is not known.

Available Forms, Dosage, and Administration Guidelines
Preparations: Tea, tincture, EO
Typical Dosage
- *Tea:* 0.5 tsp dried herb in 8 oz hot water, steep 15 minutes (covered); take 4 oz twice daily. Take for no more than a few days a month.
- *Tincture* (1:5, 35% alcohol): Avoid
- *EO:* Toxic; do not use

Pharmacokinetics—If Available (form or route when known): Metabolized by the liver, where pulegone is converted by cytochrome P450 enzymes into menthofuran, a proximate hepatotoxic metabolite of pulegone

Toxicity: Causes uterine contractions. The EO is associated with seizures, respiratory depression, liver failure, and death.

Contraindications: Pregnancy, menorrhagia, liver disease, kidney disease, seizure disorders

Side Effects: Some pregnant women become nauseated just from smelling pennyroyal.

Long-Term Safety: Use only the tea in healthy adults and on a short-term basis. Not recommended for regular use (Bruneton, 1999).

Use in Pregnancy/Lactation/Children: Avoid in all

Drug/Herb Interactions and Rationale (if known): None known

Special Notes: Do not use the EO topically or orally. Pet owners who have heard that the oil repels mosquitoes and ticks have applied it to pets who, on licking it off, have experienced liver and kidney failure and death. N-acetylcysteine has been successfully used to treat poisoning caused by ingestion of pennyroyal EO.

BIBLIOGRAPHY

Anderson IB, et al. (1996). Pennyroyal toxicity: Measurement of toxic metabolite levels in two cases and review of the literature. *Annals of Internal Medicine.* 124(8):726–734.

Bakerink JA, et al. (1996). Multiple organ failure after ingestion of pennyroyal oil from herbal tea in two infants. *Pediatrics.* 98(5):944–947.

Bruneton J. (1999). *Pharmacognosy, Phytochemistry, Medicinal Plants* (p. 547). Paris: Lavoisier.

Khojasteh-Bakht S, et al. (1999). Metabolism of (R)-(+)-pulegone and (R)-(+)-menthofuran by human liver cytochrome P-450s: Evidence for formation of a furan epoxide. *Drug Metabolism and Disposition.* 28(5):574–580.

Newall C, et al. (1996). *Herbal Medicines* (p. 208). London: Pharmaceutical Press.

Sudekum M, et al. (1992). Pennyroyal oil toxicosis in a dog. *Journal of the American Veterinary Medical Association.* 200(6):817–818.

Sullivan JB Jr, et al. (1979). Pennyroyal oil poisoning and hepatotoxicity. *Journal of the American Medical Association.* 242(26):2873–2874.

Tisserand R, Balacs T. (1995). *Essential Oil Safety* (pp. 159–160). Edinburgh: Churchill Livingstone.

Yang YC, et al. (2004). Insecticidal activity of plant essential oils against *Pediculus humanus capitis* (Anoplura: Pediculidae). *Journal of Medical Entomology.* Jul;41(4):699–704.

NAME: Peppermint *(Mentha piperita)* (hybrid of spearmint [*M. spicata*] and water mint [*M. aquatica*])

Common Names: Peppermint

Family: *Lamiaceae*

Description of Plant

- Aromatic perennial member of the mint family with square purple-green stems and leaves and small, lilac-colored flowers
- Plant is sterile and spreads through rhizomes underground.
- Many varieties of peppermint exist and are cultivated worldwide.

Medicinal Part: Dried herb, EO

Constituents and Action (if known)

- More than 100 components have been identified.
- Volatile oils
  - Menthol (35%–55%): antispasmodic in the colon, calcium antagonist effect, reduces abdominal pain, smooth muscle relaxant, decongestant, topical analgesic (ESCOP, 2003)
  - Menthone (10%–35%), isomenthone (1.5%–10%), menthyl acetate (2.8%–10%), limonene (1%–5%)
- Flavonoids (luteolin, rutin, hesperidin, erioeitrin): bile-stimulating activity in doses of 0.1 to 50 mg/kg (dogs and guinea pigs) but 25 to 50 mg/kg constricted the sphincter; antiviral, antioxidant, antiallergic (McKay & Blumberg, 2006).
- Phenolic acids: rosmarinic acid—antioxidant

Other Actions

- Peppermint EO stimulated bile secretion.
- EO and menthol have antibacterial activity.
- EO has antiviral activity against herpes simplex virus types 1 and 2 (Schumacher et al., 2003).

Nutritional Ingredients: Flavoring for mouthwashes, teas, candies; fresh leaves are used in Middle Eastern cuisine

Traditional Use

- Carminative, GI antispasmodic, choleretic, antipruritic (menthol), nervine, topical analgesic, antiemetic
- Used with elderflower for fevers in children
- Used to treat digestive upsets, including flatulence, nausea, borborygmus, and intestinal cramps
- Used to relieve colic in infants in combination with chamomile; often given to breast-feeding mothers: the oils pass into the breast milk, relieving gas in the infant

Current Use

- Enteric-coated capsules containing peppermint EO are used as a smooth muscle relaxant for irritable bowel syndrome (Grigoleit et al., 2005). The enteric-coated capsules have also been used successfully as an antispasmodic for double-contrast barium meal examinations (Mizuno et al., 2006), for upper GI endoscopy (Hiki et al., 2003), and for endoscopic retrograde cholangiopancreatography (Yamamoto et al., 2006).

- The EO is used as an inhalation for congestion, cough, and colds, usually combined with eucalyptus, thyme, or tea tree EO.
- The tea is effective for digestive disturbances: dyspepsia, flatulence, nausea, biliousness, and stress-induced GI disturbance (combined with valerian, catnip, or chamomile). The EO combined with caraway EO was as effective as cisapride for functional dyspepsia (Freise & Kohler, 1999; Madisch et al., 1999). The EO of peppermint was also useful for postoperative nausea (Tate, 1997).
- The EO is used as a counterirritant in topical analgesics for rheumatic pain, toothache, headache and postherpetic neuralgia (Davies et al., 2002).
- Antipruritic in topical creams (EO or menthol) for symptomatic relief of itching caused by poison ivy, insect bites, and dry skin.
- A tea of peppermint leaf mixed with linden flower, chamomile, or lemon balm is flavorful and relaxing for minor stress, insomnia, or tension headaches.

Available Forms, Dosage, and Administration Guidelines

Preparations: Dried herb, tea, capsules, tincture, EO, ointment (semisolid preparation containing 5%–20% EO in base of beeswax and olive oil)

Typical Dosage

- *Infusion:* 2 tsp dried herb in 8 oz of hot water, steep covered 15 to 20 minutes; take two to four cups a day
- *Tincture* (1:5, 30% alcohol): 60 to 120 gtt (3–6 mL) two or three times daily
- *EO:* 6 to 12 gtt a day for internal and external use, unless otherwise prescribed. Average single dose for internal use is 0.2 to 0.4 mL of EO diluted in carrier oils. For IBS, the average daily dose is 0.6 mL of EO in the enteric-coated capsules or 1 to 2 capsules TID.
- *Inhalant:* Add 3 to 4 gtt EO to hot water; deeply inhale the steam vapor

- *External use:* Rub a few drops of EO into the affected skin areas. Should be diluted with a carrier such as apricot, olive, or sesame oil.
- *Ointment or unguent:* Apply locally by massage

Pharmacokinetics—If Available (form or route when known): Menthol and other terpenes are fat soluble and rapidly absorbed by the small intestine. Excretion by the kidney peaks in 3 hours.

Toxicity: None known

Contraindications: Hiatal hernia and GERD, because it relaxes the GI smooth muscle and may worsen symptoms. Do not use EO on the face or mucous membranes (conjunctiva, vagina).

Side Effects: Menthol component may cause allergic reaction and contact dermatitis.

Long-Term Safety: Safe

Use in Pregnancy/Lactation/Children: No restrictions of the tea for pregnant or breast-feeding women. Avoid using the EO internally while pregnant. Do not give to or apply directly to the nasal or chest area of infants and small children because there is a risk of laryngeal or bronchial spasms. Give the tea to the mother, and the oils will pass through the breast milk.

Drug/Herb Interactions and Rationale (if known): Peppermint EO enhanced the bioavailability of felodipine and simvastatin and inhibited CYP 3A4 in vitro and in vivo. (Dresser et al., 2002).

Special Notes: Peppermint EO has low toxicity compared with many other essential oils; however, it is still a highly concentrated substance and should be diluted before use and used with caution.

BIBLIOGRAPHY

Davies SJ, et al. (2002). A novel treatment of postherpetic neuralgia using peppermint oil. *Clinical Journal of Pain.* May-Jun;18(3): 200–202.

Dresser GK, et al. (2002). Peppermint oil increases the oral bioavailability of felodipine and simvastatin. American Society for Clinical Pharmacology and Therapeutics Annual Meeting, March 24–28;TPII-95.

European Scientific Cooperative on Phytotherapy. (2003). *ESCOP Monographs* (pp. 329–336). New York: Thieme.

Freise J, Kohler S. (1999). Peppermint oil–caraway oil fixed combination in non-ulcer dyspepsia: Comparison of the effects of enteric preparations. *Pharmazie*. 54(3):210–215.

Grigoleit HG, et al. (2005). Peppermint oil in irritable bowel syndrome. *Phytomedicine*. Aug;12(8):601–606.

Hiki N, et al. (2003). Peppermint oil reduces gastric spasm during upper endoscopy: A randomized, double-blind, double-dummy controlled trial. *Gastrointestinal Endoscopy*. Apr;57(4):475–482.

Kingham JGC. (1995). Commentary: Peppermint oil and colon spasm. *Lancet*. 346:986.

Madisch A, et al. (1999). Treatment of functional dyspepsia with a fixed peppermint oil and caraway oil combination preparation as compared to cisapride. A multicenter, reference-controlled double-blind equivalence study. *Arzneimittelforschung*. 49(11):925–932.

McKay DL, Blumberg JB. (2006). A review of the bioactivity and potential health benefits of peppermint tea (*Mentha piperita* L.). *Phytotherapy Research*. Aug;20(8):619–633.

Mizuno S, et al. (2006). Oral peppermint is a useful antispasmodic for double-contrast barium meal examination. *Journal of Gastroenterology and Hepatology*. Aug;21(8):1297–1301.

Pittler MH, Ernst E. (1998). Peppermint oil for irritable bowel syndrome: A critical review and meta-analysis. *American Journal of Gastroenterology*. 93(7):1131–1135.

Schumacher A, et al. (2003). Virucidal effect of peppermint oil on the enveloped viruses herpes simplex virus type 1 and type 2 in vitro. *Phytomedicine*. 10(6-7):504–510.

Tate S. (1997). Peppermint oil: A treatment for postoperative nausea. *Journal of Advanced Nursing*. 26(3):543–549.

Weiss RF, Fintelmann V. (2000). *Herbal Medicine* (2nd ed.; pp. 45–46). Stuttgart: Thieme.

Yamamoto N, et al. (2006). Efficacy of peppermint oil as an antispasmodic during endoscopic retrograde cholangiopancreatography. *Journal of Gastroenterology and Hepatology*. Sep;21(9):1394–1398.

NAME: Picrorrhiza (*Picrorrhiza kurroa,*
P. scrophulariiflora)

Common Names: Katuki

Family: *Scrophulariaceae*

Description of Plant: A small perennial herb native to the northwestern Himalayas, from Kashmir to Sikkim

Medicinal Part: Root

Constituents and Action (if known)
- Iridoid glycosides (picoside I, II, III, kutkoside): hepatoprotective (Bone, 1994)
- Triterpenes (cucurbitacin glycosides)
- Bitter substances (apocynin, androsin)

Other Actions: Antioxidant

Nutritional Ingredients: None

Traditional Use
- Anti-inflammatory, bitter tonic, choleretic, hepatoprotective, laxative
- Used in Ayurvedic medicine as a liver and bowel stimulant, for constipation, and for periodic fevers (malaria), to treat hepatitis A with jaundice, and used topically for snake bites and scorpion stings

Current Use
- Hepatoprotective agent: used to prevent and treat liver damage caused by hepatitis A, B, or C; industrial chemicals (carbon tetrachloride); aflatoxin B(1); pharmaceutical drugs; and *Entamoeba histolytica* (Singh et al., 2005) by inhibiting lipid peroxidation of liver microsomes, increasing free radical scavenging activity, and increasing nucleic acid and protein synthesis (in rat livers). Reduces elevated liver enzymes; reduces nausea, vomiting, and anorexia; and has shown superior activity to the well-researched herb milk thistle (Saraswat et al., 1999; Lee et al., 2006).
- Used for treating asthma: stabilizes mast cells and inhibits allergen and PAF-induced bronchial obstruction by a nonspecific anti-inflammatory effect (Williamson, 2002)

- Immune potentiation and modulator: an ethanotic extract of this herb increased T-cell, B-cell, and phagocytic function. Oral administration of the standardized Picroliv at 10 mg/kg for 7 days stimulated antigen-specific and nonspecific immune response; there was a 10-fold increase in antibody production and a 77.5% increase in activated lymphocytes (Bone, 1996; Williamson, 2002).
- In a 7-year study, picrorrhiza combined with psoralens and light therapy dramatically decreased the number and size of depigmented skin patches in vitiligo.
- Vitiligo and other autoimmune diseases (rheumatoid arthritis, ankylosing spondylitis, and psoriasis) have shown improvement with picrorrhiza treatment.
- Lowers cholesterol levels in animal studies (Lee et al., 2006)

Available Forms, Dosage, and Administration Guidelines
Preparations: Dried root, tea, tincture, standardized extract (60% picroside I and kutkoside)
Typical Dosage
- *Dried root:* 300 to 500 mg, up to 2 g a day
- *Tea:* 0.5 tsp dried root in 8 oz hot water, decoct 15 to 20 minutes, steep 15 minutes; take 4 oz three times a day. Use with other herbs; the intensely bitter taste will reduce compliance significantly.
- *Tincture* (1:5, 30% alcohol): 10 to 40 gtt (0.5–2 mL) three times a day
- *Standardized extract (Picroliv):* Follow manufacturer's recommended dosage

Pharmacokinetics—If Available (form or route when known): Not known

Toxicity: Low potential for toxicity

Contraindications: Pregnancy

Side Effects: Nausea, diarrhea and intestinal cramping (at higher doses), skin rash

Long-Term Safety: Safe when used in recommended doses. Animal studies have found no chronic toxicity.

Use in Pregnancy/Lactation/Children: Avoid in all

Drug/Herb Interactions and Rationale (if known): None known

Special Notes: It is an important ingredient in many Ayurvedic preparations. Most studies are of poor quality, so it is difficult to determine efficacy.

BIBLIOGRAPHY

Bone K. (1994). Picrorrhiza: Important modulator of immune function. *Mediherb Professional Newsletter*. #40–#41.

Bone K. (1996). *Clinical Applications of Ayurvedic and Chinese Herbs* (pp. 126–130). Queensland, Australia: Phytotherapy Press.

Joy KL, et al. (2000). Effect of *Picrorrhiza kurroa* extract on transplanted tumours and chemical carcinogenesis in mice. *Journal of Ethnopharmacology*. 71(1–2):261–266.

Joy KL, Kuttan R. (1999). Antidiabetic activity of *Picrorrhiza kurroa* extract. *Journal of Ethnopharmacology*. 67(2):143–148.

Lee HS, et al. (2006). Hypolipemic effect of water extracts of *Picrorrhiza rhizoma* in PX-407 induced hyperlipemic ICR mouse model with hepatoprotective effects: A prevention study. *Journal of Ethnopharmacology*. May 24;105(3):380–386.

Saraswat B, et al. (1999). Ex vivo and in vivo investigations of picroliv from *Picrorrhiza kurroa* in an alcohol intoxication model in rats. *Journal of Ethnopharmacology*. 66(3):263–270.

Singh M, et al. (2005). Protective activity of picroliv on hepatic amoebiasis associated with carbon tetrachloride toxicity. *Indian Journal of Medical Research*. May;121(5):676–682.

Williamson E. (2002). *Major Herbs of Ayurveda* (pp. 220–224). Edinburgh: Churchill Livingstone.

 NAME: Plantain (*Plantago lanceolata, P. major*)

Common Names: English plantain, broadleaf plantain (*P. major*), buckhorn, common plantain, greater plantain, white man's foot, lanceleaf plantain (*P. lanceolata*)

Family: *Plantaginaceae*

Description of Plant

- Small, weedy perennial plant with a rosette of basal leaves and inconspicuous flowers in heads or spikes
- The genus contains up to 270 species throughout the world.

Medicinal Part: Leaves and root

Constituents and Action (if known)
Leaves
- Iridoid glycosides
  - Aucubin: anti-inflammatory, spasmolytic, hepatoprotective, antibacterial (Samuelson, 2000), immune stimulant (Chiang et al., 2003b)
  - Catapol, gardoside, geniposidic acid, mayoroside, melittoside
- Terpenoids: ursolic acid (anti-inflammatory), oleanolic acid (antihyperlipidemic, tumor inhibitor, hepatoprotective activity) (Samuelson, 2000)
- Caffeic acid derivatives: caffeic acid, chlorogenic acid (immune stimulant; Chiang et al., 2003a,b), plantamajoside R (anti-inflammatory, antioxidant), aceteoside R (antibacterial, antioxidant, inhibits lipid peroxidation, immunosuppressant, analgesic) (Samuelson, 2000)
- Polysaccharides: plantaglucide, glucomannon, PMII, PMIa (activates human monocytes in vitro for increased production of tumor necrosis factor)
- Alkaloids: indican, plantagonin
- Polyholozide: gastroprotective, laxative (Hriscu et al., 1990)
- Flavonoids and flavone glucosides: luteolin-7 glucoside, hispidulin 7-glucuronide, apigenin, balcalein, scutallarin, plantaginin: antioxidant, free radical scavengers, inhibit lipid peroxidation, anti-inflammatory, antiallergic (Samuelson, 2000)

Seeds
- Tannins
- *P. major* seeds contain polysaccharides but are much less mucilaginous than its relative psyllium.
- Fatty acids

Nutritional Ingredients: Young leaves can be cooked and eaten as greens. They contain vitamin C, K, carotenoids, zinc, and potassium.

Traditional Use
- Astringent, vulnerary, anti-inflammatory, expectorant, topical analgesic, antibacterial, styptic

- The tea of the leaf and root was used for hemoptysis, hematuria, sore throats, coughs, diarrhea, and dysentery.
- Local application for hemorrhoids (baths), cervicitis (vaginal douche), rectal fissures (suppository)
- Vulnerary for insect bites, snake bites, cuts, bruises, and boils

Current Use
Oral Use
- Gastroprotective: heals gastric and intestinal inflammation (gastritis, gastric and duodenal ulcers, mild colitis) (Winston, 2006)
- Bronchial irritation and coughs: reduces upper respiratory tract irritation and bronchitis (Wegener & Kraft, 1999)
- Irritation and minor infections of the urinary tract (interstitial cystitis, hematuria, cystitis) (Winston, 2006).

Topical Use
- Astringent and vulnerary for burns, cuts, wounds, cervical erosion, rectal fissures, hemorrhoids, and episiotomy incisions
- Reduces inflammation and pain of insect bites and stings (bee, wasp, spider, scorpion, ant) and poison ivy

Available Forms, Dosage, and Administration Guidelines
Preparations: Dried herb, tea, capsules, tincture
Typical Dosage
- *Tea:* Steep 2 tsp dried herb in 1 cup hot water for 10 to 15 minutes; take 8 oz three or four times a day as needed.
- *Tincture* (1:2, 30% alcohol): 60 to 120 gtt (3–6 mL) three times a day
- Or follow manufacturer or practitioner recommendations

Pharmacokinetics—If Available (form or route when known): None known

Toxicity: None known

Contraindications: None known

Side Effects: None

Long-Term Safety: Safe. Long-term human use as a food and medicine and animal studies show no toxicity.

Use in Pregnancy/Lactation/Children: Safe

Drug/Herb Interactions and Rationale (if known): None known

Special Notes: Be sure that the suppliers of the dried herb use guaranteed botanical identification. In the past few years, plantain was accidentally adulterated with foxglove (digitalis), with one known death.

BIBLIOGRAPHY

Chiang LC, et al. (2003a). In vitro cytotoxic, antiviral and immunomodulatory effects of *Plantago major* and *Plantago asiatica*. *American Journal of Chinese Medicine*. 31(2): 225–234.

Chiang LC, et al. (2003b). Immunomodulatory activities of flavonoids, monoterpenoids, triterpenoids, iridoid glycosides and phenolic compounds of *Plantago* species. *Planta Medica*. Jul;69(7): 600–604.

Hriscu A, et al. (1990). A pharmacodynamic investigation of the effect of polyholozidic substances extracted from *Plantago* sp. on the digestive tract. *Revista Medico-Chirurgicala a Societatii de Medici si Naturalisti Din Iasi*. 94(1):165–170.

Mauri M, et al. (1995). Phenylethanoids in the herb of *Plantago lanceolata* and inhibitory effect on arachidonic acid-induced mouse ear edema. *Planta Medica*. 61(5):479–480.

Ringbom T, et al. (1998). Ursolic acid from *Plantago major*, a selective inhibitor of cyclooxygenase-2 catalyzed prostaglandin biosynthesis. *Journal of Natural Products*. 61(10):1212–1215.

Samuelson AB. (2000). The traditional uses, chemical constituents, and biological activities of *Plantago major*: A review. *Journal of Ethnopharmacology*. 71(1–2):1–22.

Wegener T, Kraft K. (1999). Plantain (*Plantago lanceolata* L.): Anti-inflammatory action in upper respiratory tract infections. *Wien Medizinische Wochenschrift*. 149(8–10): 211–216.

Wichtl M, Bisset NG. (1994). *Herbal Drugs and Phytopharmaceuticals* (pp. 378–381). Stuttgart: Medpharm.

Winston D. (2006). *Winston's Botanic Materia Medica*. Washington, NJ: DWCHS.

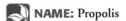 **NAME:** Propolis

Common Names: Bee glue, propolium

Family: None

Description of Plant

- Propolis is a resin collected by bees from leaf buds of a variety of trees, including Balm of Gilead (*Populus*), birch, alder, pines, and other conifers.
- Bees mix tree resins with their salivary and enzymatic secretions; propolis is used to seal the cracks in the hive, prevent fungal and bacterial growth in the hive, and to embalm invading insects or rodents (Borrelli & Izzo, 2002).

Medicinal Part: Bee-gathered tree resin

Constituents and Action (if known): Constituents can vary depending on the plant source of the propolis. Major constituents include:

- Caffeic acid phenethyl ester (CAPE): immune regulatory, anti-inflammatory (Ansorge et al., 2003), antioxidant (Russo et al., 2002), hepatoprotective (Kus et al., 2004), antitumor (Chung et al., 2004), neuroprotective (Noelker et al., 2005)
- Cinnamic acid and cinnamic acid derivatives (drupanin, baccharin, artepillin C): antitumor (Akao, 2003)
- Flavonoids
  ○ Hesperidin: radioprotective (Hosseinimehr & Nemati, 2006), antioxidant (Cirico & Omaye, 2006), anti-inflammatory (Ansorge et al., 2003)
  ○ Quercitin: antioxidant (Paulikova & Berczeliova, 2005), antiviral (Lyu et al., 2005), antitumor, immune stimulant (Orsolic & Basic, 2005), anti-inflammatory (Ansorge et al., 2003)
  ○ Chrysin: antiviral (Lyu et al., 2005), antitumor, immune stimulant (Orsolic & Basic, 2005)
  ○ Galangin: antifungal (Quiroga et al., 2006), antioxidant (Paulikova & Berczeliova, 2005), antibacterial (Cushnie & Lamb, 2006)
  ○ Naringenin: antiviral (Lyu et al., 2005), immune stimulant, antitumor (Orsolic & Basic, 2005)

- Other actions: antiherpetic (Huleihel & Isanu, 2002), anticandidal (Santos et al., 2005), antibacterial (*Helicobactor pylori*) (Nostro et al., 2006), antiprotozoal—*Giardia*

Nutritional Ingredients: Propolis is used in medicinal lozenges and candies for treating sore throats and gum disease.

Traditional Use

- Antibacterial, antifungal, antioxidant, antiviral, antioxidant, anti-inflammatory, antiamoebic, immune modulator, vulnerary
- Propolis was used in ancient times for embalming the dead and to fill cavities in the teeth.
- Propolis has a long history of use for treating topical, oral, and gastric infections, including thrush, bedsores, aphthous stomatitis, wounds, periodontal disease, sore throats, and gastric ulcers.

Current Use

- Propolis has strong antibacterial, antiviral, and antifungal activity and has been successfully used clinically and in human studies to treat oral candidiasis (Santos et al., 2005), upper respiratory tract infections (Cohen et al., 2004), oral herpes (Huleihel & Isanu, 2002), esinophilic ulcers (Kiderman et al., 2001), and chronic vaginitis (Imhof et al., 2005)
- Additional studies indicate that propolis may be of benefit as a sterilizing agent for root canal surgery (Oncag et al., 2006), for immune enhancement, and radioprotective activity (Takagi et al., 2005) as well as an antitumor agent, to protect against chemotherapy-induced cytopenia (Suzuki et al., 2002), and for atherosclerosis (Borrelli & Izzo, 2002)
- Several studies from Cuba indicate that propolis has benefits for treating the early stages (1–2 years' duration) of Peyronie's disease. Over 6 months, the patients taking propolis (propolium) had reduced curvative angle and plaque (Lemourt et al., 2005).
- In patients with mild to moderate asthma, adding propolis to theophylline control therapy had significant benefits. In

patients taking the propolis, there was a marked reduction in the incidence and severity of nighttime asthma attacks and improvement in pulmonary function (Khavyal et al., 2003).

- Animal and in vitro studies indicate that propolis has hepatoprotective (Seo & Park, 2003), antiulcer (Nostro et al., 2006), anti-inflammatory, antiarthritic (Ansorge et al., 2003), and immune modulating effects (Takagi et al., 2005).

Available Forms, Dosage, and Administration Guidelines

Preparations: Capsules, tincture, lozenges, suppositories

Typical Dosage

- *Capsules:* Two to three 300- to 500-mg capsules a day
- *Tincture* (1:5, 80% alcohol): 20 to 30 gtt (1.0–1.5 mL) three times a day
- *Lozenges:* As needed
- *Suppositories:* Once daily

Pharmacokinetics—If Available (form or route when known): Not known

Toxicity: There are multiple cases of propolis ointments, lip balms, vaginal suppositories, and throat sprays causing contact dermatitis, ulceration of mucous membranes, and even anaphylaxis (Walgrave et al., 2005). It is a good idea to do a skin test before using propolis in a patient with no history of use of this product.

Contraindications: Propolis allergy or sensitivity. Use cautiously in patients with allergic asthma and severe pollen allergies.

Side Effects: Beyond allergic response, none known

Long-Term Safety: Safe

Use in Pregnancy/Lactation/Children: In one case report (Kiderman et al., 2001), a 13-month-old female infant with bilateral esinophilic ulcers of the mouth was successfully treated using a lanolin-based propolis ointment. It is vital to test infants and children for reactivity to propolis before using it.

Drug/Herb Interactions and Rationale (if known): Propolis enhanced the activity of clarithromycin in inhibiting

Helicobacter pylori. It also enhanced the protective effects of paclitaxel against DMBA-induced breast cancers in rats (Padmavathi et al., 2006). One of the major constituents of propolis, caffeic acid phenethyl ester (CAPE), protected rats against renal toxicity caused by carbon tetrachloride (Ogeturk et al., 2005) and cyclosporine-A–induced cardiotoxicity (Rezzani et al., 2005).

Special Notes: There are very significant variations in constituents in propolis from different regions of the world. A significant amount of the propolis in the marketplace is contaminated with lead (from lead paint in bee hives). Be sure that any propolis product is tested by the manufacturer and is certified to have safe levels of this toxic metal.

BIBLIOGRAPHY

Akao Y, et al. (2003). Cell growth inhibitory effect of cinnamic acid derivatives from propolis on human tumor cell lines. *Biological & Pharmaceutical Bulletin.* Jul;26(7):1057–1059.

Ansorge S, et al. (2003). Propolis and some of its constituents down-regulate DNA synthesis and inflammatory cytokine production but induce TGF-beta1 production of human immune cells. *Zeitschrift fur Naturforschung [C].* Jul-Aug;58(7–8):480–489.

Biomedical Papers of the Medical Faculty of the University Palaky, Olomouc. Czechoslovakia.

Borrelli F, Izzo A. (2002). Propolis: Chemical and pharmacological aspects. *Fitoterapia.* Nov;73(31):S1–S64.

Chung TW, et al. (2004). Novel and therapeutics effect of caffeic acid phenyl ester on hepatocarcinoma cells: Complete regression of hepatome growth and metastasis by dual mechanism. *FASEB Journal.* Nov;18(14):1670–1681.

Cirico TL, Omaye ST. (2006). Additive or synergetic effects of phenolic compounds on human low density lipoprotein oxidation. *Food and Chemical Toxicology.* Apr;44(4):510–516.

Cohen HA, et al. (2004). Effectiveness of an herbal preparation containing echinacea, propolis, and vitamin C in preventing respiratory tract infections in children: A randomized, double-blind, placebo-controlled, multicenter study. *Archives of Pediatric and Adolescent Medicine.* Mar;158(3):217–221.

Cushnie TP, Lamb AJ. (2006). Assessment of the antibacterial activity of galangin against 4-quinolone resistant strains of *Staphylococcus aureus. Phytomedicine.* Feb;13(3):187–191.

Hosseinimehr SJ, Nemati A. (2006). Radioprotective effects of hesperidin against gamma irradiation in mouse bone marrow cells. *British Journal of Radiology.* May;79(941):415–418.

Huleihel M, Isanu V. (2002). Anti-herpes simplex virus effect of an aqueous extract of propolis. *Israel Medical Association Journal.* Nov;4[11 Suppl.]:923–927.

Imhof M, et al. (2005). Propolis solution for the treatment of chronic vaginitis. *International Journal of Gynaecology and Obstetrics.* May;89(2):127–132.

Khavyal MT, et al. (2003). A clinical pharmacological study of the potential beneficial effects of a propolis food product as an adjuvant in asthmatic patients. *Fundamental and Clinical Pharmacology.* Feb;17(1):93–102.

Kiderman A, et al. (2001). Bi-lateral eosinophilic ulcers in an infant treated with propolis. *Journal of Dermatological Treatment.* Mar;12(1):29–31.

Kus I, et al. (2004). Protective effects of caffeic acid phenethyl ester (CAPE) on carbon tetrachloride induced hepatotoxicity in rats. *Acta Histochemica.* 106(4):289–297.

Lemourt OM, et al. (2005). Peyronie's disease. Evaluation of 3 therapeutics modalities: Propoleum, laser and simultaneous propoleum-laser. *Archivos Espanoles de Urologia.* Nov;58(9):931–935.

Lyu SY, et al. (2005). Antiherpetic activities of flavonoids against herpes simplex virus type 1 (HSV-1) and type 2 (HSV-2) in vitro. *Archives of Pharmacal Research.* Nov;28(11):1293–1301.

Noelker C, et al. (2005). The flavonoide caffeic acid phenthyl ester blocks 6-hydroxydopamine-induced neurotoxicity. *Neuroscience Letters.* Jul 22–29;383(1–2):39.

Nostro A, et al. (2006). Effects of combining extracts (from propolis or *Zingiber officinale*) with clarithromycin on *Helicobacter pylori.* *Phytotherapy Research.* Mar;20(3):187–190.

Ogeturk M, et al. (2005). Caffeic acid phenethyl ester protects kidneys against carbon tetrachloride toxicity in rats. *Journal of Ethnopharmacology.* Feb 28;97(2):273–280.

Oncag O, et al. (2006). Efficacy of propolis as an intracanal medicament against *Enterococcus faecalis.* *General Dentistry.* Sep-Oct;54(5):319–322.

Orsolic N, Basic I. (2005). Water soluble derivative of propolis and its polyphenolic compounds enhance tumoricidal activity of macrophages. *Journal of Ethnopharmacology.* Oct 31;102(1):37–45.

Padmavathi R, et al. (2006). Therapeutic effect of paclitaxel and propolis on lipid peroxidation and antioxidant system in 7,12 dimethyl benz(a)anthracene-induced breast cancer in female sprague dawley rats. *Life Sciences.* May 8;78(24):2820–2825.

Paulikova H, Berczeliova E. (2005). The effect of quercetin and galangin on glutathione reductase. Dec;149(2):497–500.

Quiroga EN, et al. (2006). Propolis from the northwest of Argentina as a source of antifungal principles. *Journal of Applied Microbiology.* Jul;101(1):103–110.

Rezzani R, et al. (2005). The protective effect of caffeic acid phenethyl ester against cyclosporine A-induced cardiotoxicity in rats. *Toxicology.* Sep 1;212(2–3):155–164.

Russo A, et al. (2002). Antioxidant activity of propolis: Role of caffeic acid phenethyl ester and galangin. *Fitoterapia.* Nov;73[Suppl. 1]: S21–S29.

Santos VR, et al. (2005). Oral candidiasis treatment with Brazilian ethanol propolis extract. *Phytotherapy Research.* Jul;19(7):652–654.

Seo KW, Park M. (2003). The protective effects of propolis on hepatic injury and its mechanism. *Phytotherapy Research.* Mar;17(3):250–253.

Sobocanec S, et al. (2006). Oxidant/antioxidant properties of Croatian native propolis. *Journal of Agricultural and Food Chemistry.* Oct 18;54(21):8018–8026.

Suzuki I, et al. (2002). Antitumor and anticytopenic effects of aqueous extracts of propolis in combination with chemotherapeutic agents. *Cancer Biotherapy and Radiopharmaceuticals.* Oct;17(5):553–662.

Takagi Y, et al. (2005). Immune activation and radioprotection by propolis. *American Journal of Chinese Medicine.* 33(2):231–240.

Volpi N. (2004). Separation of flavonoids and phenolic acids from propolis by capillary zone electrophoresis. *Electrophoresis.* Jun;25(12):1872–1878.

Walgrave SE, et al. (2005). Allergic contact dermatitis from propolis. *Dermatitis.* Dec;16(4):209–215.

Winston D. (2006). *Winston's Botanic Materia Medica.* Washington, NJ: DWCHS.

 NAME: Psyllium Seed (*Plantago psyllium, P. ovata*)

Common Names: Black psyllium (*P. psyllium*), blonde psyllium (*P. ovata*), ispaghula

Family: *Plantaginaceae*

Description of Plant
- Black psyllium is native to the Mediterranean.
- Blonde psyllium is native to the Mediterranean, North Africa, and Western Asia.

Medicinal Part: Seeds and husks

Constituents and Action (if known)

- Soluble fiber (47%), mucilage (10%–30%): when soaked in water, increases greatly in volume, adding bulk to the stool (ESCOP, 2003; McRorie et al., 1998)
  - May be able to reduce diarrhea in patients receiving enteral feedings (Belknap et al., 1997; Olson et al., 1997)
  - Lowers cholesterol (Anderson et al., 2000); reduces the ratio of LDL to HDL (Jenkins et al., 1997)
  - Reduces glucose absorption, improving postprandial glucose in persons with type 1 and 2 diabetes (Anderson et al. 1999; Frati Munari et al., 1998; Rodriguez-Moran et al., 1998)
- Insoluble fiber (53%)
- Fixed oils and unsaturated fatty acids
- Trisaccharide (planteose)

Nutritional Ingredients: Protein (15%–20%)

Traditional Use

- Tea (mucilage) used for sore throats, dry coughs, and gastric irritation
- Bulk laxative
- Topically used as a poultice for styes, boils, and sores

Current Use

- Increases fiber in stool
- Short-term (3–4 days) treatment of nonspecific diarrhea and amoebic diarrhea/dysentery (Zaman et al., 2002)
- Reduces cholesterol (Larkin, 2000); binds bile acids and increases their fecal excretion, which in turn stimulates further bile salt synthesis from cholesterol (ESCOP, 2003)
- Bulk laxative and stool softener for habitual constipation, especially in patients with anal fissures, hemorrhoids, after rectal surgery, and during pregnancy (ESCOP, 2003)
- Reduces symptoms of irritable bowel syndrome; psyllium decreases B-glucuronidase activity of intestinal bacteria, inhibiting cleavage of toxic compounds from their liver conjugates
- Short-chain fatty acids (acetate, proprionate, butyrate) that are released from the digestible part of the fiber by bacterial

fermentation have a normalizing effect on mucosal cells (ESCOP, 2003). Psyllium is superior to bran in maintaining stool frequency without producing flatulence (Blumenthal et al., 2000).

- May reduce blood sugar by slowing glucose absorption in gut (Frati Muneri et al., 1998) and decreases glycosylated hemoglobin in diabetic patients (Ziai et al., 2005)

Available Forms, Dosage, and Administration Guidelines

- A single dose usually contains 1.7 g of soluble fiber. Unless otherwise prescribed, take 10 to 30 g a day of whole or ground seeds or other galenical preparations for oral use.
- *Seed:* 5 to 10 g seed, two or three times daily. Presoak seeds in 100 to 200 mL warm water for several hours. Follow each dose by drinking at least another 200 mL water. WHO recommends an average dose of 7.5 g dissolved in 240 mL water or juice, one to three times daily. Children 6 to 12 years should take half the adult dosage.

Pharmacokinetics—If Available (form or route when known): Not known

Toxicity: None known

Contraindications: Psyllium allergies, bowel obstruction, stenosis of the esophagus or GI tract

Side Effects: Allergic reactions may occur, with rare reports of severe allergies and anaphylaxis with repeated inhalation of psyllium dust (Khalili & Bardana, 2003).

Long-Term Safety: Safe

Use in Pregnancy/Lactation/Children: Safe

Drug/Herb Interactions and Rationale (if known): Separate by 2 hours from all other drugs. If taken with diabetic drugs, the dose may need to be reduced because blood sugar can be reduced.

Special Notes: Always take with sufficient fluids to ensure that the seeds do not cause bowel obstruction.

BIBLIOGRAPHY

Anderson JW, et al. (1999). Effects of psyllium on glucose and serum lipid responses in men with type 2 diabetes and hypercholesterolemia. *American Journal of Clinical Nutrition*. 70(4):466–473.

Anderson JW, et al. (2000). Cholesterol-lowering effects of psyllium intake adjunctive to diet therapy in men and women with hypercholesterolemia: Meta-analysis of 8 controlled trials. *American Journal of Clinical Nutrition*. 71(2):472–479.

Belknap D, et al. (1997). The effects of psyllium hydrophilic mucilloid on diarrhea in enterally fed patients. *Heart and Lung*. 26(3):229–237.

Blumenthal M, et al. (2000). *Herbal Medicine Expanded Commission E Monographs* (pp. 316–321). Austin, TX: American Botanical Council.

European Scientific Cooperative on Phytotherapy. (2003). *ESCOP Monographs* (pp. 388–390). New York: Thieme.

Frati Munari AC, et al. (1998). Lowering glycemic index of food by acarbose and *Plantago psyllium* mucilage. *Archives of Medical Research*. 29(2):137–141.

Jenkins DJ, et al. (1997). Effect of psyllium in hypercholesterolemia at two monounsaturated fatty acid intakes. *American Journal of Clinical Nutrition*. 65(5):1524–1533.

Khalili B, Bardana EJ Jr. (2003). Psyllium-associated anaphylaxis and death: A case report and review of the literature. *Annals of Allergy, Asthma, and Immunology*. Dec;91(6):579–584.

Larkin M. (2000). Functional foods nibble away at serum cholesterol concentrations. *Lancet*. 355(9203):555.

McRorie JW, et al. (1998). Psyllium is superior to docusate sodium for treatment of chronic constipation. *Alimentary Pharmacology and Therapeutics*. 12(5):491–497.

Olson BH, et al. (1997). Psyllium-enriched cereals lower blood total cholesterol and LDL cholesterol, but not HDL cholesterol, in hypercholesterolemic adult: Results of a meta-analysis. *Journal of Nutrition*. 127(10):1973–1980.

Rodriguez-Moran M, et al. (1998). Lipid and glucose-lowering efficacy of *Plantago psyllium* in type I diabetes. *Journal of Diabetes Complications*. 12(5):273–278.

Sierra M, et al. (2002). Therapeutic effects of psyllium in type 2 diabetic patients. *European Journal of Clinical Nutrition*. Sep;56(9):830–842.

Zaman V, et al. (2002). The presence of antiamoebic constituents in psyllium husk. *Phytotherapy Research*. Feb;16(1):78–79.

Ziai SA, et al. (2005). Psyllium decreased serum glucose and glycosylated hemoglobin significantly in diabetic outpatients. *Journal of Ethnopharmacology*. Nov 14;102(2):202–207.

NAME: Pygeum (*Prunus africana*)

Common Names: African plum, African prune

Family: *Rosaceae*

Description of Plant
- An evergreen tree 30 to 70' high native to southern and central Africa
- Grows in highland mountain forests above 2500'. Much of its natural habitat has been lost to clear-cutting.

Medicinal Part: Bark

Constituents and Action (if known)
- Fatty acids
  - Decrease inflammation in prostate by antagonizing 5-lipoxygenase (Bruneton, 1999; Levin et al., 1997)
  - Reduce hormonal level in prostate (Edgar et al., 2007)
  - Increase bladder elasticity (Levin et al., 1997)
  - Histologically modify glandular cells (Levin et al., 1997)
  - Increase prostatic secretions (Mathe et al., 1995; Yablonski et al., 1997)
- Phytosterols (beta-sitosterol, beta-sitosterone, campesterol)
  - Reduce inflammation and edema in and near prostate (Melo et al., 2002)
  - Inhibit prostaglandin biosynthesis (Schulz et al., 1998)
  - Inhibit 5-alpha-reductase, an enzyme that increases the production of DHT (Bruneton, 1999)
- Triterpenoid pentacyclic acids (ursolic, oleanolic): anti-inflammatory
  - Ferulic acid esters (n-docosanol and n-tetracosanol): lower testosterone and prolactin levels
- Organic acids (hydrocyanic acid)

Nutritional Ingredients: None

Traditional Use: Used to treat intercostal pain, improve kidney function, improve difficult urination; taken in milk for dysuria, stomachache

Current Use

- Relieves symptoms of BPH, including dysuria, nocturia, pollakiuria, and volume of residual urine (Chatelain et al., 1999; Ishani et al., 2000)
- Commonly used in Germany, Italy, and France for BPH along with saw palmetto, nettle root, and rye pollen
- May reverse impotence and sterility associated with a reduction in prostatic secretions and improve seminal fluid composition (Anonymous, 2002)
- Also used to treat prostatitis and may inhibit prostatic cancer (Edgar et al., 2007)

Available Forms, Dosage, and Administration Guidelines

Preparations: Dried bark, capsules, tablets, tinctures. Some products are standardized to 14% beta-sitosterol and/or 12% to 13% phytosterols and 0.5% n-docosanol.

Typical Dosage: For standardized products, take 100 to 200 mg a day or follow manufacturer or practitioner recommendations. Take with meals. Take in 6- to 8-week cycles with at least 1 week in between. May be started at half the therapeutic dose to prevent gland enlargement. Men should start therapy in their early 40s.

Pharmacokinetics—If Available (form or route when known): Not known

Toxicity: None known

Contraindications: None known

Side Effects: Nausea, stomach pain

Long-Term Safety: Safe

Use in Pregnancy/Lactation/Children: Do not use

Drug/Herb Interactions and Rationale (if known): None known

Special Notes: In comparative studies, pygeum was less effective than saw palmetto and less well tolerated by patients (Winston, 1999). Pygeum is often combined with saw palmetto, nettle root, or pumpkinseed oil to treat BPH, because each herb has a slightly different mechanism of action and the combinations have a synergistic effect superior to any one single treatment. Patients should be seen by a medical practitioner first for baseline studies, including prostatic-specific antigen. Use only cultivated bark; pygeum has been drastically overharvested in the wild.

BIBLIOGRAPHY

Anonymous. (2002). *WHO Monographs on Selected Medicinal Plants* (pp. 246–258). Geneva: World Health Organization.

Bruneton J. (1999). *Pharmacognosy, Phytochemistry, Medicinal Plants* (pp. 161–162). Paris: Lavoisier.

Chatelain C, et al. (1999). Comparison of once- and twice-daily dosage forms of *Pygeum africanum* extract in patients with benign prostatic hyperplasia: A randomized, double-blind study, with long-term open label extension. *Urology.* 54(3):473–478.

Edgar AD, et al. (2007). A critical review of the pharmacology of the plant extract of *Pygeum africanum* in the treatment of LUTS. *Neurourology and Urodynamics.* 26(4):458–463.

Hutchings A, et al. (1996). *Zulu Medicinal Plants: An Inventory* (p. 118). Scottsville, South Africa: University of Natal Press.

Ishani A, et al. (2000). *Pygeum africanum* for the treatment of patients with benign prostatic hyperplasia: A systematic review and quantitative meta-analysis. *American Journal of Medicine.* Dec 1;109(8):654–664.

Levin R, et al. (1997). Cellular and molecular aspects of bladder hypertrophy. *European Urology.* 32[Suppl. 1]:15–21.

Mathe G, et al. (1995). The so-called phyto-estrogenic action of *Pygeum africanum* extract. *Biomedical Pharmacotherapeutics.* 49(7–8):339–343.

Melo EA, et al. (2002). Evaluating the efficacy of a combination of *Pygeum africanum* and stinging nettle (*Urtica dioica*) extracts in treating benign prostatic hypoplasia (BPH): double-blind, randomized, placebo controlled trial. *International Brazilian Journal of Urology.* Sept-Oct;28(5):418–425.

Schulz V, et al. (1998). *Rational Pytotherapy.* Berlin: Springer-Verlag.

Winston D. (1999). *Saw Palmetto for Men and Women* (p. 66). Pownal, VT: Storey Publishing.

Yablonski F, et al. (1997). Antiproliferative effect of *Pygeum africanum* extract on rat prostatic fibroblasts. *Journal of Urology.* June;157(6): 2381–2387.

NAME: Raspberry (*Rubus idaeus, R. stryosus*)

Common Names: Red raspberry, raspberry leaf

Family: *Rosaceae*

Description of Plant
- Cultivated throughout the world as a food plant for its berries
- Plant has thorny canes with three- to five-toothed leaflets
- Fruit is usually red but can also be yellow

Medicinal Part: Leaves, fruit

Constituents and Action (if known)
- Gallo- and elligitannins: astringent properties for diarrhea or as mouthwash antiviral activity
- Flavonoids (rutin, kaemferol, quercitin): antioxidants, anti-inflammatory
- Volatile oils (monoterpenes): geraniol, linolool

Other Actions
- Raspberry leaf may lower blood glucose (Briggs & Briggs, 1997) and has antispasmodic activity (Rojas-Vera et al., 2002) and in vitro antileukemic activity (Skupien et al., 2006).

Nutritional Ingredients: The fruit is a source of vitamin C, flavonoids, pectin, and fructose. The leaves contain calcium, magnesium, and flavonoids.

Traditional Use
- Astringent, uterine tonic, styptic, mild antispasmodic
- As an astringent to treat diarrhea, hematuria, and enuresis
- Pregnancy tonic, as a tea, to strengthen the uterus, reduce morning sickness, and prevent miscarriage
- As a uterine tonic for a boggy atonic uterus, uterine prolapse, and menorrhagia
- As an astringent gargle for inflammation of the mouth, gums, and throat
- Dried raspberry fruit (*fu pen zi*) is used in TCM for frequent urination, bedwetting, and impotence.

Current Use

- Pregnancy tonic. Two studies found that raspberry leaf used throughout pregnancy did not shorten the first stage of labor but did shorten the second stage. An unexpected finding in both studies was that women who took this herb had reduced need for artificial rupture of their membranes, cesarean sections, or forceps delivery than the control groups (Parsons et al., 1999; Simpson et al., 2001).
- Astringent tea to treat mild diarrhea and mouth sores
- Mild uterine tonic for women in their 40s and 50s with uterine prolapse, menorrhagia, worsening dysmenorrhea, and pelvic congestion. Preliminary studies suggest that the leaves may have antispasmodic activity (Rojas-Vera et al., 2002).

Available Forms, Dosage, and Administration Guidelines

Preparations: Dried herb, tea, tincture, capsules
Typical Dosage
- *Dried herb:* 4 to 8 g
- *Tea:* 1 to 2 tsp herb in 8 oz hot water, steep half-hour; take one to three cups a day
- *Tincture* (1:5, 30% alcohol): 60 to 100 gtt (3–5 mL) three times a day
- *Capsules:* One or two 300- to 400-mg capsules twice a day

Pharmacokinetics—If Available (form or route when known): Not known

Toxicity: None known

Contraindications: None known

Side Effects: None known

Long-Term Safety: Safe

Use in Pregnancy/Lactation/Children: Used for millennia as a pregnancy tonic; empirical use as well as clinical use by midwives suggests safety. In two clinical trials, no adverse effects were seen (Parsons et al., 1999; Simpson et al., 2001).

Drug/Herb Interactions and Rationale (if known): None known

Special Notes: There is little scientific information on this herb because of a lack of studies. Ethnobotanical and empirical use suggests numerous benefits, and studies of related species suggest that this herb may have anti-inflammatory, antiviral, and antioxidant activity.

BIBLIOGRAPHY

Briggs CJ, Briggs K. (1997). Raspberry. *Canadian Pharmaceutical Journal.* 130:41–43.

McIntyre A. (1995). *The Complete Woman's Herbal* (p. 25). New York: Henry Holt Co.

Parsons M, et al. (1999). Raspberry leaf and its effect on labour: Safety and efficacy. *Australian College of Midwives Journal.* Sep;12(3):20–25.

Patel AV, et al. (2004). Therapeutics commission and actions of *Rubus* species. *Current Medicinal Chemistry.* Jun;11(11): 1501–1512.

Rojas-Vera J, et al. (2002). Relaxant activity of raspberry (*Rubus idaeus*) leaf extract in guinea-pig ileum in vitro. *Phytotherapy Research.* Nov;16(7):665–668.

Simpson M, et al. (2001). Raspberry leaf in pregnancy: Its safety and efficacy in labor. *Journal of Midwifery and Women's Health.* Mar-Apr;46(2):51–59.

Skupien K, et al. (2006). In vitro antileukemic activity of extracts from berry plant leaves against sensitive and multidrug resistant HL60 cells. *Cancer Letters.* May 18;236(2):282–291.

Wichtl M, Bisset NG. (1994). *Herbal Drugs and Phytopharmaceuticals* (pp. 434–436). Stuttgart: Medpharm.

NAME: Red Clover (*Trifolium pratense*)

Common Names: Meadow clover, purple clover, wild clover, beebread

Family: *Fabiaceae*

Description of Plant
- Native to Europe but naturalized in the United States
- Low-growing perennial with trifoliate leaves and purplish flowers

Medicinal Part: Flowering tops

Constituents and Action (if known)

- More than 125 phytochemicals have been isolated from red clover.
- Flavone glycosides, including genistein, diadzen, biochanin A, and formononetin, are responsible for weak estrogen-like actions (Hidalgo et al., 2005).
  - Anticancer activity: enhances apoplasis inhibits angiogenesis and cancer cell adhesion in prostate cancer (Jarred et al., 2002).
  - Increase follicle-stimulating hormone and alter luteinizing hormone, therefore helping to decrease many menopausal signs and changes (Zava et al., 1998); inhibit oxidation of steroid hormones and increase production of sex hormone–binding globulin (Kelly et al., 1998)
  - Increases arterial compliance, which may assist with blood pressure control (Nestel et al., 1999)
  - Promote calcium storage and maintain bone density (Kelly et al., 1998)
- Coumarins (medicagol) may affect platelet activity; antioxidant, lipid-reducing, reduces triglycerides, increases HDL (Geller & Studee, 2006) and antitumor activity (McCaleb et al., 2000)
- Saponins
- Minerals: calcium, iron, magnesium, manganese, potassium, copper
- May have antitumor activity; is part of the controversial Hoxsey formula used to treat cancer in Mexico (Cassady et al., 1988). Used in more than 30 countries to treat cancer (McCaleb et al., 2000).
- Reduces insulin-like growth factor

Nutritional Ingredients: Florets can be added to salads and used as edible garnishes. They are rich in minerals (potassium, iron, magnesium, calcium, manganese). Widely grown as animal fodder.

Traditional Use

- Alterative, anticancer remedy, expectorant, vulnerary
- The herb is used as an "alterative or blood cleanser" for cancer, especially breast, lymph, and lung cancers

- Topical use: chronic skin conditions including skin cancer (Samuel Thomson's Cancer Salve), eczema, and dermatitis
- Used as a tea and cough syrup to suppress coughs; useful for colds, bronchitis, and pertussis
- Lymph tonic for chronic lymphatic congestion associated with skin problems, mastitis, and arthritis
- There is no traditional use for extracted red clover isoflavones.

Current Use

- Standardized isoflavone extracts made from red clover are used as a "natural hormone replacement" therapy to control menopausal symptoms and changes (hot flashes, night sweats, vaginal dryness) (Hidalgo et al., 2005; van de Weijer & Barentsen, 2002).
- Red clover–derived isoflavone supplements (RCDIS) reduced bone loss in 49- to 65-year-old women (Atkinson et al., 2004), lowered blood pressure and enhanced endothelial function in postmenopausal women with type 2 diabetes (Howes et al., 2003), lowered triglycerides in menopausal women (Hidalgo et al., 2005), and a biochanin-enhanced isoflavone extract lowered LDL cholesterol in men (Nestel et al., 2004).
- Further research should be done to assess this plant's possible activity for treating human cancers.

Available Forms, Dosage, and Administration Guidelines

Preparations: Dried flowering tops, tea, tincture, capsules. Promensil is a widely used standardized product for control of menopausal symptoms.

Typical Dosage

- *Standardized tablets:* Two a day, each containing 40 mg isoflavones
- *Capsules:* Up to five 500-mg capsules a day
- *Tea:* 1 to 2 tsp dried flowering tops in 8 oz hot water, steep half-hour; take two or three cups a day
- *Tincture* (1:5, 30% alcohol): 60 to 100 gtt (3–5 mL) up to three times a day

• Or follow manufacturer or practitioner recommendations

Pharmacokinetics—If Available (form or route when known): Metabolized in liver, excreted in bile (Moon et al., 2006).

Toxicity: None

Contraindications: Use cautiously in patients with bleeding disorders. Use of phytoestrogens is controversial in patients with estrogen-positive cancers. Some researchers speculate that these substances may stimulate estrogen-sensitive tumor growth. Studies show that genistein and biochanin prevent the growth of cancer cell lines (prostate, stomach) in vitro and inhibit breast cancer in rats.

Side Effects: Theoretical possibility of decreased clotting; animals (cows, sheep) who eat large quantities of this plant are much more sensitive to isoflavones than humans and become infertile.

Long-Term Safety: Safe; FDA GRAS list

Use in Pregnancy/Lactation/Children: Avoid using the standardized isoflavone products during pregnancy. Long history of use of the herb with children; no adverse effects expected.

Drug/Herb Interactions and Rationale (if known)
• Use cautiously with anticoagulants (warfarin) and antiplatelet agents (ASA, ticlopidine): theoretical possibility of effects on platelets and an increase of bleeding. Obtain prothrombin time and INR to assess possible interactions.
• May interfere with effectiveness of oral contraceptives (North American Menopause Society, 2005) avoid concurrent use.

Special Notes: There is a major difference between red clover as an herb or crude extract and the standardized preparations, which are highly concentrated for isoflavones. Epidemiologists believe cultures that eat food rich in isoflavones have a lower incidence of cancer. Population studies clearly show that in

Asian cultures where daily consumption of isoflavones is usually 40 mg (vs. 2–5 mg in the United States), there is a lower incidence of prostate cancer in men and breast cancer in women.

BIBLIOGRAPHY

Atkinson C, et al. (2004). The effects of phytoestrogen isoflavones on bone density in women: A double-blind, randomized, placebo-controlled trial. *American Journal of Clinical Nutrition.* Feb;79(2):326–333.

Geller SE, Studee L. (2006). Soy and red clover for mid-life and aging. *Climacteric.* Aug;9(4):245–263.

Hidalgo LA, et al. (2005). The effect of red clover isoflavones on menopausal symptoms, lipids, and vaginal cytology in menopausal women: A randomized, double-blind, placebo-controlled study. *Gynecological Endocrinology.* Nov;21(5):325–332.

Howes JB, et al. (2003). Effects of dietary supplementation with isoflavones from red clover on ambulatory blood pressure and endothelial function in postmenopausal type 2 diabetes. *Diabetes, Obesity and Metabolism.* Sep;5(5):325–332.

Jarred RA, et al. (2002). Induction of apoptosis in low to moderate-grade human prostate carcinoma by red clover-derived dietary isoflavones. *Cancer Epidemiol Biomarkers Prev.* Dec;11(12):1689–1696.

McCaleb R, et al. (2000). *Encyclopedia of Popular Herbs* (pp. 317–324). Roseville, CA: Prima Publishers.

Moon YJ, et al. (2006). Pharmacokinetics and bioavailability of the isoflavone biochanin A in rats. *AAPS J.* Jul 7;8(3):E433–442.

Nachtigall L, et al. (1999). *The effects of isoflavone derived from red clover on vasomotor symptoms, endometrial thickness, and reproductive hormone concentrations in menopausal women.* Endocrine Society 81st annual meeting, June 12–15, 1999.

Nestel P, et al. (2004). A biochanin-enriched isoflavone from red clover lowers LDL cholesterol in men. *European Journal of Clinical Nutrition.* Mar;58(3):403–408.

Nestel PJ, et al. (1999). Isoflavones from red clover improve systemic arterial compliance but not plasma lipids in menopausal women. *Journal of Clinical Endocrinology and Metabolism.* 84(3):895–899.

North American Menopause Society. (2004). Treatment of menopause-associated vasomotor symptoms: position statement of The North American Menopause Society. *Menopause.* 11:11–33.

van de Weijer PH, Barentsen R. (2002). Isoflavones from red clover (Promensil) significantly reduce menopausal hot flush symptoms compared with placebo. *Maturitas.* Jul 25;42(3):187–193.

Yanagihara K, et al. (1993). Antiproliferative effects of isoflavones on human cancer cell lines established from the gastrointestinal tract. *Cancer Research.* 53:5815–5821.

Zava DT, et al. (1998). Estrogen and progestin bioactivity of foods, herbs and spices. *Proceedings of the Society for Experimental Biology and Medicine.* 217:369–378.

 NAME: Reishi (*Ganoderma lucidum*)

Common Names: Varnish shelf fungus, *ling zhi* or *ling chih* (Chinese)

Family: *Polyporaceae*

Description of Plant
- A woody shelf fungus (polypore) with a shiny red or reddish-brown upper surface
- The mushroom grows on oak trees in China, Japan, Russia, and the eastern United States.

Medicinal Part: Fruiting body and mycelium

Constituents and Action (if known)
- Polysaccharides
  - Beta-D-glucans: enhance protein synthesis and nucleic acid metabolism
  - Ganoderans A, B, and C: hypoglycemic
  - GL-1: antitumor, immunostimulating (Yue et al., 2006)
  - FA, F1, F1-1a: antitumor, immunostimulating (Yue et al., 2006)
  - Other polysaccharides have shown cardiotonic activity.
- Triterpenes
  - Ganoderic acids A, B, C, D: inhibit histamine release
  - Ganoderic acids R and S: antihepatotoxin
  - Ganoderic acids B, D, F, H, K, S, Y: antihypertensive, inhibit angiotensin-converting enzyme
  - Ganoderic acids B and M: inhibit cholesterol synthesis
  - Ganodermadiol: antihypertensive, inhibit angiotensin-converting enzyme
- Protein (ling-zhi-8): antiallergic, immunomodulator (Yue et al., 2006)

- Steroid (ganodosterone): hepatoprotective
- Whole ganoderma extracts have also shown anti-inflammatory, antioxidant, expectorant, adrenal stimulant, radiation protective, antiulcer, and antitumor activity (Hobbs, 1995).
- Protects against ultraviolet and x-ray radiation in mice (Kim & Kim, 1999)

Nutritional Ingredients: Black ganoderma (*G. sinensis*) has been used for millennia to make a stock for soups.

Traditional Use

- Adaptogen, immune amphoteric, hepatoprotective, nervine, cardiotonic
- The Chinese considered *ling zhi* a profoundly powerful tonic remedy; it was rare and reserved for the emperor and his court.
- In TCM, *ling zhi* is used to tonify the blood and vital energy. It is also used to calm disturbed *shen* (nervousness, insomnia) and as an antitussive for coughs. Ganoderma is used in formulas for insomnia, palpitations, anxiety, impaired memory, general weakness and debility, heart disease, cancer, allergies, and hypertension.

Current Use

- Immune amphoteric: normalizes immune response and can be used for immune deficiency and hyperimmune response (autoimmune conditions [rheumatoid arthritis, lupus, scleroderma, ankylosing spondylitis, multiple sclerosis] and allergies) (Stamets, 2002)
- Immunostimulant: enhances NK cells, interleukin 1 and 2, and interferon production in vitro and in vivo. Has been used clinically for HIV/AIDS, herpes virus, hepatitis B and C, CFS, fibromyalgia, acute myeloid leukemia, and recurrent nasopharyngeal carcinomas. In an in vivo study, ganoderma extracts inhibited estrogen-sensitive breast cancer growth by modulating the estrogen receptor and NF-KappaB signaling (Jiang et al., 2006).
- Use is sanctioned by the Japanese Health Ministry as an adjunct treatment for cancer. Increases the activity of chemotherapeutic agents and reduces adverse effects such as nausea, decreased white blood cell counts, and cachexia. A ganoderma polysaccharide extract was found to enhance

immune responses in late-stage cancer patients (Gao et al.,
2003).

- Inhibits breast, colorectal and prostate cancers (Jiang et al.,
2006; Xie et al., 2006).
- Hepatoprotective: used to protect the liver against damage
caused by viral, drug, or environmental liver toxins. Used
with vitamin C for treating hepatitis B and C; also effective
for treating toxipathic hepatitis caused by ingestion of
poisonous mushrooms, hepatodynia, and hyperlipidemia.
- Fourteen patients with mushroom poisoning (*Russula
subnigricans*) had much lower mortality rates when given
ganoderma decoction than did 11 patients given
conventional treatment (Xiao et al., 2003).
- Useful as a cardiotonic; enhances myocardial metabolism
and improves coronary artery hemodynamics. Symptoms
that showed improvement include palpitations, dyspnea,
arrhythmias, elevated cholesterol, and high blood pressure
(Hobbs, 1995).
- In Chinese clinical trials, tablets were given to more than 2,000
patients with chronic bronchitis. In 2 weeks, 60% to 90% of
the patients had improvement of symptoms and increased
appetite. Also beneficial for allergic asthma and allergic rhinitis
because of its ability to inhibit histamine release.
- Prevention and possibly treatment of atherosclerosis
- Treatment of altitude sickness: use with ginkgo, cordyceps,
and rhodiola
- Effective for treating the symptoms of a rare genetic disease,
myotonia dystrophica (Hobbs, 1995)
- Useful as an adaptogen for reducing the effects of chronic stress.
Improves adrenal function, sleep quality, appetite; acts as an
antioxidant; reduces anxiety and inflammation. In a
randomized, double-blind, placebo-controlled study, ganoderma
polysaccharide extract significantly improved symptoms of
fatigue in patients with neurasthenia (Tang et al., 2005).

Available Forms, Dosage, and Administration
Guidelines
Preparations: Dried mushroom, tea, tincture, spray-dried extract
Typical Dosage
- *Dried mushroom* (finely ground): 3 to 12 g a day

- *Tea:* 2 tsp ground mushroom in 16 oz water, decoct slowly until the water is reduced by half (8 oz); take two or three cups a day
- *Tincture* (1:5, 30% alcohol): 80 to 160 gtt (4–8 mL) three times a day
- *Spray-dried extract* (5:1): Three 300-mg capsules three times a day

Pharmacokinetics—If Available (form or route when known): Not known

Toxicity: None

Contraindications: Mushroom allergies

Side Effects: Diarrhea (large doses) and GI upset

Long-Term Safety: Safe

Use in Pregnancy/Lactation/Children: Safe

Drug/Herb Interactions and Rationale (if known): None known

Special Notes: Other species of ganoderma mushroom (*G. sinensis, G. tsugae, G. applanatum, G. tenue, G. capense, G. japonicum*) have been shown to have antioxidant, antitumor, hepatoprotective, anti-inflammatory, and antiviral activity.

BIBLIOGRAPHY

el-Mekkawy S, et al. (1998). Anti-HIV-1 and anti-HIV-1-protease substances from *Ganoderma lucidum. Phytochemistry.* 49(6):1651–1657.

Gao Y, et al. (2003). Effects of ganopoly (a *Ganoderma lucidum* polysaccharide extract) on the immune functions in advanced-stage cancer patients. *Immunological Investigations.* Aug;32(3):201–215.

Hijikata Y, Yamada S. (1998). Effect of *Ganoderma lucidum* on postherpetic neuralgia. *American Journal of Chinese Medicine.* 26(3–4):375–381.

Hobbs C. (1995). *Medicinal Mushrooms* (2nd ed.; pp. 96–107). Santa Cruz, CA: Botanica Press.

Jiang J, et al. (2006). *Ganoderma lucidum* inhibits proliferation of human breast cancer cells by down-regulation of estrogen receptor and NF-KappaB signaling. *International Journal of Oncology.* Sep;29(3):695–703.

Jones K. (1996). *Reishi: Ancient Herb for Modern Times*. Seattle: Sylvan Press.

Kim DH, et al. (1999). Beta-glucuronidase-inhibitory activity and hepatoprotective effect of *Ganoderma lucidum*. *Biological Pharmacy Bulletin*. 22(2):162–164.

Kim KD, Kim IG. (1999). *Ganoderma lucidum* extract protects DNA from strand breakage caused by hydroxyl radical and UV irradiation. *International Journal of Molecular Medicine*. 4(3):273–277.

Patocka J. (1999). Anti-inflammatory triterpenoids from mysterious mushroom *Ganoderma lucidum* and their potential possibility in modern medicine. *Acta Medica (Hradec Kralove)*. 42(4):123–125.

Seong-Kug E, et al. (1999). Antiherpetic activities of various protein-bound polysaccharides isolated from *Ganoderma lucidum*. *Journal of Ethnopharmacology*. 68:175–181.

Stamets, P. (2002). *MycoMedicinals* (pp. 24–29). Olympia, WA: MycoMedia Productions.

Tang W, et al. (2005). A randomized, double-blind and placebo-controlled study of a *Ganoderma lucidum* polysaccharide extract in neurasthenia. *Journal of Medicinal Food*. Spring;8(1):53–58.

Xiao FL, et al. (2003). Clinical observation on treatment of *Russula subnigricans* poisoning patients by *Ganoderma lucidum* decoction. *Zhongguo Zhong Xi Yi Jie He Za Zhi*. Apr;23(4):278–280.

Xie JT, et al. (2006). Ganoderma extract inhibits proliferation of SW 480 human colon cancer cells. *Experimental Oncology*. Mar; 28(1):25–29.

Yue GG, et al. (2006). Comparative studies of various ganoderma species and their different parts with regard to their antitumor and immunomodulating activites in vitro. *Journal of Alternative and Complementary Medicine*. Oct;12(8):777–789.

Yuen JW, Gohel MD. (2005). Anticancer effects of *Ganoderma lucidum:* A review of scientific evidence. *Nutrition and Cancer*. 53(1):11–17.

Zhu M, et al. (1999). Triterpene antioxidants from *Ganoderma lucidum*. *Phytotherapy Research*. 13(6):529–531.

 NAME: Rhodiola Root (*Rhodiola rosea*)

Common Names: Rose root, golden root

Family: *Crassulaceae*

Description of Plant

- Rose root grows in the northern circumpolar regions of Russia, Scandinavia, Canada as well as in mountainous regions of Europe

- It is a small, succulent plant with yellow flowers related to the ornamental sedums
- The root has a lovely "rose-like" odor, hence its common name

Medicinal Part: Dried root

Constituents and Action (if known)
- Rosavins (cinnamyl-alcohol-glycosides)
  - Rosavin: adaptogenic (Panossian & Wagner, 2005)
  - Rosin: adaptogenic (Panossian & Wagner, 2005)
  - Rosarin: adaptogenic (Panossian & Wagner, 2005)
- Salidroside (rhodioloside): cytoprotective (Cao et al., 2006), antioxidant (Zhang et al., 2005), enhances recovery of hematopoietic function (Zhang et al., 2005)
- p-Tyrosol: antioxidant, protected against lead-induced cell damage (Pashkevich et al., 2003)
- Flavonoids
  - Rodiolin: antioxidant (Kwon et al., 2006)
  - Rodionin: antioxidant (Kwon et al., 2006)
  - Rodiosin: antioxidant (Kwon et al., 2006)
- EO
  - Geraniol: antitumor, CNS stimulant (Duke, 2006)

Other Actions: ACE inhibitory effects (Kwon et al., 2006), antibacterial (Ming et al., 2005), anti-inflammatory (Abidov et al., 2004)

Nutritional Ingredients: In Ukraine, a medicinal liquor, Nastoyka, is made with rhodiola and vodka. It is reputed to promote energy and resistance to illness (Winston & Maimes, 2007).

Traditional Use
- Adaptogen, antidepressant, antioxidant, antiarrythmic, astringent. Mild CNS stimulant, cardioprotective, neuroprotective.
- Rhodiola was used as a strengthening tonic by the Vikings. It remained a popular tonic remedy in Scandinavia and was listed as an officinal medicine in the first Swedish *Pharmacopoeia* published in 1755 (Winston & Maimes, 2007).
- Several rhodiola species (*R. rosea, R. sacra, R. wallichianum, R. crenulata, R. imbricata, R. saccharinensis,* etc.) have been

used in traditional Chinese and Tibetan medicine to reduce fevers, relieve altitude sickness, enhance energy, and treat coughs and asthma (Winston & Maimes, 2007).

Current Use

- Rhodiola is a mildly stimulating adaptogen, antidepressant, and nootropic agent that has been accepted in the Russian *Pharmacopoeia* since 1969.
- There have been a number of human studies showing that ingestion of this herb can improve exercise endurance (De Bock et al., 2004), reduce mental fatigue, and enhance cognitive function (Darbinyan et al., 2000, Spasov et al., 2000, Shevtsov et al., 2003); lower levels of C-reactive protein and creatine kinase (Abidov et al., 2004); and benefits work performance (Panossian & Wagner, 2005). It should be noted that there are also two very small negative studies, both of a short duration, using a rhodiola/cordyceps formula that failed to improve exercise performance or muscle tissue oxygen saturation (Colson et al., 2005; Earnest et al., 2004). There are several possible issues with these last two studies, including the small sample size, the short period of use of the product(s), and possibly the quality of the products.
- Adaptogens help to re-regulate the HPA axis and sympathoadrenal system (SAS). These control systems maintain normal endocrine, immune, and nervous system function. This makes these herbs useful for treating chronic stress, elevated cortisol levels, depression, insulin resistance, and chronic fatigue immune deficiency syndrome (CFIDS) (Winston & Maimes, 2007)
- Rhodiola has immunomodulating effects, and in a study of women with advanced ovarian cancer, a combination of rhodiola, rhaptonicum, eleuthero, and schisandra enhanced immune function while undergoing chemotherapy (Kormosh et al., 2006).
- In a Chinese study, 40 patients with severe pulmonary hypertension were pretreated with rhodiola before having cardiopulmonary bypass surgery. Another 36 patients who acted as the control had identical preoperative treatment and surgery, except they did not receive rhodiola. The occurrence

rate of acute lung injury and its mortality in the rhodiola group were 7.5% and 0%; in the control group, 19.4% developed lung injury and 43% died (Xu et al., 2003).
- A number of in vitro and in vivo studies show that rhodiola is cardioprotective (Maslova et al., 1994), antiarrythmic, reduces stress-induced cardiac damage, and decreases myocardial catecholamine levels (Brown et al., 2002). It also reduces C-reactive protein levels (Abidov et al., 2004), a major risk factor for heart disease and atherosclerosis.
- This herb has also been shown to help re-regulate menstrual cycles in women with amenorrhea (Brown et al., 2002), relieve erectile dysfunction in 26 out of 35 men (Brown et al., 2002), and enhance thyroid function without causing hyperthyroidism (Maslova et al., 1994).

Available Forms, Dosage, and Administration Guidelines
Preparations: Tea, tincture, standardized extract (SHR-5)/capsules
Typical Dosage:
- *Tea:* 1 to 2 tsp dried root in 8 oz hot water, decoct 15 minutes; take one to three cups a day
- Standardized extract/*Capsules:* 500 mg standardized 3% to 6% rosavins and 1% salidroside, one to two a day
- *Tincture* (1:5, 30% alcohol): 80 to 120 gtt (4–6 mL) TID

Pharmacokinetics—If Available (form or route when known): Not known

Toxicity: None known

Contraindications: Do not use in patients with bipolar disorder, mania, or paranoid anxiety (Skenderi, 2003).

Side Effects: It can, on rare occasion, cause overstimulation and insomnia in sensitive people.

Long-Term Safety: Safe

Use in Pregnancy/Lactation/Children: There is no animal or human evidence of toxicity or teratogenicity.

Drug/Herb Interactions and Rationale (if known): Animal studies show that rhodiola decreases the toxicity of chemotherapy agents (cyclophosphamide, doxorubicin) while enhancing their anticancer effects (Brown et al., 2002).

Special Notes:

- There are many species of rhodiola, and while several have shown activity, only *R. rosea* contains the highly active rosavins and has extensive clinical research to back up claims made for this herb. Many of the studies use a proprietary extract (SHR-5) of rhodiola sold as Arctic root.
- Rhodiola is a slow-growing plant and has been overharvested in the wild. Purchase only cultivated rhodiola. It is being cultivated on a large scale in Scandinavia and Russia.

BIBLIOGRAPHY

Abidov M, et al. (2004). Extract of *Rhodiola rosea* radix reduces the level of C-reactive protein and creatinine kinase in the blood. *Bulletin in Experimental Biology and Medicine.* Jul;138(1):63–64.

Brown R, et al. (2002). *Rhodiola rosea*, a phytomedicinal overview. *Herbalgram.* 56:40–52.

Cao LL, et al. (2006). The effect of salidroside on cell damage induced by glutamate and intracellular free calcium PC12 cells. *Journal of Asian Natural Products Research.* Jan-Mar;8(1–2):159–165.

Colson SN, et al. (2005). *Cordyceps sinensis*– and *Rhodiola rosea*–based supplementation in male cyclists and its effect on muscle tissue oxygen saturation. *Journal of Strength and Conditioning Research.* May;19(2):358–363.

Darbinyan V, et al. (2000). *Rhodiola rosea* in stress induced fatigue— A double blind cross-over study of a standardized extract SHR-5 with a repeated low-dose regimen on the mental performance of healthy physicians during night duty. *Phytomedicine.* Oct;7(5):365–371.

De Bock K, et al. (2004). Acute *Rhodiola rosea* intake can improve endurance exercise performance. *International Journal of Sport Nutrition and Exercise Metabolism.* Jun;14(3):298–307.

Duke J. Dr. Duke's phytochemical and ethnobotanical databases. Retrieved October 30 2006, from www.ars-grin.gov/cgi-bin/duke/chemactivities.

Earnest CP, et al. (2004). Effects of a commercial herbal-based formula on exercise performance in cyclists. *Medicine and Science in Sports and Exercise.* Mar;36(3):504–509.

Kormosh N, et al. (2006). Effect of a combination of extracts from several plants on cell-mediated and humoral immunity of patients with advanced ovarian cancer. *Phytotherapy Research.* May;20(5): 424–425.

Kwon YI, et al. (2006). Evaluation of *Rhodiola crenulata* and *Rhodiola rosea* for management of type II diabetes and hypertension. *Asian Pacific Journal of Clinical Nutrition.* 15(3):425–432.

Maslova LV, et al. (1994). The cardioprotective and antiadrenergic activity of an extract of *Rhodiola rosea* in stress. *Eksperimentalnaia I Klinicheskaia Farmakologiia.* 57(6):61–63.

Ming DS, et al. (2005). Bioactive compounds from *Rhodiola rosea* (Crassulaceae). *Phytotherapy Research.* Sep;19(9):740–743.

Panossian A, Wagner H. (2005). Stimulating effect of adaptogens: An overview with particular reference to their efficacy following singe dose administration. *Phytotherapy Research.* Oct;19(10): 819–838.

Pashkevich IA, et al. (2003). Comparative evaluation of effects of p-Tyrosol and *Rhodiola rosea* extract on bone marrow cells in vivo. *Eksperimentalnaia I Klinicheskaia Farmakologiia.* Jul-Aug;66(4): 50–52.

Shevtsov VA, et al. (2003). A randomized trial of two different doses of a SHR-5 *Rhodiola rosea* extract versus placebo and control of capacity for mental work. *Phytomedicine.* 10(2–3):95–105.

Skenderi G. (2003). *Herbal Vade Mecum* (pp. 85–86). Rutherford, NJ: Herbacy Press.

Spasov AA, et al. (2000). A double-blind, placebo-controlled pilot study of the stimulating and adaptogenic effect of *Rhodiola rosea* SHR-5 extract on the fatigue of students. *Phytomedicine.* 7(2):85–89.

Xu KJ, et al. (2003). Preventive and treatment effect of composite Rhodiolae on acute lung injury in patients with severe pulmonary hypertension during extracorporeal circulation. *Zhongguo Zhong Xi Yi Jie He Za Zhi.* Sep;23(9):648–650.

Winston D. (2006). *Winston's Botanic Materia Medica.* Washington, NJ: DWCHS.

Winston D, Maimes S. (2007). *Adaptogens, Herbs for Strength, Stamina, and Stress Relief* (pp. 191–194). Rochester, VT: Inner Traditions.

Zhang XS, et al. (2005). Effect of salidroside on bone marrow cell cycle and expression of apoptosis-related proteins in bone marrow cells of bone marrow depressed anemia mice. *Sichuan Da Zue Xue Bao Yi Xue Ban.* Nov;36(6):820–823, 846.

Zhang Y, Liu Y. (2005). Study on effects of salidroside on lipid peroxidation on oxidative stress in rat hepatic stellate cells. *Zhong Yao Cai.* Sep;28(9):794–796.

NAME: Rosemary (*Rosmarinus officinalis*)

Common Names: Garden rosemary

Family: *Lamiaceae*

Description of Plant

- A highly aromatic member of the mint family with waxy linear leaves and pale blue flowers
- A small, bushy shrub native to the southern Mediterranean; now commonly cultivated throughout the world
- Leaves are harvested and can be used fresh or dried.

Medicinal Part: Leaves, flowering tops, EO

Constituents and Action (if known)

- Volatile oils (0.5%–2.5%): monoterpenes: camphor (15%–25%), cineole (15%–50%), alpha-pinene (10%–25%), camphene, and borneol (spasmolytic): antibacterial, antiviral, and antifungal activity (Prabuseenivasan et al., 2006)
- Flavonoids (diosmin, diosmetin, genkwanin, luteolin, apigenin)
  - May reduce capillary permeability and fragility
  - Antioxidant and antimicrobial activity
  - Anti-inflammatory activity
- Phenolic acids
  - Rosmarinic acid: anti-inflammatory, antioxidant; radio-protective, antimutagenic (Del Bano et al., 2006), antimicrobial (Moreno & Scheyer, 2006), reduces smooth muscle activity (in vitro); suppresses release of thromboxane A_2, prostacyclin (al-Sereiti et al., 1999), photogenic acid (Bruneton, 1999)
  - Caffeic acid: antioxidant (al-Sereiti et al., 1999)
  - Phenolic compounds inhibit cancers by inhibiting activation of phase I enzymes (cyclic P450) and stimulating phase II enzymes (glutathione S-transferase). In laboratory animals, adding 1% rosemary extract to the diet reduced the incidence of experimentally caused mammary tumors by 47%. Skin tumors were also inhibited by topical application.
- Tricyclic diterpenes
  - Carnosolic (carnosic) and labiatic acids: antioxidant and anticancer properties; carnosol (radio-protective, antimutagenic) (Del Bano et al., 2006), protects against

rotenone-induced neurotoxicity (Kim et al., 2006);
rosmanol, rosmariquinone, rosmadial: anti-inflammatory,
antioxidant, antiviral (ESCOP, 2003)
  ○ Inhibitory against HIV-1 protease (Paris et al., 1993)

Other Actions
- Rosemary extracts have a strong antiviral activity.
- Extracts have a topical anti-inflammatory activity.
- May have potential as a chemoprotectant (more studies in
  humans are needed) (Offord et al., 1997) and
  hepatoprotective agent
- In mice, it reduced symptoms of morphine withdrawal
  (Hosseinzadeh & Nourbakhsh, 2003)

Nutritional Ingredients: A versatile spice that can be used to
flavor meat, fish, and fowl; can also be used in rolls and bread

Traditional Use
- Astringent, antioxidant, carminative, antispasmodic,
  choleretic, circulatory tonic
- Digestive tonic for flatulence, borborygmus, eructations,
  nausea, and biliousness
- Tea used as a hair rinse to stimulate hair growth and prevent
  baldness
- Used to strengthen the memory and cerebral circulation
- Used in Europe for headaches, hypotension, and impaired
  circulation
- EO in a carrier oil is used as a massage oil for arthritic pain
  and muscle spasms.

Current Use
Internal
- Liver/gallbladder tonic for impaired fat digestion,
  biliousness, nausea, and biliary dyskinesia. Rosemary
  enhanced the activity of two liver enzymes (GSH-transferase,
  NAD(P)H-quinone reductase) when included at very low
  levels in the diet of rats.
- Reduces GI upset, gas, and abdominal distention
- Powerful dietary antioxidant that may reduce the risk of
  cancers, arteriosclerosis, and other oxidative diseases
- It is a mild circulatory tonic for hypotension, impaired
  memory, and age-related depression.

- In human trials, inhalation of rosemary EO enhanced memory and mood (Moss et al., 2003).

Topical: Topical application of rosemary EO in carrier oils or liniments is useful for muscle pain and arthralgias and may inhibit risk of skin cancers.

Available Forms, Dosage, and Administration Guidelines

Preparations: Dried herb, tincture, capsules, EO, ointment (semisolid preparation containing 6%–10% EO in base of beeswax and vegetable oil)

Typical Dosage

- *Dried herb:* 4 to 6 g per day
- *Infusion:* 1 tsp dried herb in 8 oz hot water, steep covered 15 to 20 minutes; take two cups a day
- *Tincture* (1:5, 40% alcohol): 40 to 80 gtt (2–4 mL) three times a day
- *Capsules:* One or two 500-mg capsules three times a day
- *EO:* 1 to 2 gtt two times a day (short-term use only)
- *Bath additive:* Infuse 2 oz leaf in 1 qt water, let stand covered for 15 to 30 minutes, strain, and add to one full bath
- *Ointment:* Massage into affected areas

Pharmacokinetics—If Available (form or route when known): Not known

Toxicity: Herb: none known; EO: overdoses can cause irritation of the stomach and intestines and kidney damage

Contraindications: Avoid internal use of EO in patients with seizures.

Side Effects: Contact dermatitis with external use (Fernandez et al., 1997); GI disturbances with large internal doses of the tea

Long-Term Safety: Safe; long history of human consumption as a spice and medicine

Use in Pregnancy/Lactation/Children: Avoid in pregnancy; may have adverse effects on fetus and uterus. No restrictions during lactation.

Drug/Herb Interactions and Rationale (if known): None known

Special Notes: Rosemary EO, like all EOs, is highly concentrated and should be used internally in very minute amounts, if at all. Topically, the EO should be diluted before being applied to the skin.

BIBLIOGRAPHY

al-Sereiti MR, et al. (1999). Pharmacology of rosemary (*Rosmarinus officinalis* Linn.) and its therapeutic potentials. *Indian Journal of Experimental Biology.* 37(2):124–130.

Bruneton J. (1999). *Pharmacognosy, Phytochemistry, Medicinal Plants* (2nd ed.;pp. 249–250). Paris: Lavoisier.

Correa Dias P, et al. (2000). Antiulcerogenic activity of crude hydroalcoholic extract of *Rosmarinus officinalis* L. *Journal of Ethnopharmacology.* 69(1):57–62.

Del Bano MJ, et al. (2006). Radioprotective-antimutagenic effects of rosemary phenolics against chromosomal damage induced in human lymphocytes by gamma-rays. *Journal of Agricultural and Food Chemistry.* Mar 22;54(6):2064–2068.

European Scientific Cooperative on Phytotherapy. (2003). *ESCOP Monographs* (pp. 429–436). New York: Thieme.

Fahim FA, et al. (1999). Allied studies on the effect of *Rosmarinus officinalis* L. on experimental hepatotoxicity and mutagenesis. *International Journal of Food Science and Nutrition.* 50(6): 413–427.

Fernandez L, et al. (1997). Allergic contact dermatitis from rosemary (*Rosmarinus officinalis* L). *Contact Dermatitis.* 37(5): 248–249.

Hjorther AB, et al. (1997). Occupational allergic contact dermatitis from carnosol, a naturally-occurring compound present in rosemary. *Contact Dermatitis.* 37(3):99–100.

Hosseinzadeh H, Nourbakhsh M. (2003). Effect of *Rosmarinus officinalis* L. aerial parts extract on morphine withdrawal syndrome in mice. *Phytotherapy Research.* Sep;17(8): 938–941.

Kim SJ, et al. (2006). Carnosol, a component of rosemary (*Rosmarinus officinalis* L.) protects nigral dopaminergic neuronal cells. *Neuroreport.* Nov 6;17(16):1729–1733.

Moreno S, Scheyer T. (2006). Antioxidant and antimicrobial activities of rosemary extracts linked to their polyphenol composition. *Free Radical Research.* Feb;40(2):223–231.

Moss M, et al. (2003). Aromas of rosemary and lavender essential oils differently affect cognition and mood in healthy adults. *International Journal of Neuroscience.* Jan;113(1):15–38.

Offord EA, et al. (1997). Mechanisms involved in the chemoprotective effects of rosemary extract studied in human liver and bronchial cells. *Cancer Letters.* 114:275–281.

Paris A, et al. (1993). Inhibitory effect of carnosic acid on HIV-1 protease in cell-free assays. *Journal of Natural Products.* 56(8): 1426–1430.

Prabuseenivasan S, et al. (2006). In vitro antibacterial activity of some plant essential oils. *Complementary and Alternative Medicine.* Nov 30;6(1):39.

Tisserand R, Balacs T. (1995). *Essential Oil Safety* (p. 165). Edinburgh: Churchill Livingstone.

 NAME: Sage (*Salvia officinalis*)

Common Names: Garden sage, Dalmatian sage

Family: *Lamiaceae*

Description of Plant
- Sage is a small perennial in the mint family with a highly aromatic odor and grayish-green leaves.
- It is native to the Mediterranean region of Europe but is winter hardy to zone 6.

Medicinal Part: Dried herb

Constituents and Action (if known)
- EOs
  - 1,8-cineole: cytokine inhibitor (Juergens, 1998), anti-inflammatory (Juergens, 2003)
  - α and β thujone: neurotoxic
  - Camphor: antioxidant, antibacterial, antifungal (Jutea et al., 2002)
  - β-carophyllene: anti-inflammatory (Duke, 2006), antifungal, antioxidant, antibacterial (Jutea et al., 2002)
- Other effects of EO: antimutagenic (Vukovic-Gacic et al., 2006)

- Diterpenes
  - Carnosic acid: antioxidant (Matsingou et al., 2003), anti-inflammatory, hypoglycemic (Rau et al., 2006), hypolipidemic (Ninomiya et al., 2004)
  - Carnasol: antioxidant (Matsingou et al., 2003), anti-inflammatory, hypoglycemic (Rau et al., 2006)
  - Rosmanol: antioxidant (Matsingou et al., 2003)
  - Galdosol: antioxidant (Matsingou et al., 2003), benzodiazepine receptor ligand (Kavvadias et al., 2003)
- Triterpenoids
  - Oleanolic acid: antioxidant, antiviral, antiallergic, immunomodulator (Duke, 2006)
- Ursolic acid: anti-inflammatory (Baricevic et al., 2001)
- Phenolic compounds
  - Rosmarinic acid: antioxidant, anti-inflammatory, antibacterial, antiviral (Peterson et al., 2003), neuroprotective (Iuvone et al., 2006)
- Flavonoids

Nutritional Ingredients: Sage is a common culinary spice used in making poultry stuffing and sausage.

Traditional Use

- Antibacterial, antiviral, antifungal, astringent (mild), anti-inflammatory, antioxidant, carminative, antiperspirant, antigalactogogue
- Sage has a long history of use as a carminative and GI antibacterial for treating diarrhea, dysentery, digestive upset, nausea, vomiting, and gas.
- It also makes an excellent gargle for sore throats, thrush, periodontal disease, and aphthous stomatitis.
- For millennia, women have taken sage tea to dry up breast milk when weaning their children.
- The tea is effective for treating colds, sinusitis (use as a nasal wash), and postnasal drip (use as a nasal wash).

Current Use

- Most of the traditional uses for this herb are still valid today. The antibacterial EOs make sage tea (or tincture) an effective treatment for bacterial food poisoning, diarrhea, and gastritis (Winston, 2006).

- Sage reduces excessive secretions from the sinus and upper respiratory tract mucous membranes as well as excessive sweating. It is used to reduce menopausal sweating and nightsweats. A sage throat spray was found to be effective for treating pain caused by acute pharyngitis (Hubbert et al., 2006).
- Recent research has found that sage has a benefit for relieving symptoms of mild to moderate Alzheimer's disease. It reduced agitation and improved cognitive function over a four-month trial (Akhondzadeh et al., 2003). A second study of healthy young people found that a single dose of sage improved mood and cognitive performance (Kennedy et al., 2006).
- A topical ointment of sage moderately inhibited *Herpes labialis* lesions; a combined product made from sage and rhubarb root was as effective as topical acyclovir for reducing the pain and length of a herpes outbreak (Saller et al., 2001).

Available Forms, Dosage, and Administration Guidelines
Preparations: Tea, capsules, tincture
Typical Dosage
- *Tea:* 1 tsp dried herb to 8 oz hot water, steep 15 to 20 minutes; take 4 oz three times a day
- *Capsules:* One 250- to 300-mg capsule, once or twice a day
- *Tincture* (1:5, 35% alcohol): 30 to 40 gtt (1.5–2.0 mL TID)

Pharmacokinetics—If Available (form or route when known): Not known

Toxicity: The EO thujone in high doses over a prolonged period of time is neurotoxic. The levels of thujone in tea would be limited, but an alcohol tincture or sage EO would have considerably higher levels of this compound.

Contraindications: Breast-feeding

Side Effects:: None known

Long-Term Safety: The tea is safe when taken in normal therapeutic amounts. The tincture should be used for short periods of time (4 weeks or less). Avoid using sage EO internally.

Use in Pregnancy/Lactation/Children: Avoid use during pregnancy and lactation.

Drug/Herb Interactions and Rationale (if known): None known

Special Notes: Several other species of *Salvia* are used medicinally, including Dan Shen (*S. miltiorrhiza*) (see p. 153), white sage (*S. apiana*), Greek sage (*S. triloba*), and Spanish sage (*S. lavandufolia*). With the exception of Dan Shen, which is used quite differently from garden sage, most other medicinal sages are used for their carminative and antibacterial activity.

BIBLIOGRAPHY

Akhondzadeh S, et al. (2003). *Salvia officinalis* extract in the treatment of patients with mild to moderate Alzheimer's disease: A double blind, randomized and placebo-controlled trial. *Journal of Clinical Pharmacy and Therapeutics.* Feb;28(1):53–59.

Baricevic D, et al. (2001). Topical anti-inflammatory activity of *Salvia officinalis* L. leaves: The relevance of ursolic acid. *Journal of Ethnopharmacology.* May;75(2–3):125–132.

Brinker F. (2001). *Herb Contraindications & Drug Interactions* (3rd ed.; p. 171). Sandy, OR: Eclectic Medical Publications.

European Scientific Cooperative on Phytotherapy. (2003). *ESCOP Monographs*—(2nd ed.; pp. 174–177). Stuttgart: Thieme.

Hubbert M, et al. (2006). Efficacy and tolerability of a spray with *Salvia officinalis* in the treatment of acute pharyngitis—A randomised, double-blind, placebo-controlled study with adaptive design and interim analysis. *European Journal of Medical Research.* Jan 31;11(1):20–26.

Iuvone T, et al. (2006). The spice sage and its active ingredient rosmarinic acid protect PC12 cells from amyloid-beta peptide-induced neurotoxicity. *Journal of Pharmacology and Experimental Therapeutics.* June;317(3):1143–1149.

Jutea F, et al. (2002). Antibacterial and antioxidant activities of *Artemisia annua* essential oil. *Fitoterapia.* Oct;73(6):532–535.

Juergens UR, et al. (1998). Inhibition of cytokine production and arachidonic acid metabolism by eucalyptol (1.8-cineole) in human blood monocytes in vitro. *European Journal of Medical Research.* Nov 17;3(11):508–510.

Juergen UR, et al. (2003). Anti-inflammatory activity of 1.8-cineole (eucalyptol) in bronchial asthma: a double-blind placebo controlled trial. *Respiratory Medicine.* Mar;97(3):250–256.

Kavvadias D, et al. (2003). Constituents of sage (*Salvia officinalis*) with in vitro affinity to human brain benzodiazeprine receptor. *Planta Medica.* Feb;69(2):113–117.

Kennedy DO, et al. (2006). Effects of cholinesterase inhibiting sage (*Salvia officinalis*) on mood, anxiety, and performance on a psychological stressor battery. *Neuropsychopharmacology.* Apr;31(4):845–852.

Lima CF, et al. (2005). The Drinking of a *Salvia officinalis* infusion improves liver antioxidant status in mice and rats. *Journal of Ethnopharmacology.* Feb 28;97(2):383–389.

Matsingou TC, et al. (2003). Antioxidant activity of organic extracts from aqueous infusions of sage. *Journal of Agricultural and Food Chemistry.* Nov 5;51(23):6696–6701.

Ninomiya K, et al. (2004). Carnosic acid, a new class of lipid absorption inhibitor from sage. *Bioorganic and Medicinal Chemistry Letters.* Apr 19;14(8):1943–1946.

Petersen M, et al. (2003). Rosmarinic acid. *Phytochemistry.* Jan;62(2): 121–125.

Rau O, et al. (2006). Carnosic acid and carnosol, phenolic diterpene compounds of the labiate herbs rosemary and sage, are activators of the human perioxisome proliferator-activated receptor gamma. *Planta Medica.* Aug;72(10):881–887.

Saller R, et al. (2001). Combined herbal preparation for topical treatment of *Herpes labialis. Forschende Komplementarmedizin und Klassische Naturheilkunde.* Dec;8(6):373–382.

Skenderi G. (2003). *Herbal Vade Mecum* (p. 328). Rutherford, NJ: Herbacy Press.

Vukovic-Gacic B, et al. (2006). Antimutagenic effect of essential oil of sage (*Salvia officinalis* L.) and its monoterpenes against uv-induced mutations in *Escherichia coli* and *Saccharomyces Cerevisiae. Food and Chemical Toxicology.* Oct;44(10):1730–1708.

Winston D. (2006). *Winston's Botanic Materia Medica.* Washington, NJ: DWCHS.

 NAME: Sarsaparilla (*Smilax* species)

Common Names: Honduras or brown sarsaparilla (*S. regelii*), Mexican or gray sarsaparilla (*S. medica*), Jamaican or red sarsaparilla (*S. ornata*), Ecuadorian sarsaparilla (*S. febrifuga*), Tu Fu Ling or Chinese sarsaparilla (*S. glabra*), Jing Gang Ten (*S. china*)

Family: *Liliaceae*

Description of Plant
- Woody, trailing vine that can grow to 150' long
- Numerous species are used, and many are similar in appearance.
- Cultivated in Mexico, Jamaica, and Central and South America and China

Medicinal Part: Rhizome

Constituents and Action (if known)
- Steroidal saponins
  - Sarsaponin, sarasapogenin, smilagenin, smilasaponin: have ability to bind endotoxins, so may be beneficial in liver disease, psoriasis, fever, and inflammatory processes (Li et al., 2006)
  - Diosgenin, tigogenin, and asperagenin (Li et al., 2006)
- Phytosterols (sitosterol, stigmasterol, pollinastanol) (Li et al., 2006)
- Other constituents include starch (50%), resin (2.5%), kaempferol, quercetin; have anticancer activity.
- Minerals: potassium (diuretic), chromium, magnesium, selenium, calcium, and zinc

Nutritional Ingredients: Root has mild spicy-sweet taste and has been used as a natural flavoring in medicines, foods, and nonalcoholic beverages.

Traditional Use
- Anti-inflammatory, alterative, diuretic, hepatoprotective, antisyphylitic, and rheumatic
- It was used with guaiac to treat syphilis. A Chinese species, *S. glabra*, along with five other herbs, has been reported to be 90% effective in curing acute syphilis and 50% effective in treating chronic cases (confirmed by blood tests).
- For red, hot, and inflamed skin and connective tissue conditions (psoriatic and rheumatoid arthritis and psoriasis), use with gotu kola (Winston, 2006).
- Systemic anti-inflammatory for arthralgias

Current Use
- Reduces inflammation in arthritis, bursitis, rheumatoid arthritis, and gout. Increases uric acid excretion and binds

endotoxins, reducing the oxidative load in the bowel. Combine with additional anti-inflammatory herbs, such as turmeric, bupleurum, or boswellia. In animal studies, *S. glabra* downregulated overactive macrophages and upregulated dysfunctional T-lymphocytes in rheumatoid arthritis (Jiang J et al., 2003). *Smilax china* has been shown to have anti-inflammatory activity equal to aspirin, and it downregulates COX-2 activity (Shu et al., 2006).
- Moderate hepatoprotective activity (Leung & Foster, 1996)
- Anti-inflammatory to the large and small intestines; a useful therapy for dysbiosis, leaky gut syndrome, and irritable bowel syndrome. Use with yarrow, chamomile, turmeric, or marshmallow (Winston, 2006).
- Adjunctive therapy for leprosy

Available Forms, Dosage, and Administration Guidelines
Preparations: Dried root, capsules, tablets, tincture
Typical Dosage
- *Dried root:* 6 to 10 g
- *Capsules:* Up to six 500-mg capsules a day
- *Tea:* 2 tsp powdered root, decoct in 10 oz hot water for 10 to 15 minutes, steep half-hour; take two or three cups a day
- *Tincture* (1:5, 30% alcohol): 60 to 100 gtt (3–5 mL) three times a day
- Or follow manufacturer or practitioner recommendations

Pharmacokinetics—If Available (form or route when known): None known

Toxicity: None known

Contraindications: None known

Side Effects: GI irritation and nausea in large doses; asthma may occur from exposure to sarsaparilla dust (Vandenplas et al., 1996)

Long-Term Safety: Long history of human use in beverages and as a medicine; no adverse effects expected in normal therapeutic dosage

Use in Pregnancy/Lactation/Children: No known problems, but no research to establish safety

Drug/Herb Interactions and Rationale (if known): Separate from all other oral drugs by 2 hours; saponins may affect absorption. Sarsaparilla has been reported to change digoxin absorption and increase elimination of sedatives (Leung & Foster, 1996).

Special Notes: Advertising claims suggest that sarsaparilla is a natural source of testosterone (this is false) and that it enhances exercise performance (this is unsubstantiated). Few studies are available on the Western species of *Smilax*, but the Chinese species, *S. glabra*, has been well studied and is shown to be effective in treating rheumatoid arthritis and leptospirosis.

BIBLIOGRAPHY

Bernardo RR, et al. (1996). Steroidal saponins from *Smilax officinalis*. *Phytochemistry*. 43(20):465–469.

Der Marderosian A, Beutler J. [Eds.]. (2004). *The Review of Natural Products*. St. Louis, MO: Facts and Comparisons.

Jiang J, et al. (2003). Immunomodulatory activity of the aqueous extract from rhizome of *Smilax glabra* in the later phase of adjuvant-induced arthritis in rats. *Journal of Ethnopharmacology*. Mar;85(1):53–59.

Leung A, Foster S. (1996). *Encyclopedia of Common Natural Ingredients* (2nd ed.; pp. 462–463). New York: John Wiley & Sons.

Li et al. (2006). Steroidal glycosides and aromatic compounds from *Smilax riparia*. *Chemical and Pharmaceutical Bulletin*. Oct;54(10): 1451–1454.

Shu XS, et al. (2006). Anti-inflammatory and anti-nociceptive activities of *Smilax china* L. aqueous extract. *Journal of Ethnopharmacology*. Feb 20;103(3):327–332.

Vandenplas O, et al. (1996). Occupational asthma caused by sarsaparilla root dust. *Journal of Allergy and Clinical Immunology*. 97(6):1416–1418.

Winston D. (2006). *Winston's Botanic Materia Medica*. Washington, NJ: DWCHS.

NAME: Sassafras (*Sassafras albidum*)

Common Names: Ague tree, cinnamon wood, lignum floridium

Family: *Lauraceae*

Description of Plant
- Common deciduous tree found growing throughout the eastern United States
- Leaves have three distinct forms (entire, mitten, and trident)

Medicinal Part: Root bark

Constituents and Action (if known)
- Volatile oils (5%–9%): safrole (80%), alpha-pinene, alpha- and beta-phellandrene, camphor, methyleugenol
- Sesquiterpenes
- Tannins

Nutritional Ingredients: Commonly used as a beverage tea throughout the southeastern and south-central United States. The leaf is dried and powdered and sold as filé, a spice and thickener in Creole cooking. A safrole-free extract is used for flavoring root beer.

Traditional Use
- Carminative, diaphoretic, diuretic
- Used for digestive disturbances (gas, nausea, vomiting, borborygmus)
- Taken as a hot tea to stimulate sweating and break fevers
- A spring tonic or "blood purifier" used to stimulate elimination of wastes by the kidney, liver, and skin

Current Use: Not commonly used, except as a home remedy and beverage tea. The purported toxicity of sassafras as a tea is overstated, and its occasional ingestion in small amounts is not a cause for serious concern. The carcinogen safrole is poorly water-soluble, so very little is consumed in a tea. Avoid the EO, capsules, and tincture because of their high safrole content.

Available Forms, Dosage, and Administration Guidelines
Preparations: Dried root bark, tea

Typical Dosage
- *Tea:* 1 tsp dried root bark in 8 oz water, steep covered 5 minutes, take 4 oz, twice a day
- *Tincture:* Not recommended
- *EO:* Toxic; avoid

Pharmacokinetics—If Available (form or route when known): Safrole is broken down to 1-hydroxysafrole, a potent hepatic carcinogen.

Toxicity: Safrole, a component of the EO, is a potential carcinogen and is banned in the United States, even as a flavoring or fragrance. However, it is still sold and labeled "not for human consumption."

Contraindications: Pregnancy

Side Effects: Nausea or vomiting in large doses. The hot tea may cause excess sweating, especially in obese or menopausal patients.

Long-Term Safety: Avoid regular long-term use.

Use in Pregnancy/Lactation/Children: Avoid in all.

Drug/Herb Interactions and Rationale (if known): Safrole inhibits many CYP450 isoforms, especially CYP1A2, CYP2A6, and CYP2E1 (Ueng et al., 2005).

Special Notes: Studies in mice clearly show the toxicity of safrole. There are no known cases of human toxicity from consuming the tea.

BIBLIOGRAPHY

Bruneton J. (1999). *Pharmacognosy, Phytochemistry, Medicinal Plants* (2nd ed.; p. 552). Paris: Lavoisier.

DeSmet PAGM. (1997). *Adverse Effects of Herbal Drugs, Vol. 3* (pp. 123–127). Berlin: Springer-Verlag.

Kamdem DP, Gage DA. (1995). Chemical composition of essential oil from the root bark of *Sassafras albidum*. *Planta Medica.* Dec;61(6):574–575.

Leung A, Foster S. (1996). *Encyclopedia of Common Natural Ingredients* (2nd ed.; p. 463–465). New York: John Wiley & Sons.

Tisserand R, Balacs T. (1995). *Essential Oil Safety* (p. 168). Edinburgh: Churchill Livingstone.

Ueng YP, et al. (2005). Inhibition of human cytochrome P450 enzymes by the natural hepatotoxin safrole. *Food and Chemical Toxicology.* May;43(5):707–712.

NAME: Saw Palmetto (*Serenoa repens*)

Common Names: Dwarf palmetto, fan palm

Family: *Palmae*

Description of Plant

- Small palm tree native to the Atlantic and Gulf coasts of North America, from South Carolina to Florida, west to Georgia
- Grows 6' to 10' high, with 2' to 4' spiny-toothed leaves that form a circular fan shape
- Berries are blue-black with an oily texture and a pungent, cheesy aroma.

Medicinal Part: Berries (drupes)

Constituents and Action (if known)

- Fatty acids (63%–65%) (lauric, capric, caproic, caprylic, oleic, linoleic, linolenic, myristic, palmitic and stearic acids): reduce the formation of dihydrotestosterone by being a weak inhibitor of 5-alpha-reductase (Goepel et al., 1999; Marks & Tyler, 1999; McKinney, 1999); anti-inflammatory for prostatic tissue (Gerber et al., 1998)
- High-molecular-weight alcohols (n-docosanol, n-octacosanol, n-tricosanol, and hexacosanol): inhibit both subtypes of 5-alpha-reductase (Weisser et al., 1996); inhibit prolactin (Plosker & Brogden, 1996) and growth-factor-induced prostatic cell proliferation (Plosker & Brogden, 1996)
- Fatty acids (ethyl esters and sterols: beta-sitosterol, stigmasterol): anti-inflammatory, antitumor; lupeol, campesterol: anti-inflammatory
- Diterpenes (geranylgeraniol, phytol)
- Triterpenes (cycloartenal): bactericide, hypocholesterolemic

- Polysaccharides (S1, S2, S3, S4): immunostimulating; found in herb, not in standardized extracts (Winston, 1999)

Nutritional Ingredients: Used by the native people of Florida as a food; used as a flavoring in cognac; in the early part of the 20th century, it was used to flavor a soft drink called Metto.

Traditional Use
- Nutritive tonic, anti-inflammatory, diuretic, demulcent, immune amphoteric, urinary antiseptic
- Used by native people as a food; there is no history of them using the berries as a medicine
- Introduced into Western medical practice in 1877 as a digestive tonic and nutritive and to relieve irritation of the mucous membranes and upper respiratory tract. Was used for anorexia, pertussis, laryngitis, chronic coughs, tuberculosis, bronchitis, asthma, and weakness and deficiency after a serious illness (Winston, 1999).
- The eclectic physicians popularized *Serenoa* as a urinary tract and reproductive remedy and used it for orchitis, epididymitis, ovarian pain, prostatic hypertrophy, pelvic congestion, and atrophy of the testes and ovaries.

Current Use
- For mild to moderate BPH—improves urine flow rate, relieves nocturia by up to 73%, reduces residual urine volume, decreases dysuric pain and pollakiuria. Reduces prostatic swelling, prevents further progression of the condition (reducing the need for later surgery), and does not affect prostatic-specific antigen levels (Debruyne et al., 2002; Pytel et al., 2002; Pytel'Iu et al., 2004). Saw palmetto has also been found to relieve symptoms of chronic prostatitis (Wu et al., 2004). It decreased postoperative bleeding, inflammation, and the duration of postoperative catheterization in men who have had transurethral resection of the prostate (Pecoraro et al., 2004), and it does not cause sexual dysfunction, which can occur with pharmaceutical medications for BPH (Ziotta et al., 2005).
- A valuable upper respiratory herb (capsule, tea, tincture) useful for chronic irritable coughs, laryngitis, chronic bronchitis, and asthma (Winston, 2006)

- The tea or encapsulated herb is an immune tonic and adaptogen and can be used for patients with immune deficiency, frequent colds, cachexia, anorexia, and allergies.
- A mild, nonirritating diuretic, the berries can be beneficial for interstitial cystitis, UTIs, and scalding urine.
- Reduces symptoms of pelvic congestion syndrome (Winston, 1999)
- Useful along with chaste tree, licorice, and white peony for treating polycystic ovarian disease, ovarian pain, and female infertility caused by excessive androgens (Winston, 2006)
- Can be beneficial for deep cystic acne, combined with red alder or Oregon grape root, and chaste tree

Available Forms, Dosage, and Administration Guidelines

Preparations: Dried herb, capsules, tinctures, standardized soft gels, tea

Typical Dosage

- *Dried herb:* 2 to 6 g a day
- *Capsules (nonstandardized):* Six to nine 500-mg capsules a day
- *Tincture* (1:3, 70% alcohol): 60 to 100 gtt (3–5 mL) up to four times a day, or follow manufacturer or practitioner recommendations
- *Standardized preparations* (85%–95% fatty acids and sterols): Once or twice a day for a daily dose of 320 mg
- *Tea:* 1 tsp crushed berries to 8 oz hot water, decoct 15 minutes, steep half-hour; take two or three cups a day. The taste is horrible and will severely limit patient compliance.

Pharmacokinetics—If Available (form or route when known): Metabolized in the liver

Toxicity: There is one case report of supposed saw palmetto–induced hepatitis. In extensive animal studies and many human trials, no evidence of hepatotoxicity has emerged (Singh et al., 2007).

Contraindications: None known

Side Effects: GI upset (take with meals to minimize), diarrhea, headache (rare)

Long-Term Safety: Very safe

Use in Pregnancy/Lactation/Children: Used as a food by native people so it is probably safe, but because there is no current research, it is best to avoid. Avoid in breast-feeding women, because it inhibits prolactin and may interfere with lactation.

Drug/Herb Interactions and Rationale (if known): Saw palmetto did not affect CYP-450 (CYP2D6, CYP3A4) activity in a human study (Markowitz et al., 2003).

Special Notes: A medical diagnosis of BPH before starting treatment with saw palmetto and appropriate medical follow-up are recommended. A recent well-publicized study published in the *New England Journal of Medicine* (Bent et al., 2005) found that saw palmetto was not effective for treating BPH. The results were trumpeted loudly as another example of "herbs don't work." There was one serious flaw in this study—virtually all previous studies found that *Serenoa* was useful for mild to moderate BPH symptoms. Rarely mentioned in media reports, the *NEJM* study was on men with moderate to severe BPH. What the reports should have said is not that saw palmetto is not effective for BPH, but that it is not effective for more advanced (stage 3 and 4) BPH.

BIBLIOGRAPHY

Bach D, Ebeling L. (1996). Long-term drug treatment of benign prostatic hyperplasia: Results of a three-year multicenter study. *Phytomedicine*. 3(2):105–111.

Bach D, et al. (1997). Phytopharmaceutical and synthetic agents in the treatment of benign prostatic hyperplasia. *Phytomedicine*. 3(4):309–313.

Bennett BC, Hicklin JR. (1998). Uses of saw palmetto (*Serenoa repens, Arecaceae*) in Florida. *Economic Botany*. 52(4):381–393.

Bent S, et al. (2005). Saw palmetto for benign prostatic hyperplasia. *New England Journal of Medicine*. Feb 9;354(6):557–566.

Bombardelli E, Morazzoni P. (1997). *Serenoa repens* (Bartram). *Fitoterapia*. 68(2):99–114.

Debruyne F, et al. (2002). Comparison of a phytotherapeutic agent (Permixon) with an alpha-blocker (Tamsulosin) in the treatment of benign prostatic hyperplasia: A 1-year randomized international study. *European Urology*. May;41(5):497–506; discussion 506–507.

Gerber GS, et al. (1998). Saw palmetto (*Serenoa repens*) in men with lower urinary tract symptoms: Effects on urodynamic parameters and voiding symptoms. *Urology*. 51:1003–1007.

Goepel M, et al. (1999). Saw palmetto extracts potently and noncompetitively inhibit human alpha 1-adrenoceptors in vitro. *Prostate*. 38(3):208–215.

Markowitz JS, et al. (2003). Multiple doses of saw palmetto (*Serenoa repens*) did not alter cytochrome P450 2D6 and 3A4 activity in normal volunteers. *Clinical Pharmacology and Therapeutics*. Dec;74(5):536–542.

Marks LS, et al. (2000). Effects of a saw palmetto herbal blend in men with symptomatic benign prostatic hyperplasia. *Journal of Urology*. 163(5):1451–1456.

Marks LS, Tyler VE. (1999). Saw palmetto extract: Newest (and oldest) treatment alternative for men with symptomatic benign prostatic hyperplasia. *Urology*. 53(3):457–461.

McKinney DE. (1999). Saw palmetto for benign prostatic hyperplasia. *Journal of the American Medical Association*. 281(18): 1699.

McPartland JM, Pruitt PL. (2000). Benign prostatic hyperplasia treated with saw palmetto: A literature search and an experimental case study. *Journal of the American Osteopathic Association*. 100(2): 89–96.

Pecoraro S, et al. (2004). Efficacy of pretreatment with *Serenoa repens* on bleeding associated with transurethral resection of prostate. *Minerva Urologica e Nefrologica*. Mar;56(1):73–78.

Plosker GL, Brogden RN. (1996). *Serenoa repens* (Permixon): A review of its pharmacology and therapeutic efficacy in benign prostatic hyperplasia. *Drugs in Aging*. 9:379–395.

Pytel YA, et al. (2002). Long-term clinical and biologic effects of the lipidosterolic extract of *Serenoa repens* in patients with symptomatic benign prostatic hyperplasia. *Advances in Therapy*. Nov-Dec;19(6): 297–306.

Pytel'Iu A, et al. (2004). The results of long-term permixon treatment in patients with symptoms of lower urinary tracts dysfunction due to benign prostatic hyperplasia. *Urologila*. Mar-Apr;(2):3–7.

Singh YN, et al. (2007). Hepatotoxicity potential of saw palmetto (*Serenoa repens*) in rats. *Phytomedicine*. Feb;14(2–3):204–208. Epub 2006 July 18.

Weisser H, et al. (1996). Effects of the *Sabal surrulata* extract IDS 89 and its subfractions on 5-alpha-reductase activity in human benign prostatic hyperplasia. *Prostate*. 28:300–306.

Wilt TJ, et al. (1998). Saw palmetto extracts for treatment of benign prostatic hyperplasia: A systematic view. *Journal of the American Medical Association.* 280(18):1604–1609.

Winston D. (1999). *Saw Palmetto for Men and Women.* Pownal, VT: Storey Publishing.

Winston D. (2006). *Winston's Botanic Materia Medica.* Washington, NJ: DWCHS.

Wu T, et al. (2004). Effects of prostadyn sabale capsules on chronic prostatitis. *Zhonghua Nan Ke Xue.* May;10(5):337–339.

Ziotta AR, et al. (2005). Evaluation of male sexual function in patients with lower urinary tract symptoms (LUTS) associated with benign prostatic hyperplasia (BPH) treated with a phytotherapeutic agent (permixon), tamsulosin or finasteride. *European Urology.* Aug;48(2):269–276.

NAME: Schisandra (*Schisandra chinensis*)

Common Names: Schizandra, *gomishi* (Japanese), *wu-wei-zi* (Chinese), Chinese magnolia vine

Family: *Schisandraceae*

Description of Plant
- Climbing woody vine with white to pink flowers producing purple-red globular fruits with kidney-shaped seeds
- Native to China, Russia, Korea, and Japan
- Fruit is harvested in autumn.

Medicinal Part: Dried fruit

Constituents and Action (if known)
- Dibenzo[a,c] cycloactadiene lignans (18% of seeds): approximately 40 have been identified
  - Gomisins D, E, F, G, H, J, N; schizandrol A, B; schisandrin A, B; schisantherin A, B, C; gomisins D-O
  - PAF antagonist activity (Lee et al., 1999)
  - May have cardioprotective activity (in rats) and protect from hypoxia (Li et al., 1996), antioxidants (Bone, 1996)
  - Enhance glutathione protection in liver (Ko et al., 1995), stimulate liver glycogen and protein synthesis, inhibit lipid peroxidation; enhanced survival in experimental fulminant

hepatitis from 7.5% to 80% and prevented liver cell necrosis (Bone, 1996)
  ○ Gomisin N, schisandrin B, schizandrol B protect the liver against halothane-induced hepatitis, carbon tetrachloride, and hepatic failure induced by bacteria (Ip et al., 1996; Ko et al., 1995; Upton, 1999)
- Gomisin A (schizandrol B)
  ○ May improve bile acid metabolism
  ○ Improves liver regeneration and hepatic blood flow (in rats) as well as inhibiting hepatocarcinogenesis
  ○ May decrease amphetamine-induced motor activity
  ○ May reduce multi-drug resistance in HIV treatment (Wan et al., 2006)
  ○ Anti-inflammatory
  ○ Propinguanin is cytotoxic to tumor cells. Enhances apoptosis (Xu et al., 2006)
- N granoic acid may inhibit HIV-1 reverse transcriptase replication (Sun et al., 1996)
- Volatile oils: monoterpenes (borneal, 1,8-cineol, citral) and sesquiterpenes (sesquicarene, ylangene, chamigrenol)
- Vitamins A, C, E (Upton, 1999)
- Organic acids (10% by weight): malic, citric, tartaric
- Fixed oils (38%): linoleic, oleic, linolenic, lauric, and palmitic acids

Other Actions
- Nervous system stimulant, enhances memory in humans (Nishiyama et al., 1995), antidepressant (Bone, 1996), anticonvulsant
- May enhance neuron growth and prevent neuron atrophy
- Used to treat insomnia (You-Ping, 1998)

Nutritional Ingredients: Fresh berry juice with sugar and water has been used as a beverage ("sandra berry" juice).

Traditional Use
- Adaptogen, anti-inflammatory, astringent, hepatoprotective, antiasthmatic
- Commonly used in TCM; the berries are used in formulas to calm *shen* (insomnia, palpitations, impaired memory) and

to astringe the *jing* (frequent urination, spermatorrhea, leukorrhea, night sweats, early morning diarrhea)
- Relieves dry coughs, dyspnea, asthma

Current Use

- Tonic and restorative herb (adaptogen); effective for deficiency conditions such as neurasthenia, CFS, insomnia, impaired memory, fatigue, chronic stress, and depression (Panossian & Wagner, 2005; Upton, 1999)
- Human athletes and race horses improved performance, displayed accelerated recovery after exercise, and had greater stamina after taking schisandra for 2 weeks (Hancke et al., 1996).
- Hepatoprotective; use with milk thistle, turmeric, or picrorrhiza to prevent or treat liver damage caused by alcohol, industrial solvents, viruses, or pharmaceutical medications. In one controlled study of 189 patients with hepatitis B and elevated SGPT levels, levels returned to normal in 68% of patients after 4 weeks of taking schisandra (Upton, 1999).
- To treat respiratory conditions such as allergic asthma with wheezing, dyspnea, and chronic coughs (You-Ping, 1998)
- Cardiac antioxidant: in animal studies, the berries reduced ischemic myocardial damage, reduced stress-induced palpitations, and protected against doxorubicin-induced cardiotoxicity (You et al., 2006)

Available Forms, Dosage, and Administration Guidelines

Preparations: Dried fruit, tea, capsules, tinctures

Typical Dosage

- *Dried berry:* 1.5 to 6 g a day
- *Capsules:* Up to six 500-mg capsules a day
- *Tea:* Steep 1 tsp dried fruit in 1 cup hot water, decoct for 10 to 15 minutes, steep 15 minutes; take 4 oz three times a day
- *Tincture* (1:5, 35% alcohol): 40 to 80 gtt (2–4 mL) three times a day, or follow manufacturer or practitioner recommendations

Pharmacokinetics—If Available (form or route when known):

Metabolized in liver. Competitively inhibits and irreversibly inactivates CYP 3A4

Toxicity: Experimental overdose in mice caused decreased activity, apathy, and increased body weight.

Contraindications: Epilepsy, pregnancy

Side Effects: Acid indigestion and GI upset, urticaria

Long-Term Safety: Safe. Very low toxicity when used in normal therapeutic doses.

Use in Pregnancy/Lactation/Children: Avoid during pregnancy; may stimulate uterine contractions (Bone, 1996). No adverse reactions expected during lactation (Upton, 1999).

Drug/Herb Interactions and Rationale (if known): Use cautiously with pentobarbitol and barbitol; may potentiate action. May antagonize the CNS-stimulatory effect of caffeine and amphetamines. In rats, schisandra activated the pregnane X receptor and increased warfarin clearance (Mu et al., 2006). Use cautiously with blood thinners (do regular PT and INR to rule out possible interactions).

Special Notes: Lignan content has been well studied, and it seems to be responsible for schisandra's hepatoprotective effects.

BIBLIOGRAPHY

Bone K. (1996). *Clinical Applications of Ayurvedic and Chinese Herbs* (pp. 69–74). Queensland, Australia: Phytotherapy Press.

Hancke J, et al. (1996). Reduction of serum hepatic transaminases and CPK in sports horses with poor performance treated with a standardized *Schisandra chinensis* fruit extract. *Phytomedicine*. 3(3):237–240.

Ip SP, et al. (1996). Effect of a lignan-enriched extract of *Schisandra chinensis* on aflatoxin B1 and cadmium chloride-induced hepatotoxicity in rats. *Pharmacology and Toxicology*. 78(6):413–416.

Jung KY, et al. (1997). Lignans with platelet activating factor antagonist activity from *Schisandra chinensis* (Turcz.) Baill. *Phytomedicine*. 4(3):229–232.

Lee IS, et al. (1999). Structure-activity relationships of lignans from *Schisandra chinensis* as platelet activating factor antagonists. *Biologic Pharmacy Bulletin*. 22(3):265–267.

Li PC, et al. (1996). *Schisandra chinensis*-dependent myocardial protective action of sheng mai-san in rats. *American Journal of Chinese Medicine.* 24(3–4):255–262.

Mu Y, et al. (2006). Traditional chinese medicines wu wei zi (*Schisandra chinensis* Baill) and gan cao (*Glycyrrhiza uralensis* Fisch) activate pregnane x receptor and increase warfarin clearance in rats. *Journal of Pharmacology and Experimental Therapeutics.* Mar;316(3):1369–1377.

Nishiyama N, et al. (1995). Beneficial effects of S-113m, a novel herbal prescription, on learning impairment model in mice. *Biologic Pharmacy Bulletin.* 18(11):1498–1503.

Panossian A, Wagner H. (2005). Stimulant effect of adaptogens: An overview with particular reference to their efficacy following single dose administration. *Phytotherapy Research.* Oct;19(10): 819–838.

Sun HD, et al. (1996). Nigranoic acid, a triterpenoid from *Schisandra sphaerandra* that inhibits HIV-1 reverse transcriptase. *Journal of Natural Products.* 59(5):525–527.

Upton R. [Ed.]. (1999). *American Herbal Pharmacopoeia and Therapeutic Compendium—Schisandra.* Santa Cruz, CA: AHP.

Wan CK, et al. (2006). Gomisin A alters substrate interaction and reverses P-glycoprotein-mediated multidrug resistance in HepG2-DR cells. *Biochemistry and Pharmacology.* Sept 28;72(7):824–837.

Xu Q, et al. (2007). Investigation on influencing factors of 5 MF content of schisandra. *Journal of Zhejiang University. Science.* June 8;8(6):439–445.

You JS, et al. (2006). *Schisandra chinensis* protects against Adriamycin-induced cardiotoxicity in rats. *Chang Gung Medical Journal.* Jan-Feb;29(1):63–70.

You-Ping Z. (1998). *Chinese Materia Medica: Chemistry, Pharmacology and Applications* (pp. 653–654). Amsterdam: Harwood.

 NAME: Scullcap (*Scutellaria lateriflora*)

Common Names: Mad dog, skullcap, blue skullcap, skullcap

Family: *Lamiaceae*

Description of Plant

- A small (1'–2' tall) nonaromataic perennial member of the mint family
- It prefers to grow in damp areas.

Medicinal Part: Fresh or freeze-dried herb

Constituents and Action (if known)

- Flavonoid glycosides (scutellarein, scutellarin, ikonnikoside 1, lateriflorin, baicalin, baicalein) bind to benzodiazepine site in GABA receptors (Awad et al., 2003)
- Diterpenoid (scuterivulaetone)
- Bitter iridoid (catapol)

Nutritional Ingredients: None

Traditional Use

- Antispasmodic, nervine, anticonvulsant, anxiolytic
- Used for nervous exhaustion with spasms, tics, and palsies
- Mild antispasmodic useful for controlling tremors, stress headaches, back spasms, and facial tics

Current Use

- Useful in nervine formulas with chamomile, lemon balm, fresh oat, and St. John's wort for nervous exhaustion (neurasthenia), insomnia, anxiety with muscle tightness, and mild forms of obsessive-compulsive disorder (Winston, 2006; Wolfson & Hoffmann, 2003)
- A useful antispasmodic that can be effective for reducing or controlling tremors (Parkinson's disease), restless legs syndrome, Lyme's neuralgias, TMJ pain, mild Tourette's syndrome, and bruxism. In rats, scullcap inhibited drug-induced seizures (Peredery & Persinger, 2004).

Available Forms, Dosage, and Administration Guidelines

Preparations: Fresh plant tincture, freeze-dried capsules. Dried *S. lateriflora* has very little activity. Another species, *S. galericulata*, is reported to maintain activity when dried (Winston, 2006).

Typical Dosage

- *Fresh plant tincture* (1:2, 30% alcohol): 60 to 120 gtt (3–6 mL) three times a day
- *Freeze-dried capsules:* Two capsules three times a day

Pharmacokinetics—If Available (form or route when known): Not known

Toxicity: Intentional overdoses of the alcoholic tincture from homeopathic provings caused giddiness, stupor, confusion, slowed pulse, and twitching of the limbs.

Contraindications: None

Side Effects: None at normal therapeutic doses

Long-Term Safety: Unknown

Use in Pregnancy/Lactation/Children: Best to avoid due to lack of studies and history of adulteration

Drug/Herb Interactions and Rationale (if known): None known

Special Notes: Be sure of suppliers and botanical identification of all scullcap products. As a result of adulteration with the hepatotoxic herb germander, scullcap has falsely been accused of being hepatotoxic (De Smet et al., 1993; McGuffin et al., 1997).

BIBLIOGRAPHY

Awad R, et al. (2003). Phytochemical and biological analysis of skullcap (*Scutellaria lateriflora* L.): A medicinal plant with anxiolytic properties. *Phytomedicine*. Nov;10(8):640–649.

Der Marderosian A, Beutler J. [Eds.]. (2004). *The Review of Natural Products*. St. Louis, MO: Facts and Comparisons.

De Smet PAGM, et al. (1993). *Adverse Effects of Herbal Drugs, Vol. 2* (pp. 289–296). Berlin: Springer-Verlag.

Gafner S, Bergeron C. (2003). Inhibition of [3H]-LSD binding to 5-HT7 receptors by flavonoids from *Scutellaria lateriflora*. *Journal of Natural Products*. Apr;66(4):535–537.

Garner S, et al. (2003). Analysis of *Scutellaria lateriflora* and its adulterants *Teucrium canadense* and *Teucrium chamaedrys* by LC-UV/MS, TLC, and digital photomicroscopy. *Journal of AOC International*. May-Jun;86(3):453–460.

McGuffin M, et al. (1997). *American Herbal Products Association's Botanical Safety Handbook* (p. 105). Boca Raton, FL: CRC Press.

Peredery O, Persinger MA. (2004). Herbal treatment following post-seizure induction in rats by lithium pilocarpine: *Scutellaria lateriflora* (Skullcap), *Gelsemium sempervirens* (Gelsemium) and *Datura stramonium* (Jimson Weed) may prevent development of spontaneous seizures. *Phytotherapy Research*. Sep;18(9):700–705.

Winston D. (2006). *Winston's Botanic Materia Medica*. Washington, NJ: DWCHS.

Wolfson P, Hoffmann DL. (2003). An investigation into the efficacy of *Scutellaria lateriflora* in healthy volunteers. *Alternative Therapies in Health and Medicine*. Mar-Apr;9(2):74–78.

NAME: Senna Leaf (*Cassia senna,* syn. *C. angustifolia*)

Common Names: Cassia senna, *fan xie ye* (Chinese), Alexandrian senna

Family: *Fabiaceae*

Description of Plant
- It is a weedy perennial that grows in the Middle East, Africa, India, and China.
- An American species, *C. marilandica,* is rarely used but has similar activity.

Medicinal Part: Dried leaves, pods

Constituents and Action (if known)
- Anthraquinone glycosides
  - Sennosides A-D-laxative (ESCOP, 2003), cathartic
  - Aloe: emodin dianthrone—stimulated release of platelet activating factor in vitro (ESCOP, 2003), antibacterial, cytotoxic, laxative (Duke, 2006)
  - Rhein: laxative (ESCOP, 2003), antibacterial, antiviral, purgative (Duke, 2006)
- Flavonoids

Nutritional Ingredients: None

Traditional Use
- Antibacterial, laxative
- In Chinese medicine, senna leaves are used as a laxative as well as for headaches with red, painful eyes.
- In India, senna leaves are used topically for dermatosis.

Current Use: Senna is a strong stimulant laxative that can, with regular use, cause bowel dependence. It is appropriate for short-term use for occasional situational constipation (travel, stress, etc.). Use it with antispasmodic carminatives such as ginger, caraway seeds, or fennel to prevent bowel spasms.

Available Forms, Dosage, and Administration Guidelines
Preparations: Tea, capsules/tablets, tincture
Typical Dosage
- *Tea:* 1 to 2 tsp dried herb, 8 oz hot water, steep 20 minutes; take 4 oz twice a day (short-term use only)

- *Capsules/tablets:* 1 to 2 tablets a day or as recommended (short-term use)
- *Tincture* (1:5, 40% alcohol): 20 to 30 gtt twice a day (short-term use only)

Pharmacokinetics—If Available (form or route when known): After oral administration of sennosides, 3% to 6% are excreted in the urine, some via the bile, and 90% in the feces. The laxative effect takes 6 to 12 hours.

Toxicity: There are two reports in the literature linking chronic senna ingestion with liver damage. One is a 77-year-old man who developed subacute cholestatic hepatitis, the other a 52-year-old woman who developed acute hepatic and renal impairment (Vanderperren et al., 2005). As with all reports linking herbs with hepatitis, it is absolutely necessary to botanically identify the substance to rule out possible adulterants, and it is vital to rule out other possible causes (which has more than a few times not been done) including alcohol use, hepatotoxic medications, and exposure to environmental liver toxins. Without this data, this type of single case report, while thought provoking, is not conclusive and contributes to a growing, often undeserved paranoia about the dangers of herb use.

Contraindications: IBS, IBD, including Crohn's disease and ulcerative colitis; intestinal obstruction, appendicitis

Side Effects: Diarrhea; senna should always be taken with carminative herbs to prevent bowel spasms (griping). Long-term use of senna can cause *melanosis coli*, a staining of the intestinal mucosa. There is no known health risk associated with this condition.

Long-Term Safety: Long-term use can cause bowel dependency and deplete potassium.

Use in Pregnancy/Lactation/Children: Avoid use during pregnancy (unless recommended by a health care professional), lactation, or in young children. In a study of young children (<5 years of age) who mistakenly ingested senna, 33% developed severe diaper rash and 11% had blisters or skin sloughing. Children who were still wearing diapers had more significant symptoms (Spiller et al., 2003).

Drug/Herb Interactions and Rationale (if known): Avoid concurrent use with cardiac glycosides, thiazide diuretics (Brinker, 2001), and corticosteroids due to potential for increased potassium loss.

Special Notes: In 1999, phenolphthalein was taken off the market as an over-the-counter laxative. Almost all over-the-counter laxatives now use senna as the active ingredient.

BIBLIOGRAPHY

Brinker F. (2001). *Herb Contraindications & Drug Interactions* (3rd ed.; pp. 175–177). Sandy, OR: Eclectic Medical Publications.

Duke J. Dr. Duke's phytochemical and ethnobotanical databases. Accessed November 7 2006, from www.ars-grin.gov/duke/

European Scientific Cooperative on Phytotherapy. (2003). *ESCOP Monographs* (2nd ed.; pp. 456–462). Stuttgart: Thieme.

Skenderi G. (2003). *Herbal Vade Mecum* (pp. 343–344). Rutherford, NJ: Herbacy Press.

Sonmez A, et al. (2005). Subacute cholestatic hepatitis likely related to the use of senna for chronic constipation. *Acta Gastroenterologica Belgica.* Jul-Sep;68(3):385–387.

Spiller HA, et al. (2003). Skin breakdown and blisters from senna-containing laxatives in young children. *Annals of Pharmacotherapy.* May;37(5):636–639.

Vanderperren B, et al. (2005). Acute liver failure with renal impairment related to the abuse of senna anthraquinone glycosides. *Annals of Pharmacotherapy.* Jul-Aug;39(7–8):1353–1357.

Winston D. (2006). *Winston's Botanic Materia Medica.* Washington, NJ: DWCHS.

 NAME: Shiitake (*Lentinula edodes*)

Common Names: *Hua gu* (Chinese), syn. *Lentinus edodes*

Family: *Polyporaceae*

Description of Plant
- A commonly cultivated mushroom, usually grown on oak logs
- Fungus native to Japan, China, and Korea

Medicinal Part: Mushroom, mycelium, mycelium extract (LEM)

Constituents and Action (if known)

- Polysaccharides
  - Lentinin is a highly purified high-molecular-weight polysaccharide used as an injectable medicine: antiviral, immune potentiator, activates NK cells, interleukin 1, interferon, and proliferation of PMNNs
  - LEM (lentinula edodes mycelium) extract contains a heteroglycan protein (a protein-bound polysaccharide), B vitamins, and water-soluble lignans (Hobbs, 1995): antitumor, improves macrophage activity and apoptosis, immune potentiator, antiviral
  - KS-2 is an a-mannan-peptide extract that strongly inhibits cancer cell growth orally and intraperitoneally.
- Water-soluble lignans (EP3, EPS4): antiviral, herpes simplex I and II, polio, measles, mumps, HIV, immunopotentiating
- Eritadenine: lowers cholesterol and lipids
- Tyrosinase: lowers blood pressure
- L-octen-3-ol, ethyl acetate, 2-octenol, and octylalcohol: phytochemicals responsible for the fresh shiitake odor

Nutritional Ingredients: Protein (2.0%–2.6% fresh, 25.9% dry); minerals (calcium, magnesium, zinc, potassium, phosphorus); vitamins B_2, C, and ergosterol (a vitamin D precursor)

Traditional Use: Long used in the Orient as both a food and medicine. The dry shiitake is known as black mushroom in Chinese cuisine and is considered to be a general tonic for the circulation and immune system and to improve overall health.

Current Use

- Hyperlipidemia: regular use of shiitake can lower cholesterol and blood lipids. In one study of 10 Japanese women, after 1 week of ingesting 9 g dried shiitake a day, serum cholesterol levels fell by 7% (Hobbs, 1995). Another study in a population of people 60 years or older saw cholesterol levels drop by 9% (Hobbs, 1995).
- Hepatitis B and C: antiviral and hepatoprotective effects of LEM have reduced viral load and reduced elevated liver enzyme levels (Jones, 1995). In animal studies, a mycelial extract protected against chemical-induced liver damage (Watanabe et al., 2006).

- LEM strengthens immune response; appropriate for use in patients with cancer, HIV, herpes simplex I and II, frequent colds, and bronchitis
- May be beneficial for conditions such as CFS, *Candida* overgrowth, and allergies
- Lentinin improved survival times of cancer patients when used concurrently with chemotherapy (Matsuoka et al., 1997). It also strengthened the immune function of patients with HIV and tuberculosis.

Available Forms, Dosage, and Administration Guidelines
Preparations: Fresh and dry mushroom, LEM tablets, tincture, lentinin (injectable)
Typical Dosage
- *Fresh mushrooms:* Take as a tonic; medical dosage is unrealistic in this form
- *Dried mushrooms:* 6 to 16 g three times a day
- *LEM tablets:* 2 to 6 g a day for hepatitis or cancer; 0.5 to 1 g a day as a general maintenance dosage
- *Tincture* (1:3, 25% alcohol): 80 to 120 gtt (4–6 mL) three times a day
- *Lentinin (injectable):* 1 to 5 mg intravenously or intramuscularly twice a week. This is an approved medicine in Japan but has not been approved in the United States.

Pharmacokinetics—If Available (form or route when known): Not known

Toxicity: It has been eaten as a food for thousands of years and is considered safe. Inhalation of shiitake mushroom spores has caused a case of chronic hypersensivity pneumonitis. In a small trial, daily ingestion of dried, uncooked shiitake powder caused a few cases of GI upset and eosinophilia (Levy et al., 1998). There are also reports of shiitake-induced dermatitis.

Contraindications: None known

Side Effects: LEM occasionally causes mild gastric upset or rashes.

Long-Term Safety: Safe

Use in Pregnancy/Lactation/Children: Safe

Drug/Herb Interactions and Rationale (if known):
Thyroxin and hydrocortisone inhibit the antitumor activity of lentinin. Water-soluble extracts may reduce platelet coagulation. Use cautiously with blood thinners.

Special Notes: The most effective oral form of shiitake is the LEM product. Lentinin is widely used in Japan as a prescription medication for cancer, HIV, and hepatitis B and C.

BIBLIOGRAPHY

Hobbs C. (1995). *Medicinal Mushrooms* (2nd ed.; pp. 51–54). Santa Cruz, CA: Botanica Press.

Jones K. (1995). *Shiitake: The Healing Mushroom*. Rochester, VT: Healing Arts Press.

Jong SC, Birmingham JM. (1993). Medicinal and therapeutic value of the shiitake mushroom. In: Neidlemen S, Laskin A.[Eds.]. *Advances in Applied Microbiology, Vol. 39*. New York: Academic Press.

Levy AM, et al. (1998). Eosinophilia and gastrointestinal symptoms after ingestion of shiitake mushrooms. *Journal of Allergy and Clinical Immunology*. May;101(5):613–620.

Matsuoka H, et al. (1997). Lentinin potentiates immunity and prolongs the survival time of some patients. *Anticancer Research*. 17:2751–2756.

Stamets P. (2002). *MycoMedicinals* (pp. 51–54). Olympia, WA: MycoMedia Productions.

Watanabe A, et al. (2006). Protection against D-galactosamine-induced acute liver injury by oral administration of extracts from *Lentius edodes* mycelia. *Biological and Pharmaceutical Bulletin*. Aug;29(8):1651–1654.

 NAME: Siberian Ginseng (*Eleutherococcus senticosus*)

Common Names: Eleuthero, ciwujia, *Acanthopanax senticosus*

Family: *Araliaceae*

Description of Plant: A spiny-stemmed shrub native to northeastern China, Siberia, and northern Japan

Medicinal Part: Roots, root bark

Constituents and Action (if known)

- Eleutherosides A to G (0.6%–0.9%) (Bradley, 1992)—adaptogenic hypotensive
- Eleutheroside B is identical to syringin. Syringin in powdered roots decreased by 50% after 12 months and was undetectable after 3 years (Tang & Eisenbrand, 1992).
- Eleutherans A, G (glycans)
- Lignans (sesamin)
- Coumarins (isofraxidin)

Nutritional Ingredients: None known

Traditional Use: Used in TCM as a remedy for "wind damp" arthralgias, muscle spasms, and joint pain and as a *qi* tonic for the Chinese spleen and kidney. Used for low back pain, insomnia, fatigue, and anorexia.

Current Use

- Adaptogen: increases resistance to stress (emotional, occupational, or environmental) and improves performance. While several studies confirmed these uses, other studies found no benefit in using this herb to enhance athletic performance (Goulet & Dionne, 2005).
- Improves memory and feelings of well-being; reduces fatigue; can be used for mild depression. In a study of elderly patients taking this herb, some aspects of mental health and social functioning improved over 4 weeks of use (Cicero et al., 2004). It also enhanced short-term memory in asthenic, anxious people (Arushanian et al., 2003) and enhances mental performance (Panossian & Wagner, 2005).
- Approved in Germany as a tonic for asthenic debility (CFS), impaired concentration, or during convalescence
- Eye problems: in several studies (Blumenthal et al., 2000), patients taking eleuthero showed significant improvement for primary glaucoma (102 cases), eye burns (58 cases), and myopia (122 cases)
- Normalizes immune and adrenal response; reduces effects of excessive cortisol production (Winston & Maimes, 2007)
- Supportive therapy for cancer treatment: increases natural killer and T-helper cells and reduces side effects of chemotherapy and radiation

- Ethanol extract of eleuthero dramatically improved the absolute number of immune competent cells, especially T lymphocytes (Wagner, 1999).

Available Forms, Dosage, and Administration Guidelines

Preparations: Dried root, capsules, tablets, tinctures, fluid extract

Typical Dosage

- *Tea:* 1 to 2 tsp powdered root or root bark in 8 oz water, decoct 15 to 20 minutes, steep half-hour; take two or three cups a day
- *Capsules (dried powdered root):* Three to six 500-mg capsules a day
- *Tablets:* One to three 1.25-g tablets (standardized to contain 0.7 mg eleutheroside E) a day
- *Tincture* (1:5, 30% alcohol): 80 to 120 gtt (4–6 mL) three times a day
- *Fluid extract* (1:1): 1 to 2 mL three times a day

Pharmacokinetics—If Available (form or route when known): None known

Toxicity: None known

Contraindications: Several reports suggest that eleuthero is inappropriate for patients with hypertension (especially blood pressure in excess of 180/90) (Farnsworth et al., 1985). However, the glycosides contained in this herb have been shown to reduce blood pressure (Blumenthal et al., 2000).

Side Effects: None

Long-Term Safety: Safe

Use in Pregnancy/Lactation/Children: Safe. One report implicated eleuthero in a report of a "hairy baby," but this problem was due to adulteration with another herb (*Periploca*) (Mills & Bone, 2000).

Drug/Herb Interactions and Rationale (if known): Be sure that eleuthero is from a reputable source and has been botanically authenticated. A case of elevated digoxin levels in a 74-year-old man concurrently taking Siberian ginseng has been reported (McRae, 1996). The capsules were analyzed and were

found to contain no digoxin or digitoxin. Unfortunately, the herb was not authenticated, so its actual identity is unknown. The possibility of adulteration with *Periploca*, which contains cardiac glycosides, exists. In a study of elderly patients taking digoxin and eleuthero, there were no reports of interactions (Cicero et al., 2004). A report of eleuthero being implicated in causing neonatal androgenization was discovered to be caused by an adulterant, *Periploca sepium* (Mills & Bone, 2000). In a human study, standardized extracts of eleuthero did not affect CYP2D6 or CYP3A4 (Donovan et al., 2003).

BIBLIOGRAPHY

Arushanian EB, et al. (2003). Effect of *Eleutherococcus* on short-term memory and visual perception in healthy humans. *Eksperimentalnaia i Klinicheskaia Farmakologiia*. Sep-Oct;66(5): 10–13.

Blumenthal M, et al. (2000). *Herbal Medicine: Expanded Commission E Monographs* (pp. 106–109). Austin, TX: American Botanical Council.

Bradley P. [Ed.]. (1992). *British Herbal Compendium, Vol. I* (pp. 89–91). Dorset: British Herbal Medicine Association.

Cicero AF, et al. (2004). Effects of Siberian ginseng (*Eleutherococcus sencticosus* Maxim.) on elderly quality of life: a randomized clinical trial. *Archives of Gerontology and Geriatrics Supplement*. (9):69–73.

Davydov M, Krikorian AD. (2000). *Eleutherococcus senticosus* (Rupr. & Maxim.) Maxim. (*Araliaceae*) as an adaptogen: A closer look. *Journal of Ethnopharmacology*. Oct;72(3):345–393.

Donovan JL, et al. (2003). Siberian ginseng (*Eleutherococcus senticosis*) effects on CYP2D6 and CYP3A4 activity in normal volunteers. *Drug Metabolism and Disposition*. May;3(5): 519–522.

Farnsworth NR, et al. (1985). Siberian ginseng (*Eleutherococcus senticosus*): Current status as an adaptogen. In: Wagner H, et al. [Eds.]. *Economic and Medicinal Plant Research, Vol. I*. London: Academic Press.

Goulet ED, Dionne IJ. (2005). Assessment of the effects of *Eleutherococcus senticosus* on endurance performance. *International Journal of Sport Nutrition and Exercise Metabolism*. Feb;15(1):75–83.

McRae S. (1996). Elevated serum digoxin levels in a patient taking digoxin and Siberian ginseng. *Canadian Medical Association Journal*. 155(3):293–295.

Mills S, Bone K. (2000). *Principles and Practice of Phytotherapy* (pp. 534–541). Edinburgh: Churchill Livingstone.

Panossian A, Wagner H. (2005). Stimulating effect of adaptogens: An overview with particular reference to efficacy following single dose administration. *Phytotherapy Research.* Oct;19(10): 819–838.

Tang W, Eisenbrand G. (1992). *Chinese Drugs of Plant Origin* (pp. 1–12). Berlin: Springer-Verlag.

Wagner H. [Ed.]. (1999). *Immunomodulatory Agents from Plants* (pp. 329–331). Basel: Birkhauser Verlag.

 NAME: Slippery Elm (*Ulmus rubra*)

Common Names: Red elm, Indian elm, sweet elm, syn. *Ulmus fulva*

Family: *Ulmaceae*

Description of Plant
- A deciduous tree native to eastern Canada and eastern and central United States
- Trunk is reddish-brown with gray-white bark on branches
- Can grow 50' to 60' tall

Medicinal Part: Inner bark (collected in spring or autumn)

Constituents and Action (if known)
- Mucilage (polysaccharides): hexoses, pentoses, menthypentoses, polyuronides, hexosan-demulcent
- Tannins (3.0%–6.5%): responsible for mild astringent properties (Chevallier, 1996)
- Minerals: calcium

Nutritional Ingredients: Powdered bark has been cooked as a porridge used for feeding babies and weak convalescent patients.

Traditional Use
- Antitussive, demulcent, emollient, nutritive
- Topical use: inner bark mixed with water yields a thick mucilage used as a poultice for styes, boils, carbuncles, sores, and burns

- Internally, the bark mucilage is used for irritation of the mucous membranes (throat, stomach, bowel). Used for diarrhea (solidifies the stool) and constipation (bulk laxative).

Current Use

- Protects, soothes, and heals irritated mucous membrane tissue in the esophagus, stomach, and intestinal membranes (colitis, IBS, diarrhea, leaky gut syndrome, gastric and duodenal ulcers, gastritis, ileitis)
- Local use relieves pain and decreases inflammation of abscesses, varicose ulcers, anal fissures, first-degree burns, styes, and ingrown toenails.
- Soothing demulcent: decreases throat irritation with dry and ticklish coughs, irritation of the vocal cords, and laryngitis (Winston, 2006).

Available Forms, Dosage, and Administration Guidelines

Preparations: Dried bark (cut and sifted or powdered). There are few processors of slippery elm bark because it is highly combustible. Lozenges, capsules.

Typical Dosage

- *Capsules:* Up to twelve 400-mg capsules a day
- *Tea:* 1 tsp powdered bark in 8 oz cool water, steep for 1 hour; take two or three times a day. This is the most effective dosage form.
- *Tincture:* Ineffective
- *Powdered form:* Mix with boiling water to make a poultice for skin inflammations
- Or follow manufacturer or practitioner recommendations

Pharmacokinetics—If Available (form or route when known): Not known

Toxicity: None known

Contraindications: None known

Side Effects: Allergic reaction (rare)

Long-Term Safety: Safe

Use in Pregnancy/Lactation/Children: Safe; long history of use as a food and medicine

Drug/Herb Interactions and Rationale (if known): For all drugs, separate by at least 2 hours when a mucilage preparation is used.

Special Notes: FDA has stated that slippery elm is a safe and effective oral demulcent.

BIBLIOGRAPHY

Anonymous. (2000) *Integrative Medicine Access: Professional Reference to Conditions, Herbs & Supplements.* Newton, MA: Integrative Medicine Communications.

Bradley PR. (1992). *British Herbal Compendium, Vol. 1* (p. 204). Bournemouth: British Herbal Medicine Association.

Bradley PR.[Ed.]. (1996). *British Herbal Pharmacopoeia* (4th ed.; p. 81). Guildford, UK: Biddles Ltd.

Chevallier A. (1996). *Encyclopedia of Medicinal Plants* (p. 144). New York: DK Publishing.

Der Marderosian A, Beutler J. [Eds.]. (2004). *The Review of Natural Products.* St. Louis, MO: Facts and Comparisons.

Morton JF. (1993). Mucilaginous plants and their use in medicine. *Biological and Pharmalogic Bulletin.* 16:735–739.

Newall C, et al. (1996). *Herbal Medicines* (p. 248). London: Pharmaceutical Press.

Winston D. (2006). *Winston's Botanic Materia Medica.* Washington, NJ: DWCHS.

 NAME: Soy (*Glycine max*)

Common Names: Soya, soybeans

Family: *Fabiaceae*

Description of Plant: Legume that has been cultivated for its edible beans in China for more than 2,000 years

Medicinal Part: Beans and food/nutritional products soy protein and soy isoflavone extracts

Constituents and Action (if known)

• Isoflavones (phytoestrogens): genistein, daidzein, glycetein; similar in structure to estradiol, with weak estrogenic and antiestrogenic effects

- ○ Reduce menopausal symptoms such as hot flashes (Albertazzi et al., 1999; Burke et al., 2003; Chiechi, 1999; Colacurci et al., 2004; Duncan et al., 1999; Setchell, 1998)
  - ○ Increase bone density in some women by up to 6% (Newton et al., 2006, Ye et al., 2006)
- Genistein
  - ○ Reduces risk of tumor formation, inhibits protein tyrosine kinase (PTK), topoiomerase II and matrix metalloprotein (MMPQ), which downregulates cell growth and proliferation (Ravindranath et al., 2004)
  - ○ Boosts immune system function by increasing the phagocytic response of macrophages (Fiedor et al., 1998)
  - ○ Lowers risk of prostatic enlargement and cancer, possibly due to antiestrogen and weak estrogen effect (Geller et al., 1998; Moyad, 1999)
  - ○ Lowers risk of colon and other cancer (Messina & Bennink, 1998)
  - ○ Lowers risk of breast cancer (Messina, 1999; Shao et al., 1998)
  - ○ Antiproliferation effect on breast (Brzezinski & Debi, 1999)
  - ○ Lowers cholesterol and lowers risk of cardiovascular disease (25 g a day is necessary) (Clarkson & Anthony, 1998); improved arterial elasticity by 26% (Der Marderosian & Beutler, 2004).
  - ○ Antioxidant to protect cells from oxygen free radicals (King & Bursill, 1998)
  - ○ Decreases blood clotting
- Fatty acids (25%): linoleic, palmitic, stearic acids
- Phytates: antinutrients

Nutritional Ingredients: Source of protein, vitamin E, minerals (calcium, iron, potassium), isoflavones, and fatty acids. Generally unaffected by cooking, but extensive processing lowers the medicinal value. Some soy products, such as tamari (soy sauce), contain substantial amounts of added sodium. Traditionally made tofu is high in calcium.

Traditional Use: In the Orient, soy has long been a popular food. Most soy products were traditionally fermented (miso, tempeh, natto) or processed (tofu) to make them more digestible and to remove phytates.

Current Use

- Controls mild to moderate menopausal symptoms such as hot flashes (takes 4 to 5 weeks to notice activity) (Burke et al., 2003; Colacurci et al., 2004).
- Studies show that higher intake of isoflavones prevents cancers of the prostate, breast, endometrium, and bowel (Dalais et al., 2004).
- Lowers cholesterol (Zhuo et al., 2004)
- Reduces prostatic enlargement (BPH)
- Mildly increases bone density; helps prevent bone loss; diet must also have adequate calcium, magnesium, boron (Lydeking-Olsen et al., 2004; Newton et al., 2006)
- Improves symptoms of osteoarthritis (Arimandi et al., 2004)
- Lowers blood pressure in people with prehypertension or stage I hypertension (130–159/80–99) (He et al., 2005)
- Reduced fasting blood glucose and insulin levels in postmenopausal women (Cheng et al., 2004)

Available Forms, Dosage, and Administration Guidelines

Preparations: Foods, soy protein, soy isoflavones

Typical Dosage

- 30 to 100 mg a day isoflavones or 25 to 50 g soy protein lowers cholesterol.
- Forty-five g soy flour increases bone density.
- Twenty-five to 60 g soy protein reduces menopausal signs and changes.
- Revival is a soy meal-replacement drink that tastes good. Both fat and nonfat varieties are available. Research has demonstrated this product's effectiveness. It contains 160 mg of isoflavones per serving.

Pharmacokinetics—If Available (form or route when known): The plasma half-life of genistein and daidzein is approximately 8 hours, with peak concentration in 6 to 8 hours. Elimination is by urine.

Toxicity: None

Contraindications: Soy allergies. Large doses are contraindicated if a previous estrogen-positive tumor has been

diagnosed, although it is unknown whether soy stimulates estrogen-positive receptor cells. Do not use large amounts of soy foods in patients with thyroid problems: soy isoflavones do not affect thyroid function in people who have adequate iodine intake (Bruce et al., 2003).

Side Effects: GI upset: flatulence, diarrhea

Long-Term Safety: Use organic soy products whenever possible. There are concerns about the regular use of large amounts of unfermented soy foods and soy isoflavones because of certain chemicals found in soy. Tripsin inhibitors, hemaglutinin, and phytic acid all may have long-term negative impact on health.

Use in Pregnancy/Lactation/Children: Safe, although there is concern about infants who are fed solely on soy formulas. The phytates (antinutrients) and high levels of isoflavones may have some biological impact. Additional research is needed.

Drug/Herb Interactions and Rationale (if known): None known

Special Notes: Safe for women using birth control pills and hormone replacement therapy concurrently. When buying soy protein powder, make sure that the label says "supro," because this means that the soybeans have been washed with water and the phytochemicals are intact. Otherwise, the soybeans may have been washed with alcohol, which can change the phytochemical content.

BIBLIOGRAPHY

Albertazzi P, et al. (1999). Dietary soy supplementation and phytoestrogen levels. *Obstetrics and Gynecology.* 94(2): 229–231.

Arimandi BH, et al. (2004). Soy protein may alleviate osteoarthritis symptoms. *Phytomedicine.* Nov;11(7-8):567–575.

Bruce B, et al. (2003). Isoflavone supplements do not affect thyroid function in iodine replete postmenopausal women. *Journal of Medicinal Food.* Winter;6(4):309–316.

Brzezinski A, Debi A. (1999). Phytoestrogens: The "natural" selective estrogen receptor modulators? *European Journal of Obstetrics, Gynecology, and Reproductive Biology.* 85(1):47–51.

Burke GL, et al. (2003). Soy protein and isoflavone effects on vasomotor symptoms in peri- and postmenopausal women: The Soy Estrogen Alternative Study. *Menopause*. Mar-Apr;10(2): 147–153.

Cheng SY, et al. (2004). The hypoglycemic effects of soy isoflavones on postmenopausal women. *Journal of Women's Health (Larchmont)*. Dec;13(10):1080–1086.

Chiechi LM. (1999). Dietary phytoestrogens in the prevention of long-term postmenopausal diseases. *International Journal of Gynaecology and Obstetrics*. 67(1):39–40.

Clarkson TB, Anthony MS. (1998). Phytoestrogens and coronary heart disease. *Bailliere's Clinical Endocrinology and Metabolism*. 12(4):589–604.

Colacurci N, et al. (2004). Effects of soy isoflavones on menopausal neurovegetative symptoms. *Minerva Ginecologica*. Oct;56(5): 407–412.

Dalais FS, et al. (2004). Effects of a diet rich in phytoestrogens on prostate-specific antigen and sex hormones in men diagnosed with prostate cancer. *Urology*. Sep;64(3):510–515.

Der Marderosian A, Beutler J.[Eds.]. (2004). *The Review of Natural Products—Soy Monograph*. St. Louis, MO: Facts & Comparisons.

Duncan AM, et al. (1999). Soy isoflavones exert modest hormonal effects in premenopausal women. *Journal of Clinical Endocrinology and Metabolism*. 84(1):192–197.

Fiedor P, et al. (1998). Immunosuppressive effects of synthetic derivative of genistein on the survival of pancreatic islet allografts. *Transplantation Proceedings*. 30(2):537.

Geller J, et al. (1998). Genistein inhibits the growth of human-patient BPH and prostate cancer in histoculture. *Prostate*. 34(2): 75–79.

He J, et al. (2005). Effect of soybean protein on blood pressure: A randomized, controlled trial. *Annals of Internal Medicine*. Jul 5;143(1):1–9.

Lindsay SH, Claywell LG. (1999). Considering soy: Its estrogenic effects may protect women. *Journal of Obstetrics, Gynecology, and Neonatal Nursing*. 28[6 Suppl. 1]:21–24.

Lydeking-Olsen E, et al. (2004). Soymilk or progesterone for prevention of bone loss—A 2-year randomized, placebo-controlled trial. *European Journal of Nutrition*. Aug;43(4):246–257.

Messina M. (1999). Soy, soy phytoestrogens (isoflavones), and breast cancer. *American Journal of Clinical Nutrition*. 70(4): 574–575.

Messina M, Bennink M. (1998). Soy foods, isoflavones and risk of colonic cancer: A review of the in vitro and in vivo data.

Bailliere's Clinical Endocrinology and Metabolism. 12(4): 707–728.

Moyad MA. (1999). Soy, disease prevention, and prostate cancer. *Seminars in Urology and Oncology.* 17(2):97–102.

Newton KM, et al. (2006). Soy protein and bone mineral density in older men and women: A randomized trial. *Maturitas.* Oct 20;55(3):270–277.

Potter SM. (1998). Soy protein and cardiovascular disease: The impact of bioactive components in soy. *Nutrition Review.* 56(8): 231–235.

Ravindranath MH, et al. (2004). Anticancer therapeutic potential of soy isoflavone, genistein. *Advances in Experimental Medicine and Biology.* 546:121–165.

Scambia G, et al. (2000). Clinical effects of a standardized soy extract in postmenopausal women: A pilot study. *Menopause.* 7(2): 105–111.

Setchell KD. (1998). Phytoestrogens: The biochemistry, physiology, and implications for human health of soy isoflavones. *American Journal of Clinical Nutrition.* 68[6 Suppl.]:1333S–1346S.

Ye YB.(2006). Soy isoflavones attenuate bone loss. *European Journal of Nutrition.* Sept; 45(6):327–334.

Zhuo XG, et al. (2004). Soy isoflavone intake lowers serum LDL cholesterol: A meta-analysis of 8 randomized controlled trials in humans. *Journal of Nutrition.* Sep;134(9): 2395–2400.

 NAME: Spirulina (*Spirulina maxima, S. platensis*)

Common Names: None

Family: *Oscillatoriaceae*

Description of Plant

- There are thousands of species of blue-green algae. The species known as spirulina naturally grow in warm alkaline water.
- Most blue-green algaes have cell walls made of cellulose and are difficult to digest. Spirulina's cell walls are made of complex proteins and sugars, and it is easily digestible.

- The blue-green color originates from chlorophyll (green) and phycocyanin (blue) pigments.

Medicinal Part: Dried algae

Constituents and Action (if known)
- Protein, chlorophyll, phycocyanin pigments, carotenoids, sugars
- Sulpholipids (1%)
- Calcium-spirulina (ca-sp): antiviral against HIV-1 and herpes simplex I
- Caused tumor regression in oral leukoplakia of tobacco chewers (Mathew et al., 1995)
- May increase TNF production
- Inhibits replication of several viruses—herpes simplex, cytomegalovirus, mumps, influenza, HIV, measles (Hayashi et al., 1996)
- Protects rat livers against hepatotoxicity caused by carbon tetrachloride (Torres-Duran et al., 1999)

Nutritional Ingredients: Source of protein (62%): contains 22 amino acids, B-complex vitamins (all except B_{12}), minerals (zinc, iron, manganese, selenium, potassium, calcium, magnesium), carotenoids. A rich source of GLA (25%–30%); superior to other sources such as evening primrose oil, which contains 10% to 15% GLA.

Traditional Use: Used as a food by the Aztecs and Asian and African peoples

Current Use
- Nutritional supplement with easily absorbed essential fatty acids, trace minerals, protein, and iron
- In a controlled study, spirulina significantly reduced LDL cholesterol in patients with mild hyperlipidemia and hypertension (Belay et al., 1993). It also lowered elevated blood lipids in patients with hyperlipidemia nephritic syndrome (Samuels et al., 2002).
- Rich source of GLA; may be of benefit for skin conditions such as eczema and psoriasis

- Stimulated the growth of healthy intestinal flora, especially lactobacilli and bifidobacteria
- Effective for treating iron-deficiency anemia. The iron in spirulina is absorbed 60% better than iron tablets and also promotes hematopoiesis.
- A combination of spirulina and zinc enhanced arsenic excretion in patients with chronic arsenic poisoning and reduced symptoms of keratosis (Misbahuddin et al., 2006).
- Sixty patients with chronic liver disorders were given spirulina. Physicians noted stabilization of the diseases and decreased progression to hepatocirrhosis (Gorban et al., 2000).
- Children being treated for tuberculosis were given spirulina along with conventional therapy. They experienced reduced side effects from the medication and did not need to stop the medication as frequently due to toxicity (Kostromina et al., 2003).
- A dose of 2,000 mg a day of spirulina reduced interleukin-4 levels by 32% and relieved symptoms of allergic rhinitis (Mao et al., 2005).
- In animal studies, spirulina exhibited immune-potentiating, anticancer, radiation protective, hepatoprotective, renal protective, and hypotensive activity. Rats given spirulina were protected against gentamicin, cisplatin, and cyclosporine-induced renal damage and doxorubicin-induced cardiotoxicity (Khan et al., 2005; Khan et al., 2006; Kuhad et al., 2006; Mohan et al., 2006).

Available Forms, Dosage, and Administration Guidelines
Preparations: Capsules, tablets, powders, supplemental fruit drinks
Typical Dosage: 2 to 5 g a day; four to ten 500-mg tablets a day

Pharmacokinetics—If Available (form or route when known): None known

Toxicity: None known for spirulina. Other species of wild-harvested blue-green algae may be contaminated with heavy metals or microcystins.

Contraindications: None known

Side Effects: None known

Long-Term Safety: Safe. Extensive animal studies and a long history of human use as food show no evidence of any acute or chronic toxicity.

Use in Pregnancy/Lactation/Children: Safe: no fetotoxicity or teratogenicity was found with high doses in pregnant animals.

Drug/Herb Interactions and Rationale (if known): None known

Special Notes: Promoters of spirulina have claimed that it is a diet product, but an FDA review found no such evidence. One human study found that ingestion of 2.8 g spirulina three times a day for 4 weeks resulted in a significant reduction in body weight (Belay et al., 1993). Blue-green algae is a related product gathered from the Great Klamath Lake in Oregon. It is wild harvested and may contain bacterial toxins (microcystins), which can cause liver damage. It is best to avoid any microalgae products not grown in a controlled environment.

BIBLIOGRAPHY

Belay A, et al. (1993). Current knowledge on potential health benefits of spirulina. *Journal of Applied Phycology*. 5:235–241.

Chamorro G, et al. (1996). Pharmacology and toxicology of Spirulina algae. *Revista de Investigacion Clinica*. 48:389–399.

Gorban EM, et al. (2000). Clinical and experimental study of spirulina efficacy in chronic diffuse liver diseases. *Likarska Sprava*. Sep;(6):89–93.

Hayashi T, et al. (1996). Calcium spirulin, an inhibitor of enveloped virus replication, from a blue-green algae *Spirulina palatensis*. *Journal of Natural Products*. 59(1):83–87.

Khan M, et al. (2005). Protective effect of spirulina against doxorubicin-induced cardiotoxicity. *Phytotherapy Research*. Dec;19(2):1030–1037.

Khan M, et al. (2006). Spirulina attenuates cyclosporine-induced nephrotoxicity in rats. *Journal of Applied Toxicology*. Sep-Oct; 26(5):444–451.

Kostromina VP, et al. (2003). Evaluation of the efficacy of a plant adaptogen (spirulina) in the pathogenic therapy of primary tuberculosis in children. *Likarska Sprava*. Jul-Aug;(5–6):102–105.

Kuhad A, et al. (2006). Effect of spirulina, a blue green algae, on gentamicin-induced oxidative stress and renal dysfunction in rats. *Fundamental and Clinical Pharmacology*. Apr;20(2):121–128.

Mao TK, et al. (2005). Effects of a spirulina-based dietary supplement on cytokine production from allergic rhinitis patients. *Journal of Medicinal Food.* Spring;8(1):27–30.

Mathew B, et al. (1995). Evaluation of chemoprevention of oral cancer with *Spirulina fusiformis. Nutrition and Cancer.* 24(2):197–202.

Misbahuddin M, et al. (2006). Efficacy of spirulina extract plus zinc in patients of chronic arsenic poisoning: A randomized placebo-controlled study. *Clinical Toxicology (Philadelphia).* 44(20):135–141.

Mohan IK, et al. (2006). Protection against cisplatin-induced nephrotoxicity by spirulina in rats. *Cancer Chemotherapy and Pharmacology.* Dec;58(6):802–808.

Salazar M, et al. (1998). Subchronic toxicity study in mice fed *Spirulina maxima. Journal of Ethnopharmacology.* 62(3): 235–242.

Samuels R, et al. (2002). Hypocholesterolemic effect of spirulina in patients with hyperlipidemic nephrotic syndrome. *Journal of Medicinal Food.* Summer;5(2):91–96.

Torres-Duran PV, et al. (1999). Studies on the preventative effect of *Spirulina maxima* on fatty liver development induced by carbon tetrachloride in the rat. *Journal of Ethnopharmacology.* 64(2):141–148.

 NAME: St. John's Wort (*Hypericum perforatum*)

Common Names: Klamath weed

Family: *Hypericaceae*

Description of Plant
- Shrubby perennial herb with bright-yellow flowers, grows 1' to 2' tall
- Native to Europe but now grows as a weed in many parts of the world in dry, gravelly soils with full sun
- The yellow flowers contain small black oil glands that when crushed produce a red stain; this was thought to be the blood of St. John the Baptist, hence the name St. John's wort.

Medicinal Part: Flowering tops, especially the flowers and unopened buds. Harvesting at bud stage increases hypericin levels; late harvest increases hyperforin.

Constituents and Action (if known)

- Napthodianthrones (less than 0.10%–0.15%), hypericin, pseudohypericin, isohypericin
  - Increase capillary blood flow
  - Inhibit serotonin uptake at postsynaptic receptors (Upton, 1997)
  - Inhibit reuptake of dopamine and norepinephrine
  - Block presynaptic alpha-2 receptors
  - Antiviral activity against herpes simplex virus I and II, retrovirus (HIV) in vitro and vivo, Epstein-Barr virus, influenza A and B, murine cytomegalovirus, hepatitis C (may work through protein-kinase C-mediated phosphorylation) (Schempp et al., 1999)
- Phloroglucinols
  - Hyperforin: inhibits uptake of serotonin, GABA, and L-glutamate (Chatterjee et al., 1998; Laakmann et al., 1998), antibacterial (Upton, 1997)
  - Adhyperforin
- Flavonoids and flavonol glycosides (flowers, 11.71%): kaempferol, quercetin, luteolin, amentoflavone: anti-inflammatory and antiulcerogenic activity (Upton, 1997); inhibition of benzodiazepine binding, rutin, and hyperoside/hyperin
- EOs (0.059%–0.350%): monoterpenes (pinenes) and sesquiterpenes: antiviral, antibacterial
- Tannins: astringent activity when applied topically, stimulate wound healing

Other Actions

- Inhibits catechol-o-methyl-transferase and suppresses interleukin-6 release; may affect mood through neurohormonal pathways
- Antibacterial activity against gram-positive and gram-negative bacteria
- Can stimulate and also inhibit cyclic P-450 enzyme metabolism

Nutritional Ingredients: None known

Traditional Use

- Antidepressant, antiviral, antibacterial, cholagogue, diuretic, nervine, nervous system trophorestorative, vulnerary
- Dioscorides used St. John's wort in the first century for sciatica, burns, and fevers. Gerard noted in 1633 that St. John's wort oil was excellent for wounds, bites, and burns.
- In Europe, the herb is used for depression, mental exhaustion, liver problems, nerve injuries (internally and topically), bedwetting caused by irritation of the bladder, sciatica, gastric ulcers, and topically for a wide range of skin problems and trauma injuries.

Current Use

Internal

- Mild to moderate depression (not appropriate for severe depression or bipolar disorders) (Gastpar et al., 2006; Kasper et al., 2006; Linde et al., 1996), seasonal affective disorder (Martinzez et al., 1994); use with lemon balm for greatest activity for SAD (Winston, 2006). Relieves fatigue in depressed persons (Stevinson et al., 1998). Hypericum was as effective as sertraline, citalopram, and fluoretine in human trials (Gastpar et al., 2005; Schrader et al., 2000).
- Most herbalists do not use St. John's wort as monotherapy for depression. The orthodox treatments (selective serotonin reuptake inhibitors [SSRIs] or St. John's wort alone) do not address the full spectrum of this disorder. Effective therapies may require lifestyle changes, counseling, and additional adaptogenic, antidepressant, or nervine herbs such as Siberian ginseng, schisandra, lemon balm, rosemary, basil, black cohosh, and lavender, which will improve the specificity and effectiveness of the protocol (Winston, 2006).
- Eases menopausal anxiety, nervousness, and sleep disorders; use with motherwort and blue vervain (Winston, 2006)
- Helps to heal damaged nerve tissue after cerebrovascular accident or neurologic trauma; use with ginkgo, Siberian ginseng, or bacopa
- Oral use concurrent with topical applications for sciatica, neuralgias, diabetic neuropathies, trigeminal neuralgia, and Bell's palsy (Upton, 1997)

- Several studies indicate that St. John's wort can be helpful in quitting smoking and maintaining smoking cessation (Lawvere et al., 2006).
- Antiviral activity against herpes type I and II, mononucleosis, influenza. The antiviral effect is mild when taken orally. Use St. John's wort with other antiviral herbs (basil, thyme, oregano, lemon balm, rosemary) as a supportive therapy.

Topical: Topically, *Hypericum* tincture (the undiluted tincture will cause intense burning in open lesions) or oil is effective for treating herpetic lesions and shingles. Hypericum oil speeds healing of wounds, burns, sunburn, shingles, nerve pain, and nerve damage. It can be useful for neuralgias, hemorrhoids, trauma injuries, gum disease, and painful tooth sockets after dental extractions (Upton, 1997). A *Hypericum* cream was significantly more effective than placebo for topical treatment of mild to moderate atopic dermatitis (Schempp et al., 2003).

Available Forms, Dosage, and Administration Guidelines

Preparations: Dried herb, capsules, tablets, tinctures. Most products for internal use are standardized to 0.3% hypericin, even though this is no guarantee of efficacy; some products are now standardized to include hyperforin. Well-made tinctures should be dark burgundy red and have a noticeably fragrant aroma.

Typical Dosage

- *Capsules:* For products standardized to 0.3% hypericin, take 300 mg three to four times a day
- *Tea:* Steep 1 tsp dried herb in 8 oz hot water for 15 to 20 minutes; take two cups a day
- *Tincture* (1:2 or 1:5, 40% alcohol): 40 to 80 gtt (2–4 mL) three times a day
- *Topical:* As an anti-inflammatory or for wound epithelialization, use the oil or diluted tincture and cover wound with gauze or bandage until healing is established.

Pharmacokinetics—If Available (form or route when known)

- *Onset:* Absorption 2.0 to 2.6 hours
- *Peak:* 5 hours

- *Duration:* Takes 4 to 6 weeks to be effective
- *Steady state (with long-term use):* 4 days
- *Half-life:* 24 to 48 hours
- *Metabolism and excretion:* By the CYP 3A4 System, which is responsible for more than 50% of drug interactions (Mills et al., 2004)

Toxicity: Photosensitivity may occur with high doses of hypericin-rich products, so be careful of excessive sun exposure. In a human trial using two different hypericum extracts for 14 days, there was no significant increase of photosensitivity (Schulz et al., 2006).

Contraindications: Severe depression; use of cyclosporin or other drugs to prevent organ transplant rejection

Side Effects: Headache, pruritus, and GI irritation usually subside with long-term use. If side effects occur, lower dose and then gradually increase again. Photosensitivity may occur (Golsch et al., 1997). Rash is reversible with withdrawal of herb. If nerve hypersensitivity occurs, discontinue use.

Long-Term Safety: Safe at normal therapeutic dosage

Use in Pregnancy/Lactation/Children: Use cautiously during pregnancy; safety data is positive but minimal and mostly animal studies (Dugona et al., 2006). Theoretical concern that St. John's wort may decrease production of milk by inhibiting secretion of prolactin, but evidence suggests minimal risk (Dugoua et al., 2006; Lee et al., 2003). Avoid in very young children; no research available.

Drug/Herb Interactions and Rationale (if known)
- With concurrent use of theophylline and beta-2 agonists, there is a theoretical possibility of increased anxiety, nervousness, and worsening of panic disorder (Nebel et al., 1999).
- Serotonin syndrome may occur if used with SSRIs (sweating, agitation, tremor) (Gordon, 1998).
- There has been concern about mixing St. John's wort with SSRIs. Most clinicians have not seen interactions, although there is one reported case of a possible serotonin syndrome reaction in a patient taking both medications (Gordon, 1998). Use cautiously together.

- May increase or decrease cyclic P-450 activity; St. John's wort may affect medications that are metabolized by this pathway (Wheatley, 1997; Mills et al., 2004). It induces CYP34, CYP1A2 (in females only) (Wenk et al., 2004). It did not affect CYP2D6, N-acetyltransferase 2, or xanthine oxidase (Wenk et al., 2004).
  - Protease inhibitors: one poorly done study suggests that St. John's wort may lower blood levels of indinivir in healthy individuals (Henney, 2000). More research is needed to determine whether this herb can reduce the efficacy of this type of drug in HIV-positive patients. Avoid concurrent use.
  - Cyclosporin and tacrolimus: in patients taking cyclosporin to prevent kidney and heart transplant rejection, therapeutic levels of the drug dropped when they began taking this herb. These preliminary data suggest that patients taking cyclosporin or other immunosuppressive medication should avoid taking St. John's wort (Henney, 2000).
  - There was no evidence of ovulation with concurrent use of hypericum with low dose oral contraceptives, but there was increased intracyclic bleeding and decreased 3-ketodesogestral concentrations. There was no significant change in follicle maturation, serum estradiol, or progesterone (Pfrunder et al., 2003). Use cautiously together; may increase risk of unwanted pregnancy.
- Does not potentiate alcohol; does not interfere with anesthesia
- Prolongs effects of digoxin (Mueller et al., 2004).
- A low hyperforin St. John's wort extract did not affect blood levels of alprazolam, caffeine, tolbutamide, or digoxin (Arold et al., 2005).

Special Notes: In the past, St. John's wort was believed to have monoamine oxidase inhibitor activity, but research has shown little or no such inhibition (Cott, 1997). Concerns associated with the use of monoamine oxidase inhibitors are not germane to St. John's wort (diet, anesthesia, medications).

BIBLIOGRAPHY

Arold G, et al. (2005). No relevant interaction with alprazolam, caffeine, tolbutaminde, and digoxin by treatment with a low-hyperforin St. John's wort extract. *Planta Medica.* Apr;71(4):331–337.

Bennett DA, et al. (1998). Neuropharmacology of St. John's wort. *Annals of Pharmacotherapy*. 5(4):245–252.

Chatterjee SS, et al. (1998). Hyperforin as a possible antidepressant component of hypericum extracts. *Life Science*. 63(6):499–510.

Cott JM, Fugh-Berman A. (1998). Is St. John's wort (*Hypericum perforatum*) an effective antidepressant? *Journal of Nervous and Mental Disease*. 186(8):500–501.

Dugoua JJ, et al. (2006). Safety and efficacy of St. John's wort (hypericum) during pregnancy and lactation. *Canadian Journal of Clinical Pharmacology*. Fall;13(3):e268–e276.

Gastpar M, et al. (2005). Efficacy and tolerability of hypericum extract STW3 in long-term treatment with a once-daily dosage in comparison with sertraline. *Pharmacopsychiatry*. Mar;38(2): 78–86.

Gastpar M, et al. (2006). Comparative efficacy and safety of a once-daily dosage of hypericum extract STW3-VI and citalopram in patients with moderate depression: A double-blind, randomised, multicentre, placebo-controlled study. *Pharmacopsychiatry*. Mar;39(2):66–75.

Golsch S, et al. (1997). Reversible increase in photosensitivity to UV-B caused by St. John's wort extract. *Hautarzt*. 48: 249–252.

Gordon JB. (1998). SSRIs and St. John's wort: Possible toxicity? *American Family Physician*. 57(5):950.

Henney J. (2000). Risk of interactions with St. John's wort. *Journal of the American Medical Association*. 283(13):1679.

Kasper S, et al. (2006). Superior efficacy of St. John's wort extract WS 5570 compared to placebo in patients with major depression: A randomised, double-blind, placebo-controlled, multi-center trial (ISRCTN77277298). *BMC Medicine*. Jun 23;4:14.

Laakmann G, et al. (1998). St. John's wort in mild to moderate depression: The relevance of hyperforin for the clinical efficacy. *Pharmacopsychiatry*. 31[Suppl.]:54–59.

Lawvere S, et al. (2006). A phase II study of St. John's wort for smoking cessation. *Complementary Therapies in Medicine*. Sep;14(3):175–184.

Lee A, et al. (2003). The safety of St. John's wort (*Hypericum perforatum*) during breastfeeding. *Journal of Clinical Psychiatry*. Aug;64(8):966–968.

Lenoir S, et al. (1999). A double-blind randomized trial to investigate three different concentrations of a standardized fresh plant extract obtained from the shoot tips of *Hypericum perforatum* L. *Phytomedicine*. 6(3):141–146.

Martinez B, et al. (1994). Hypericum in the treatment of seasonal affective disorders. *Journal of Geriatric Psychiatry and Neurology.* 7:S29–S33.

Miller AL. (1998). St. John's wort (*Hypericum perforatum*): Clinical effects on depression and other conditions. *Alternative Medicine Review.* 3(1):18–26.

Mills E et al.(2004). Interaction of St. John's wort with conventional drugs. *British Medical Journal.* Jul 3;329(7456):27–30.

Mueller SC et al.(2004). Effect of St. John's wort dose and preparation on pharmacokinetics of digoxin. *Clinical Pharmacology and Therapeutics.* June; 75(6):546–557.

Nathan PJ. (1999). Experimental and clinical pharmacology of St. John's wort (*Hypericum perforatum* L.). *Molecular Psychiatry.* 4:333–338.

Nebel A, et al. (1999). Potential metabolic interaction between St. John's wort and theophylline. *Annals of Pharmacotherapy.* 33(4):502.

Pfrunder A, et al. (2003). Interaction of St. John's wort with low-dose oral contraceptive therapy: A randomized controlled trial. *British Journal of Clinical Pharmacology.* Dec;56(6):683–690.

Schempp CM, et al. (1999). Antibacterial activity of hyperforin from St. John's wort, against multiresistant *Staphylococcus aureus* and gram-positive bacteria. *Lancet.* 353(9170):2129.

Schempp CM, et al. (2003). Topical treatment of atopic dermatitis with hypericum cream. A randomized, placebo-controlled, double-blind half-side comparison study. *Hautarzt.* Mar;54(3):248–253.

Schrader E, et al. (2000). Equivalence of St. John's wort extract (Ze 117) and fluoxetine: A randomised, controlled study in mild to moderate depression. *International Clinical Psychopharmacology.* 15:61–68.

Schulz HU, et al. (2006). Investigation of the effect of photosensivity following multiple oral dosing of two different hypericum extracts in healthy men. *Arzneimittelforschung.* 56(3):212–221.

Stevinson C, et al. (1998). Hypericum for fatigue: A pilot study. *Phytomedicine.* 5(6):443–447.

Upton R. [Ed.]. (1997). *American Herbal Pharmacopoeia and Therapeutic Compendium: St John's Wort.* Santa Cruz, CA: AHP.

Wenk M, et al. (2004). Effect of St. John's wort on the activities of CYP1A2, CYP3A4, Cyp2D6, N-acetyltransferase 2, and xanthine oxidase in healthy males and females. *British Journal of Clinical Pharmacology.* Apr;57(4):495–499.

Wheatley D. (1997). LI 160, an extract of St. John's wort, versus amitriptyline in mildly to moderately depressed outpatients: A controlled 6-week clinical trial. *Pharmacopsychiatry.* 30[Suppl.]:77–80.

Winston D. (2006). Differential treatment of depression and anxiety with botanical medicine. In *Proceedings of the 17th Annual American Herbalists Guild Symposium*. Cheshire, CT: AHG, 265–273.

Woelk H. (1994). Benefits and risks of the hypericum extract LI 160: Drug monitoring study with 3250 patients. *Journal of Geriatric Psychiatry and Neurology*. 7:S34–S38.

NAME: Sweet Annie (*Artemesia annua, A. apiacea, A. lancea*)

Common Names: Annual wormwood, *qing hao* (Chinese), sweet wormwood

Family: *Asteraceae*

Description of Plant
- This is a large (10'), aromatic, weedy annual that is native to southeast Asia and has become naturalized throughout much of Africa, Europe, and the United States.
- The best-quality plants are grown in Vietnam.

Medicinal Part: Dried herb, fresh juice, natural isolates (artemisinin or qinghaosu), and semisynthetic derivatives (artemether, artesunate) from the plant

Constituents and Action (if known)
- Sesquiterpene lactones
  - Artemisinin: antimalarial, antitumor (Bhakuni, 2001), antischistosomiasis (Dharmananda, 2002)
- Volatile oil (in relative % of total volatile oils in the plant, which is 0.4%–4.0%)
  - Artemesia ketone (66.7%): antioxidant, antibacterial, antifungal (Juteau et al., 2002)
  - Linalool (3.4%): antihistamine, antiviral (Duke, 2006), anti-inflammatory (Peana et al., 2004)
  - β-caryophylene (1.2%): antioxidant, antibacterial, antifungal (Juteau et al., 2002)
  - 1,8 cineole (5.5%): cytokine inhibitor (Juergens et al., 1998), anti-inflammatory (Juergens et al., 2003)

- ○ Camphor (3.3%): antioxidant, antibacterial, antifungal (Juteau et al., 2002), anti-inflammatory, antitumor (Duke, 2006)
- ○ Myrcene (3.8%)
- ○ β-pinine (0.882%)
- Various extracts (water, ether, alcohol, etc.) of the plant have been found to exhibit choleretic, antifungal, antiyeast, antiviral, antipyretic, anti-inflammatory, analgesic, cytotoxic, antimycobacterial, lymphocyte proliferation inhibition, and DNA polymerase inhibition (hepatitis B) activity.

Nutritional Ingredients: The EO is used as a flavoring in vermouth.

Traditional Use

- Antimalarial, antiprotozoal, antiamoebic, antibacterial, antitumor, antiulcerogenic, bitter tonic, cholagogue, febrifuge
- In Chinese medicine, qing hao is used to clear heat (infections). It is used for malarial fevers with alternating chills and fever; the bones feel hot, and there is little or no sweating.
- It is also used for deficient *yin* fevers with night sweats (Dengue fever) and for chronic low-grade fevers. It is used with *A. capillaris* and gardenia fruit to clear damp heat jaundice.
- The leaves have been used topically for boils and abscesses (Anonymous, 2006)

Current Use

- Trials of *A. annua* and its derivatives, artemisinin, artemether, and artesinate, have shown significant inhibitory effects for chloroquine-resistant malaria, especially *Plasmodium falciparum*. It crosses the blood—brain barrier and can treat cerebral malaria. Artemisinin has a cytotoxic effect on the malaria plasmodium. It interacts with iron and generates reactive oxygen species (ROS), which prevents the plasmodium from absorbing nutrients and replicating.
- Cancer cells have been found to have high iron levels, and artemisin's ability to induce apoptosis and have a selective cytotoxic effect on such cells has spawned a number of animal and in vitro studies on the use of this substance for

various cancers, including oral squamous cell carcinoma (Yamachika et al., 2004), fibrosarcoma, chronic myeloid leukemia, and breast cancer. There is one case of a human laryngeal squamous cell carcinoma treated with the compound artesunate (Singh & Verma, 2002). Artemisinin also seems to reduce the ability of cancer cells to become resistant to chemotherapeutic medications (Reungpatthanaphong & Mankhetkorn, 2002).

- In China, qing hao is also used to downregulate excess T-lymphocyte activity associated with autoimmune disease. The herb and artemisinin have been used for periods of 3 months to treat systemic and discoid lupus (Dharmananda, 2002).
- In a Chinese study, 61 patients who were in remission from lupus nephritis were divided into two groups. Thirty-one patients were given artemisinin and cordyceps, while the control group was given another therapy. After 5 years, 83.9% of the artemisinin/cordyceps group were still in remission compared with 50% of the control group (Lu, 2002).
- The herb and artemisinin have been used to treat *Schistosomiasis, Clonorchiasis, Leptospirosis, Leishmaniasis,* and *Babesiosis.*

Available Forms, Dosage, and Administration Guidelines

Preparations: Fresh juice, tincture, standardized extract, pharmaceutical preparations

Typical Dosage

- *Fresh juice:* 1/4 oz three times a day. This is a very effective way to take this herb, but the very bitter taste will significantly reduce patient compliance.
- *Tincture* (1:2, 30% alcohol): 60 to 80 gtt twice a day
- *Standardized extract* (30:1): One 500-mg capsule twice a day
- *Pharmaceutical preparations:* Artemisinin, 250 to 500 mg twice a day. With long-term use of artemisinin, absorption decreases. Taking artemisinin 1 week on and 1 week off may prevent this problem.

Pharmacokinetics—If Available (form or route when known): Artemisinin is actually absorbed more quickly from

the tea of the herb than from oral solid-dose forms (Rath et al., 2004). Oral artemisinin is quickly but only partially absorbed, with peak concentrations after 1 to 2 hours after ingestion (Gordi et al., 2002).

Toxicity: The pollen is allergenic. Contact with the plant or EO can cause contact dermatitis.

Contraindications: None known

Side Effects: It can cause gastric upset, nausea, diarrhea, vomiting, dizziness, and headache in some patients.

Long-Term Safety: In human and animal trials, very high doses (10 times the therapeutics dose) of isolated artemesinin caused hepatitis. All published data on the use of the herb and its derivatives in normal doses show a low level of toxicity (Dharmananda, 2002).

Use in Pregnancy/Lactation/Children: Avoid use in pregnancy, lactation, and with young children unless under a physician's care.

Drug/Herb Interactions and Rationale (if known): Azole antifungal agents (ketoconazole, griseofulvin, nystatin, fluconazole) as well as calcium channel blockers (amlodipine, diltiazem, nifedipine) can negatively affect absorption of artemisinin (Chen & Chen, 2004).

Special Notes: The World Health Organization has recommended artemisinin-based combination therapies (artemesinin combined with lumefantrine, piperaquine, or mefloquine) as the first-line treatment for *Plasmodium falciparum* infections.

BIBLIOGRAPHY

Anonymous. (2006). Plants for a future. Retrieved October 25 2006, from www.pfaf.org/database/plants.php?Arlandiatannae.

Bhakuni R, et al. (2001). Secondary metabolites of *Artemisia annua* and their biological activity. *Current Science*. 80(1):35–48.

Bone K. (2005). *Artemisia annua:* Herbal use vs. isolated active. *Townsend Newsletter for Doctors and Patients*. April:45.

Chen T, Chen T. (2004). *Chinese Medical Herbology and Pharmacology* (pp. 244–266). City of Industry, CA: Art of Medicine Press.

Dharmananda S. (2002). Ching-hao and the artemisias used in Chinese medicine. Retrieved October 25 2006, from www.itmonline.org/arts/Chinghao.htm.

Duke J. Dr. Duke's phytochemical and ethnobotanical databases. Retrieved October 25 2006, from www.ars-grin.gov/cgi-bin/duke/chemactivities.

Gordi T, et al. (2002). Artemisinin pharmacokinetics and efficacy in uncomplicated malaria patients treated with two different dosage regimens. *Antimicrobial Agents and Chemotherapy.* 46(4):1026–1031.

Hsu E. (2006). The history of qing hao in the Chinese *Materia Medica. Transactions of the Royal Society of Tropical Medicine and Hygiene.* Jun;100(6):505–508.

Juergens UR, et al. (1998). Inhibition of cytokine production and arachidonic acid metabolism by eucalyptol (1.8-cineole) in human blood monocytes in vitro. *European Journal of Medical Research.* Nov 17;3(11):508–510.

Juergens UR, et al. (2003). Anti-inflammatory activity of 1.8-cineol (eucalyptol) in bronchial asthma: A double-blind placebo-controlled trial. *Respiratory Medicine.* Mar;97(3):250–256.

Juteau F, et al. (2002). Antibacterial and antioxidant activities of *Artemisia annua* essential oil. *Fitoterapia.* Oct;73(6):432–435.

Khannan RK, et al (2005). Reaction of artemisinin with haemoglobin: Implications for antimalarial activity. *Biochemical Journal.* 385[Pt. 2]:409–418.

Lai H, et al. (2005). Targeted treatments of cancer with artemisinin and artemisinin-tagged iron-carrying compounds. *Expert Opinion on Therapeutic Targets.* 9(5):995–1007.

Lu L. (2002). Study on effect of *Cordyceps sinensis* and artemisinin in preventing recurrence of lupus nephritis. *Zhongguo Zhong Xi Yi Jie He Za Zhi.* Mar;22(3):169–171.

Messori L, et al. (2006). The reaction of artemisinins with hemoglobin: A unified picture. *Bioorganic and Medicinal Chemistry.* May;14(9):2972–2977.

Mueller MS, et al. (2004). Randomized controlled trial of a traditional preparation of *Artemisia annua* L. (annual wormwood) in the treatment of malaria. *Transactions of the Royal Society of Tropical Medicine and Hygiene.* May;98(5):318–321.

Peana AT, et al. (2004). Effects of (−)-linalool in the acute hyperalgesia induced by carrageenan, L-glutamate and prostaglandin E2. *European Journal of Pharmacology.* Aug 30;497(3):279–284.

Rath K, et al. (2004). Pharmacokinetic study of artemisinin after oral intake of a traditional preparation of *Artemisia annua* L. (annual wormwood). *American Journal of Tropical Medicine and Hygiene.* 70(2):128–132.

Reungpatthanaphong P, Mankhetkorn S. (2002). Modulation of multidrug resistance by artemisinin, artesunate and dihydroartemisinin in K562/adr and GLC4/adr resistant cell lines. *Biological and Pharmaceutical Bulletin.* 25(12): 1555–1561.

Singh N, Verma K. (2002). Case report of a laryngeal squamous cell carcinoma treated with artesunate. *Archives of Oncology.* 10(4): 279–280.

Swensson US, et al. (1998). Artemisinin induces omeprazole metabolism in human beings. *Clinical Pharmacology and Therapeutics.* 64(2):160–167.

Winston D. (2006). *Winston's Botanic Materia Medica.* Washington, NJ: DWCHS.

Yamachika E, et al. (2004). Artemisinin: An alternative treatment for oral squamous cell carcinoma. *Anticancer Research.* 24(4): 2153–2160.

T

 NAME: Tea Tree (*Melaleuca alternifolia*)

Common Names: Australian tea tree oil, Melaleuca oil

Family: *Myrtaceae*

Description of Plant
- There are many plants known as tea trees, but the species *M. alternifolia* is the source of commercial tea tree oil.
- Small, shrubby evergreen native only to the northeast coastal region of New South Wales, Australia
- It is a member of the myrtle family, grows 8' tall, and has sprays of white flowers each summer.

Medicinal Part: EO; leaves are steam-distilled to yield about 2% oil

Constituents and Action (if known)
- EOs: terpinene-4-ol (40%), alpha-terpenol, alpha-pinene, alpha-terpinene, gamma-terpinene, p-cymene, limonene; more than 100 different compounds have been identified (Bruneton, 1999)

- Antimicrobial activity against *Candida albicans*, *Escherichia coli*, *Pseudomonas aeruginosa*, *Staphylococcus aureus* (MRSA) (Chan & Loudon, 1998; Dryden et al., 2004; Gustafson et al., 1998)
- Antimicrobial activity against vancomycin-resistant enterococci (Nelson, 1997)
- Antifungal (Nenoff et al., 1996) activity against drug-resistant oral fungal and yeast infections (Bagg et al., 2006)
- Alpha-terpineol and alpha-pinene have antimicrobial activity against *S. epidermidis* and *Propionibacterium acnes* (Ramon et al., 1995).

Nutritional Ingredients: None known

Traditional Use
- Analgesic, antibacterial, antifungal, antiviral, anti-inflammatory
- Leaves used by the Aborigines of Australia as a treatment for cuts, abrasions, burns, and insect bites
- Oil used during World War II by soldiers as a disinfectant; used in the 1920s in surgery and dentistry as Australian researchers learned that it was 13 times more active as an antiseptic than carbolic acid, the common disinfectant of that time

Current Use
- Acne (as a 5% solution): in a single-blind randomized study on 124 patients with mild to moderate acne, tea tree was compared with benzoyl peroxide. Both treatments were found to be equally effective; the tea tree patients had no adverse effects (Bassett et al., 1990).
- Impetigo: apply EO undiluted two or three times a day to the lesion. May cause mild pain and irritation.
- Boils and topical infections, including MRSA: apply EO undiluted two or three times a day (Dryden et al., 2004)
- Ringworm: apply undiluted to affected area
- First- and second-degree burns: apply freely mixed with lavender EO (1–2 gtt each), in a base of fresh aloe gel (Winston, 2006)
- Mouth ulcers: apply undiluted on a cotton swab two to four times a day

- Gingivitis: use diluted in water or in commercially made mouthwashes. Swish in mouth two or three times a day (Soukoulis et al., 2004).
- Vaginal or oral candidiasis (thrush): use a vaginal suppository once or twice a day for vaginal candidiasis; use mouthwash or EO diluted in water for thrush twice a day
- Useful for fluconazole- and itraconazole-resistant oral yeast infections in patients with AIDS and late-stage cancer (Bagg et al., 2006; Vasquez & Zawawi, 2002)
- Bacterial vaginosis: use a vaginal suppository (bolus) once or twice a day
- In shampoos for dandruff: use as needed
- Herpes: apply undiluted to herpetic lesions two or three times a day; may cause irritation and mild pain
- Lung and sinus infections: use 1 to 2 gtt EO in a hot vaporizer or in hot water once or twice a day. Inhale the steam. Lavender or eucalyptus EO can be added (Winston, 2006).
- Nail fungus (onychomycosis) and athlete's foot (tinea pedis): helps control infection but rarely cures it. Apply undiluted to feet and toenails twice a day (Satchell et al., 2002).
- In dogs, topical tea tree EO cream was a useful treatment for canine localized dermatitis with pruritis (Reichling et al., 2004).

Available Forms, Dosage, and Administration Guidelines

Preparations: EO, vaginal suppositories for vaginal candidiasis, mouthwash, ointments. The Australian quality standard for tea tree oil is 30% terpinene-4-ol and less than 15% cineol.

Typical Dosage: For external use: follow manufacturer or practitioner recommendations

Pharmacokinetics—If Available (form or route when known): Not known

Toxicity: Ingestion of 0.5 tsp EO has caused symptoms including ataxia, drowsiness, petechial body rash, and neutrophil leukocytosis (Hamner et al., 2006; Tisserand & Balacs, 1995).

Contraindications: Skin hypersensitivity

Side Effects: Dermatitis, allergic contact eczema

Long-Term Safety: Safe with topical use; does not cause photosensitization, allergic sensitization, or irritation to the skin or mucous membranes

Use in Pregnancy/Lactation/Children: Safe if used topically

Drug/Herb Interactions and Rationale (if known): None known

Special Notes: Avoid using in or near the eyes. To enhance effectiveness as an antifungal, apply dimethyl sulfoxide (DMSO) immediately afterward to same area (Bucks et al., 1994). Like all EOs, tea tree is a highly concentrated product and should be used internally in very small doses. Overdoses can cause serious health problems.

BIBLIOGRAPHY

Bagg J, et al. (2006). Susceptibility to *Melaleuca alternifolia* (tea tree) oil of yeasts isolated from the mouths of patients with advanced cancer. *Oral Oncology.* May;42(5):487–492.

Bassett IB, et al. (1990). A comparative study of tea tree benzoyl peroxide oil versus benzoyl peroxide in the treatment of acne. *Medical Journal of Australia.* 153(8):455–458.

Bruneton J. (1999). *Pharmacognosy, Phytochemistry, Medicinal Plants* (p. 559). Paris: Lavoisier.

Bucks DS, et al. (1994). Comparison of two topical preparations for the treatment of onychomycosis: *Melaleuca alternifolia* (tea tree) oil and clotrimazole. *Journal of Family Practice.* 38:601–605.

Chan CH, Loudon KW. (1998). Activity of tea tree oil on methicillin-resistant *Staphylococcus aureus. Journal of Hospital Infection.* 39(3):244–245.

Dryden MS, et al. (2004). A randomized, controlled trial of tea tree topical preparations versus a standard topical regimen for the clearance of MRSA colonization. *Journal of Hospital Infection.* Apr;56(4):283–286.

Gustafson JE, et al. (1998). Effects of tea tree oil on *Escherichia coli. Letters in Applied Microbiology.* 26:194–198.

Hammer KA, et al. (1996). Susceptibility of transient and commensal skin flora to the essential oil of *Melaleuca alternifolia*. *American Journal of Infection Control*. 24(3):186–189.

Hamner KA, et al. (2006). A review of the toxicity of *Melaleuca alternifolia* (tea tree) oil. *Food and Chemical Toxicology*. May;44(5):616–625.

Nelson RRS. (1997). In vitro activities of five plant essential oils against methicillin-resistant *Staphylococcus aureus* and vancomycin-resistant *Enterococcus faecium*. *Journal of Antimicrobial Chemotherapy*. 40:305–306.

Nenoff P, et al. (1996). Antifungal activity of the essential oil of *Melaleuca alternifolia* (tea tree oil) against pathogenic fungi in vivo. *Skin Pharmacology*. 9:388–394.

Ramon A, et al. (1995). Antimicrobial effects of tea-tree oil and its major components on *Staphylococcus aureus*, *S. epidermidis* and *Propionibacterium acnes*. *Letters in Applied Microbiology*. 21(4):242–245.

Reichling J, et al. (2004). Topical tea tree oil effective in canine localised pruritic dermatitis—A multi-centre randomised double-blind controlled clinical trial in the veterinary practice. *Deutsche Tierarztliche Wochenschrift*. Oct;111(1):408–414.

Satchell AC, et al. (2002). Treatment of interdigital tinea pedis with 25% and 50% tea tree oil solution: A randomized, placebo-controlled, blinded study. *Australasian Journal of Dermatology*. Aug;43(3):175–178.

Soukoulis S, et al. (2004). The effects of a tea tree oil-containing gel on plaque and chronic gingivitis. *Australian Dental Journal*. Jun;49(2):78–83.

Tisserand R, Balacs T. (1995). *Essential Oil Safety* (p. 211). Edinburgh: Churchill Livingstone.

Vasquez JA, Zawawi AA. (2002). Efficacy of alcohol-based and alcohol-free melaleuca oral solution for the treatment of fluconazole-refractory oropharyngeal candidiasis in patients with AIDS. *HIV Clinical Trials*. Sep-Oct;3(5):379–385.

Winston D. (2006). *Winston's Botanic Materia Medica*. Washington, NJ: DWCHS.

 NAME: Thyme (*Thymus vulgaris*)

Common Names: Creeping thyme, garden thyme, wild thyme (*T. serphyllum*)

Family: *Lamiaceae*

Description of Plant
- Small, highly aromatic member of the mint family with white to pink flowers
- There are many cultivated species and varieties of thymes.

Medicinal Part: Dried herb, EO

Constituents and Action (if known)
- Volatile oils (1.0%–2.5%) (monoterpenes)
  - Thymol (30%–70%): antibacterial against *Porphyromonas gingivalis*, *Selenomonas artemidis*, and *Streptococcus sobrinus*, all of which can cause dental caries or gum disease (Mills & Bone, 2000); antibacterial and antifungal against a wide spectrum of bacteria that cause upper respiratory infections; also active against *Helicobacter pylori* and many fungi
  - Carvacrol (3%–15%): antibacterial, antifungal
- Flavonoids: luteolin (antimutagenic), thymonin, cirsilineol, 8-methoxy-cirsilineol (potent spasmolytics), eriodictyol (antioxidant)
- Phenolic acids: rosmarinic acid (antioxidant, inhibits lipid peroxidation, anti-inflammatory, antiallergenic), caffeic acid
- Tannins (10%)

Nutritional Ingredients: Fresh and dried herb commonly used as a spice in cooking

Traditional Use
- Antibacterial, antispasmodic, antifungal, antiviral, carminative, diaphoretic, expectorant, diuretic
- Spasmodic coughs: bronchitis, whooping cough, mild antibacterial/antiviral to the lungs; used for colds, influenza, chest colds, pneumonia, upper respiratory tract congestion
- Expectorant: increases and thins mucus, allowing easier elimination
- Digestive upsets with gas, nausea, vomiting, and abdominal bloating
- Mild urinary antiseptic
- Gargle for sore throats, tonsillitis, gum disease

Current Use
- Effective for spasmodic coughs (bronchospasm) associated with bronchitis, pertussis, asthma, COPD, and emphysema.

Use with wild cherry bark and licorice (Winston, 2006). A combination of thyme and primrose root (*Primula*) decreased and relieved symptoms of acute bronchitis (Gruenwald et al., 2006), as did a product with thyme and ivy (*Helix*) leaves (Kemmerich et al., 2006).

- EO (less than 1%) in mouthwashes to prevent cavities and treat gum disease (Wichtl & Bisset, 1994)
- EO diluted in a carrier base may be useful for athlete's foot (tinea pedis). Use with tea tree and lavender EOs. The EO of thyme combined with amphotericin B potentiated the antifungal effects of the pharmaceutical medication (Giordani et al., 2004).
- EO (less than 0.1%) in a cream base was successfully used to treat two cases of vulval lichen sclerosis (Mills & Bone, 2000).
- EO in a vaporizer or in hot water as an inhalation for sinusitis, *Pneumocystis carinii* pneumonia, bronchitis, and bacterial pneumonia
- EO has antiviral activity and can shorten the duration of herpes simplex I and II outbreaks (Nolkemper et al., 2006).
- Herb tea (or tincture), along with eyebright, yerba manza, or osha root, can be effective for allergic rhinitis and otitis media (Winston, 2006).
- Herb tea useful for GI tract dysbiosis with foul-smelling flatulence, abdominal bloating, and nausea; may also be beneficial for treating gastric ulcers

Available Forms, Dosage, and Administration Guidelines

Preparations: Dried herb, tea, tincture, EO

Typical Dosage

- *Dried herb:* 2 to 6 g per day
- *Tea:* 1 tsp dried herb in 8 oz hot water, steep covered 20 to 30 minutes; take up to three cups a day
- *Tincture* (1:5, 35% alcohol): 40 to 80 gtt (2–4 mL) three times a day
- *EO:* Use dilutions of 1% or less for mouthwashes or vaginal suppositories.

Pharmacokinetics—If Available (form or route when known):
After ingestion of thyme, thymol was detected in exhaled breath in 30 to 60 minutes. After 140 minutes, it was no longer detectable (ESCOP, 2003).

Toxicity: Herb is safe in normal therapeutic doses. EO is highly concentrated; do not use internally.

Contraindications: None known

Side Effects: Herb: none known. EO, undiluted or inadequately diluted, can cause irritation of the skin and especially the mucous membranes. Internal use of the EO in mice caused decreased locomotor activity and respiration (ESCOP, 2003).

Long-Term Safety: Safe

Use in Pregnancy/Lactation/Children: Herb: avoid large amounts in pregnancy, but culinary quantities are fine. No adverse effects expected in lactating women or children. Do not use the EO internally during pregnancy, lactation, or with children.

Drug/Herb Interactions and Rationale (if known): None known

Special Notes: Many chemotypes of thyme exist. The chemistry of the herb and EO can be highly variable. Good-quality thyme and thyme extracts should have a strong, aromatic fragrance and taste.

BIBLIOGRAPHY

European Scientific Cooperative on Phytotherapy. (2003). *ESCOP Monographs* (pp. 505–510). New York: Thieme.

Giordani R, et al. (2004). Antifungal effect of various essential oils against *Candida albicans*. Potentiation of antifungal action of amphotericin B by essential oil from *Thymus vulgaris*. *Phytotherapy Research*. Dec;18(12):990–995.

Gruenwald J, et al. (2006). Evaluation of the non-inferiority of a fixed combination of thyme fluid- and primrose root extract in comparison to a fixed combination of thyme fluid extract and primrose root tincture in patients with acute bronchitis. A single-blind, randomized, bi-centric clinical trial. *Arzneimittelforschung*. 56(8):574–581.

Kemmerich B et al.(2006). Efficacy and tolerability of a fluid extract combination of thyme herb and ivy leaves and matched placebo in adults suffering from acute bronchitis with productive cough. A prospective, double-blinded placebo-controlled clinical trial. *Arzneimittelforschung*. 56(9):652–660.

Mills S, Bone K. (2000). *Principles and Practice of Phytotherapy* (pp. 563–568). Edinburgh: Churchill Livingstone.

Nolkemper S, et al. (2006). Antiviral effect of aqueous extracts from species of the *Lamiaceae* family against herpes simplex virus type 1 and type 2 in vitro. *Planta Medica*. 72:1378–1382. Epub 2006 Nov 7.

Tisserand R, Balacs T. (1995). *Essential Oil Safety, a Guide for Health Care Professionals* (p. 176). Edinburgh: Churchill Livingstone.

Weiss RF. (2000). *Weiss' Herbal Medicine—Classic Edition* (pp. 208–209). New York: Thieme.

Wichtl M, Bisset NG. [Eds.]. (1994). *Herbal Drugs and Phytopharmaceuticals* (pp. 493–495). Stuttgart: Medpharm.

Winston D. (2006). *Winston's Botanic Materia Medica*. Washington, NJ: DWCHS.

NAME: Turmeric (*Curcuma longa*)

Common Names: Indian saffron, curcuma

Family: *Zingiberaceae*

Description of Plant
- Perennial member of the ginger family
- Cultivated widely throughout Asia, India, China, and other tropical countries

Medicinal Part: Dried rhizome and curcumin extracts

Constituents and Action (if known)
- Diaryheptanoids (yellow pigments)—curcumin: antioxidant properties
  - Inhibit cancer at initiation, promotion, and progression stages of development, particularly colon cancer (Chun et al., 1999; Han et al., 1999; Kawamori et al., 1999; Thangapazham et al., 2006; Plummer et al., 1999; Ranhan et al., 1999; Singhal et al., 1999) Induces apoptosis (Sharma et al., 2007)
  - May be useful in chemoprevention of cancers: tobacco smoke, benzo(alpha)pyrenes, nitrosamines (Mills & Bone, 2000; Thangapazham et al., 2006)
  - Curcumin is as effective as BHA in inhibiting lipid peroxidation; it has anti-inflammatory and antiarthritic

activity in rats and mice (Kang et al., 1999; Shah et al., 1999 Sharma et al., 2007) and is a dual inhibitor of arachidonic acid metabolism (Mills & Bone, 2000).
  ○ Strong hepatoprotective properties (Maheshwari et al., 2006)
  ○ Prevent doxorubicin (Adriamycin) nephrotoxicity in rats (Venkatesan et al., 2000)
  ○ Increase immune function, including white blood cell counts and macrophage phagocytic activity (Antony et al., 1999)
  ○ Reduce muscle injury after trauma (Thaloor et al., 1999)
  ○ Interfere with replication of viruses, including hepatitis and HIV
  ○ Antithrombotic action while preserving prostacyclin, an anti-inflammatory mediator
- EO (3%–5%): sesquiterpene ketones—ar-turmerone, zingiberene, phellandrene (antifungal, mild antibacterial, anti-inflammatory, antihistamine, choleretic) (Mills & Bone, 2000)
- Tumerin: antioxidant, antimutagen, protects DNA
- Ukonan-A: phagocytic activity (Gonda et al., 1992)
- Ukonan-D: reticuloendothelial system potentiating activity (Gonda et al., 1992); inhibits chemically induced carcinogens, which is probably the basis of anticancer treatment
- Oleo-resins: composed mostly of curcuminoids and EOs
- Extracts of whole turmeric exhibit antioxidant, antifungal, anticancer, hepatoprotective, and anti-inflammatory activity.

Nutritional Ingredients: Primary component of curry powders and some mustards; vitamin A, carotenoids, and minerals

Traditional Use
- Antioxidant, cholagogue, anti-inflammatory, antiulcerogenic, hepatoprotective
- Topical use as a poultice with neem leaves in 814 patients resulted in a 97% cure rate in patients with scabies (Mills & Bone, 2000). Turmeric is also used for skin infections, bruises, and eczema and to reduce hair growth.
- Liver problems, including hepatitis and jaundice

- Digestive tonic for impaired digestion, gas, and abdominal pain

Current Use

- Cancer prevention and possible treatment, especially bowel, cervical, and liver cancers (Cheng et al., 2001; Maheshwari et al., 2006)
- Reduces inflammation of osteoarthritis and rheumatoid arthritis as well as postsurgical inflammation; combines well with sarsaparilla, ginger, and boswellia. A combination of turmeric, ginger, and ashwagandha was significantly superior to placebo in the treatment of osteoarthritis of the knees (Chopra et al., 2004).
- Reduces cholesterol and triglyceride levels; may prevent arteriosclerosis (Williamson, 2002).
- An effective hepatoprotective agent: increases glutathione levels and glutathione-S-transferase activity. Use with milk thistle, picrorrhiza, and schisandra to prevent and treat acute and chronic liver disease (Williamson, 2002).
- Relieved stomach pain and helped heal gastric ulcers (Prucksunand et al., 2001). It also improved IBS symptomology (Bundy et al., 2004).

Available Forms, Dosage, and Administration Guidelines

Preparations: Standardized extract, powder, tea, tincture (made from fresh or dried roots)

Typical Dosage

- Unless otherwise prescribed, 1.5 to 4 g a day of the powdered rhizome as well as other equivalent galenical preparations for internal use
- *Standardized extract* (curcumin 95%): 350 mg twice a day
- *Powder:* 1 to 4 g daily or 0.5 to 1 g, several times daily (Wichtl & Biset, 1994). Taking turmeric with lecithin or black pepper increases absorption.
- *Infusion:* 0.5 tsp dried powdered rhizome in 8 oz hot water, steep for 10 to 15 minutes; take twice daily
- *Tincture* (1:2 or 1:5, 60% alcohol): 40 to 80 gtt (2–4 mL) two or three times a day

Pharmacokinetics—If Available (form or route when known): Isolated curcumin is poorly absorbed (in rats) and mostly excreted by the bowel, with only small amounts found in the bile, liver, kidneys, and adipose tissue.

Toxicity: Long history of human use as a food and medicine. Animal and human studies have revealed no acute or chronic toxicity of turmeric in normal therapeutic doses. Very high doses of curcumin and turmeric oleoresin in rats have led to physiologic and biochemical changes.

Contraindications: Ulcers (isolated curcumin product only); biliary obstruction and gallstones. In women attempting to conceive, high doses of turmeric or curcumin may inhibit fertility.

Side Effects: Allergic contact dermatitis (rare); stomach ulcers: large doses and prolonged use of the curcumin product (not the herb) may irritate the gastric mucosa and reduce mucin production

Long-Term Safety: Safe

Use in Pregnancy/Lactation/Children: Use in small dietary amounts during pregnancy; large amounts may act as an emmenagogue.

Drug/Herb Interactions and Rationale (if known): Avoid using large doses concurrently with anticoagulants and nonsteroidal anti-inflammatories; possible additive effect for bleeding.

Special Notes: It is important to differentiate between turmeric or whole turmeric extracts and standardized curcumin. Both are anti-inflammatory, hepatoprotective, and antioxidant, but the whole turmeric has a gastroprotective activity, whereas large doses of the curcumin product can irritate the gastric mucosa and suppress mucin production. It is believed that the curcumin extract is stronger (superior) to whole turmeric extracts, but there are no studies to prove this.

BIBLIOGRAPHY

Antony S, et al. (1999). Immunomodulatory activity of curcumin. *Immunologic Investigation.* 28(6-6):291–303.

Bundy R, et al. (2004). Turmeric extract may improve irritable bowel syndrome symptomology in otherwise healthy adults: A pilot study. *Journal of Alternative and Complementary Medicine.* Dec;10(6): 1015–1018.

Cheng AL, et al. (2001). Phase I clinical trial of curcumin, a chemoprotective agent, in patients with high-risk or pre-malignant lesions. *Anticancer Research.* Jul-Aug;21(4B):2895–2900.

Chopra A, et al. (2004). A 32-week randomized, placebo-controlled clinical evaluation of RA-11, an ayurvedic drug, on osteoarthritis of the knees. *Journal of Clinical Rheumatology.* Oct;10(5):236–245.

Chun KS, et al. (1999). Antitumor promoting potential of naturally occurring diaryheptanoids structurally related to curcumin. *Mutation Research.* 428(1–2):49–57.

Gonda R, et al. (1992). The core structure of ukonan A, a phagocytosis-activating polysaccharide from the rhizome of *Curcumin longa*, and immunological activities of degradation products. *Chemical and Pharmaceutical Bulletin.* 40:990.

Han SS, et al. (1999). Curcumin causes the growth arrest and apoptosis of B-cell lymphoma by downregulation of egr-1, c-myc, bcl-XL, NF-kappa and p53. *Clinical Immunology.* 93(2):152–161.

Kang BY, et al. (1999). Inhibition of interleukin-12 production in lipopolysaccharide-activated macrophages by curcumin. *European Journal of Pharmacology.* 384(2–3):191–195.

Kawamori T, et al. (1999). Chemopreventive effect of curcumin, a naturally occurring anti-inflammatory agent, during the promotion/progression stages of colon cancer. *Cancer Research.* 59(3):597–601.

Maheshwari RK, et al. (2006). Multiple biological activities of curcumin: A short review. *Life Sciences.* Mar 27;78(18):2081–2087.

Mills S, Bone K. (2000). *Principles and Practice of Phytotherapy* (pp. 569–580). Edinburgh: Churchill Livingstone.

Plummer SM, et al. (1999). Inhibition of cyclo-oxygenase 2 expression in colon cells by the chemopreventative agent curcumin involves inhibition of NF-kappa activation via the NIK/IKK signalling complex. *Oncogene.* 18(44):6013–6020.

Polasa K, et al. (1992). Effect of turmeric on urinary mutagens in smokers. *Mutagenesis.* 7:107.

Prucksunand C, et al. (2001). Phase II clinical trial on effect of the long turmeric (*Curcuma longa* Linn) on healing of peptic ulcer. *Southeast Asian Journal of Tropical Medicine and Public Health.* Mar;32(1):208–215.

Ranhan D, et al. (1999). Enhanced apoptosis mediates inhibition of EBV-transformed lymphoblastoid cell line proliferation by curcumin. *Journal of Surgical Research*. 87(1):1–5.

Shah BH, et al. (1999). Inhibitory effect of curcumin, a food spice from turmeric, on platelet-activating factor and arachidonic acid-mediated platelet aggregation through inhibition of thromboxane formation and Ca signaling. *Biochemical Pharmacology*. 58(7):1167–1172.

Sharma RA et al.(2007). Pharmacokinetics and pharmacodynamics of curcumin. *Advances in Experimental Medicine and Biology*. 595:453–470.

Singhal SS, et al. (1999). The effect of curcumin on glutathione-linked enzymes in K562 human leukemia cells. *Toxicology Letters*. 109(1–2):87–95.

Thaloor D, et al. (1999). Systemic administration of the NF-kappa B inhibitor curcumin stimulates muscle regeneration after traumatic injury. *American Journal of Physiology*. 277[2 Pt. 1]:C320–329.

Thangapazham RL et al.(2006). Multiple molecular targets in cancer chemoprevention by curcumin. *AAPS Journal*. Jul 7;8(3):E443–449.

Venkatesan N, et al. (2000). Curcumin prevents Adriamycin nephrotoxicity in rats. *British Journal of Pharmacology*. 129(2):231–234.

Williamson E. (2002). *Major Herbs of Ayurveda* (pp. 117–121). Edinburgh: Churchill Livingstone.

Wichtl M, Bisset NG. (1994). *Herbal Drugs and Phytopharmaceuticals*. Stuttgart: Medpharm.

U

 NAME: Uva Ursi (*Arctostaphylos uva ursi*)

Common Names: Bearberry, kinnikinnik, beargrape

Family: *Ericaceae*

Description of Plant
- Low-growing evergreen shrub that can form a dark-green carpet of leaves and grows up to 20" tall
- Has small, dark-green, leathery leaves and small white or pink bell-shaped flowers; blooms April to May. Produces a red, edible berry.
- Abundant throughout Northern Hemisphere.

Medicinal Part: Dried leaves

Constituents and Action (if known)

- Phenolic glycosides: arbutin (6%–10%) and methylarbutin (up to 4%)
  - Arbutin is hydrolyzed to hydroquinone, which is mildly astringent and an effective antimicrobial. Urine must be alkaline (pH 8.0) to achieve effect. Most effective against *Escherichia coli, Proteus vulgaris, Pseudomonas aeruginosa, Staphylococcus aureus*.
  - Anti-immunoinflammatory effects
- Gallotannins (6%–40%): tea can be made by soaking leaves in cold water overnight; this minimizes the extraction of tannins, which contribute to GI discomfort
- Triterpenes (0.40%–0.08%): ursolic acid, uvaole
- Monotropein (iridoid)
- Flavone glycosides: hyperin, myricitrin, isoquercitrin, quercetin

Nutritional Ingredients: None known

Traditional Use

- Diuretic, urinary antiseptic, astringent
- Used to treat urinary tract infections, especially with mucous discharge or blood in the urine
- Decreases inflammation in urinary tract (painful urination and urinary calculi)
- Gout and gouty arthritis: increases uric acid excretion

Current Use: Urinary antiseptic (cystitis, urethritis, prostatitis, pyleonephritis). Use with other urinary antiseptic herbs such as corn silk, pipsisscewa, or Oregon grape root (Winston, 2006).

Available Forms, Dosage, and Administration Guidelines

Preparations: Infusions or cold macerations; tinctures, capsules, and powdered extracts (usually put in capsules)

Typical Dosage

- Unless otherwise prescribed, 10 g a day of crushed leaf or powder corresponding to 400- to 700-mg arbutin. Medication containing arbutin should not be taken for longer than 7 to 10 days or more than 5 times a year without consulting a physician.
- *Infusion:* 1 tsp dried herb in 8 oz boiling water, steep for 15 minutes; take two or three cups a day

- *Cold maceration*: 1 tsp dried herb in 8 oz cold water, steep for several hours; take up to four times daily
- *Dry extract* (containing 100–210 mg hydroquinone derivatives calculated as water-free arbutin): Take up to four times daily
- *Capsules (ground herb):* Two 500-mg capsules two or three times a day
- *Tincture* (1:5, 30% alcohol): 40 to 60 gtt (2–3 mL) three times a day

Pharmacokinetics—If Available (form or route when known): Maximum urinary antiseptic effect occurs 3 to 4 hours after administration, with 70% to 75% of the dose excreted within 24 hours.

Toxicity: Doses up to 20 g have not caused acute toxicity in healthy adults.

Contraindications: Chronic kidney disease, pregnancy

Side Effects: GI discomfort (nausea, vomiting); urine may turn greenish

Long-Term Safety: Do not use more than 7 to 10 days and for more than 5 times a year due to concerns about possible hepatotoxic effects of hydroquinone (Skenderi, 2003). A case of bull's-eye maculopathy believed to be caused by chronic intake of uva ursi has been reported (Wang & Del Priore, 2004).

Use in Pregnancy/Lactation/Children: Large doses are oxytocic. Refrain from use in all.

Drug/Herb Interactions and Rationale (if known): Do not use with cranberry juice; it can acidify the urine and make uva ursi ineffective.

Special Notes: Urine must be alkaline for herb to be effective. Diet should include dairy products, vegetables (especially tomatoes), fruits, fruit juices, and potatoes. In addition, drink large amounts of water.

BIBLIOGRAPHY

Bruneton J. (1999). *Pharmacognosy, Phytochemistry, Medicinal Plants* (2nd ed.; pp. 243–246). Paris: Lavoisier.

Der Marderosian A, Beutler J.[Eds.].(2004). *The Review of Natural Products—Uva ursi Monograph*. St. Louis, MO: Facts and Comparisons.

European Scientific Cooperative On Phytotherapy. (2003). *ESCOP Monographs* (pp. 536–538). New York: Thieme.

Quintus J, et al. (2005). Urinary excretion of arbutin metabolites after oral administration of bearberry leaf extracts. *Planta Medica*. Feb;71(2):147–152.

Skenderi G. (2003). *Herbal Vade Mecum* (p. 283). Rutherford, NJ: Herbacy Press.

Wang L, Del Priore LV. Bull's-eye maculopathy secondary to herbal toxicity from uva ursi. *American Journal of Ophalmology*. Jun;137 (6):1135–1137.

Weiss R, Fintelmann V. (2000). *Herbal Medicine* (2nd ed.; pp. 223–224). Stuttgart: Thieme.

Winston D. (2006). *Winston's Botanic Materia Medica*. Washington, NJ: DWCHS.

Yarnell E.(2002). Botanical Medicines for the urinary tract. *World Journal of Urology*. Nov;20(5)285–293.

 NAME: Valerian (*Valeriana officinalis*)

Common Names: Great wild valerian, setwell, Indian valerian, red valerian

Family: *Valerianaceae*

Description of Plant
- Perennial plant with species native to North America, Europe, and Asia
- White to red flowers bloom June to September

Medicinal Part: Rhizome/root

Constituents and Action (if known)
- Volatile oils (monoterpenes): borneol, bornyl isovalerate, bornyl acetate, camphene—weakly antagonize benzodiazepine receptors (Wagner et al., 1998)
- Sesquiterpenes: valerenal, valerenic acid, valeranone-sedative, spasmolytic—antispasmodic properties, may cause hypotension possibly by influencing serotonin, GABA, and norepinephrine (Schultz et al., 1997)

- Iridoids: valepotriates (insoluble in water)—valtrate, didrovaltrate; bind to barbiturate and peripheral benzodiazepine receptors, resulting in sedation (Mennini et al., 1993)
- Flavonoids: diosmetin, kaempferol, luteolin
- Amino acids: GABA—calming effect
- Decomposition products (homobaldrinol, valtroxal): sedative activity, well absorbed by the gut (Houghton, 1997)
- Hydroalcoholic extracts: bind to GABA-A receptors (Mennini et al., 1993)

Nutritional Ingredients: None

Traditional Use
- Analgesic, carminative, antispasmodic, hypotensive, sedative
- Used for hundreds of years in Europe as a sedative and antispasmodic to relieve insomnia, anxiety, muscle spasms, stress-induced palpitations, gastric spasms, hysteria, nervous headaches, and menstrual pain
- Northwestern Native Americans boiled the roots of a related species, *V. sitchensis*, into a tea for calming the nerves.

Current Use
- Improves sleep quality, with no daytime sedation or impairment of concentration or performance. Those with sleep difficulties such as insomnia benefit the most. Shortens sleep latency and reduces night awakenings. In a randomized double-blind study, a valerian extract (600 mg) was as effective as oxazepam (10 mg) for improving sleep quality (Ziegler et al., 2002). Valerian is often mixed with chamomile, lemon balm, or hops. In one study, patients with insomnia took either a combination of valerian and hops, diphenhydramine, or a placebo. Both the herbs and the diphenhydramine performed better than placebo, with subjects reporting modest improvement of sleep parameters (Morin et al., 2005). Another study of valerian alone in two doses, 300 mg or 600 mg, failed to improve sleep problems compared to placebo (Diaper et al., 2004).
- Eases muscle pain and spasms: restless legs syndrome, back pain, bruxism; use with kava, black haw, or scullcap
- Acts a mild sedative; decreases tension headache, anxiety, and irritability. In a study of children, a combination of

valerian and lemon balm was effective for relieving restlessness and dyssomnia (Muller et al., 2006). A preliminary study on the use of valerian for anxiety found that valerian reduced symptoms similar to diazepam (Valium) in the psychic HAM-A factors but not in the state-trait-anxiety inventory (STAI-trait) (Andreatini et al., 2002).

- Numerous studies have looked at the combination of valerian and St. John's wort for depression and anxiety. This combination was found to be as effective as amitriptyline for depression and more effective than diazepam for anxiety. The herb combination also produced dramatically fewer side effects than the pharmaceutical medications (Mills & Bone, 2000).
- Relieves nervous stomach and other stress-induced GI symptoms
- Relieves menstrual and intestinal cramps

Available Forms, Dosage, and Administration Guidelines

Preparations: Dried root, tea, capsules, tablets, tinctures, extracts. Sometimes standardized to contain at least 0.5% EO.

Typical Dosage

- *Dried root:* 3 to 9 g per day
- *Capsules:* For products standardized to 0.5% EO, 300 to 400 mg a day. As a sleep aid, take 1 hour before bedtime. For anxiety, 150 to 500 mg a day divided into several doses.
- *Fresh tincture* (1:2, 70% alcohol): 40 to 90 gtt (2–5 mL) three times a day, or follow manufacturer or practitioner recommendations
- *Tea:* 1 tsp root in 8 oz hot water, steep for 20 to 30 minutes covered; take one to three cups daily. Patient compliance may be limited by the unpleasant taste.
- *Fluid extract* (1:1): 0.5 to 1 tsp (1–2 mL)

Pharmacokinetics—If Available (form or route when known): Valerenic acid (from valerian) reaches maximum serum concentration in 1 to 2 hours after ingestion and was measurable for 5 hours (Anderson et al., 2005).

Toxicity: A patient ingested an overdose of valerian capsules (25 g), and symptoms included fatigue, abdominal cramps, and tremor. All symptoms resolved within 24 hours (Mills & Bone, 2000). Some researchers have noted concerns that some of the valepotriates might be carcinogenic when taken orally; subsequent research showed that these compounds are unstable and are broken down by gastric HCl, forming safe decomposition products (Mills & Bone, 2000).

Contraindications: Theoretical concern that valerian may exacerbate schizophrenia or bipolar disorders (Schellenberg et al., 1993)

Side Effects: Occasionally, patients become overstimulated rather than sedated by valerian. Overdose has caused headaches, blurred vision, nausea, stupor.

Long-Term Safety: Safe and approved for food use by the FDA; nontoxic even in large doses

Use in Pregnancy/Lactation/Children: No adverse effects noted or expected

Drug/Herb Interactions and Rationale (if known): May intensify the effects of sedatives; has been shown not to potentiate effects of alcohol. In human studies, valerian did not affect CYP1A2, 2D6, 2E1, or 3A4/5 (Gurley et al., 2005).

Special Notes: Very unpleasant smell; smells like old sweaty socks. Valerian baths are commonly used in Europe (despite the odor) to relieve stress, muscle tension, anxiety, and insomnia.

BIBLIOGRAPHY

Albrecht M, et al. (1995). Phytopharmaceuticals and safety in traffic: The influence of a plant-based sedative on vehicle operation ability with or without alcohol. *Zeitschrift Allgemeinmedizin.* 71:1215–1221.

Anderson GD, et al. (2005). Pharmacokinetics of valerenic acid after administration of valerian in healthy subjects. *Phytotherapy Research.* 19(9):801–803.

Andreatini R, et al. (2002). Effect of valepotriate (valerian extract) in generalized anxiety disorder: A randomized placebo-controlled pilot study. *Phytotherapy Research.* Nov;16(7):650–654.

Diaper A, et al. (2004). A double-blind, placebo-controlled investigation of the effects of two doses of a valerian preparation on the sleep, cognitive and psychomotor function of sleep-disturbed older adults. *Phytotherapy Research.* Oct;18(1):831–836.

Donath F, et al. (2000). Critical evaluation of the effect of valerian extract on sleep structure and sleep quality. *Pharmacopsychiatry.* 33(2):47–53.

Gurley BJ, et al. (2005). In vivo effects of goldenseal, kava kava, black cohosh, and valerian on human cytochrome P450 1A2, 2D6, 2E1, and 3A4/5 phenotypes. *Clinical Pharmacology and Therapeutics.* May;77(5):415–426.

Houghton PJ. [Ed.]. (1997). *Valerian, the Genus Valeriana.* Amsterdam: Harwood.

Mennini T, et al. (1993). In vitro study on the interaction of extracts and pure compounds from *Valeriana officinalis* roots with GABA, benzodiazepine and barbiturate receptors. *Fitoterapia.* 64:291–300.

Mills S, Bone K. (2000). *Principles and Practice of Phytotherapy* (pp. 581–589). Edinburgh: Churchill Livingstone.

Morin CM, et al. (2005). Valerian-hops combination and diphenhydramine for treating insomnia: A randomized placebo-controlled clinical trial. *Sleep.* Nov 1;28(11):1465–1471.

Muller SF, et al. (2006). A combination of valerian and lemon balm is effective in the treatment of restlessness and dyssomnia in children. *Phytomedicine*, Jun;13(6):383–387.

Schultz V, et al. (1997). Clinical trials with phyto-psychopharmacological agents. *Phytomedicine.* 4(4):379–387.

Vonderheid-Guth B, et al. (2000). Pharmacodynamic effects of valerian and hops extract combination (Ze 91019) on the quantitative-topographical EEG in healthy volunteers. *European Journal of Medical Research.* 5(4):139–144.

Wagner J, et al. (1998). Beyond benzodiazepines: Alternative pharmacologic agents for the treatment of insomnia. *American Pharmacotherapy.* 32(6):680–691.

Willey LB. (1995). Valerian overdose: A case report. *Veterinary and Human Toxicology.* 37(4):364–365.

Ziegler G, et al. (2002). Efficacy and tolerability of valerian extract LI 156 compared with oxasepam in the treatment of non-organic insomnia—A randomized, double-blind, comparative clinical study. *European Journal of Medical Research.* Nov 25;7(11): 480–486.

NAME: Wild Yam (*Dioscorea villosa*)

Common Names: Wild yam root, colic root, rheumatism root

Family: *Dioscoreaceae*

Description of Plant

- More than 500 species exist worldwide; some are edible, some are medicinal, and some, like the Mexican wild yam, were used as a source of steroidal saponins, which through laboratory synthesis were turned into progesterone.
- Twining vine native to the eastern United States with ovate, heart-shaped leaves
- Inconspicuous white to greenish-yellow female flowers followed by winged seeds

Medicinal Part: Dried rhizome with rootlets

Constituents and Action (if known)

- Steroidal saponins: dioscin (anti-inflammatory activity), and gracillarin
- Tannins

Nutritional Ingredients: None

Traditional Use

- Antispasmodic, anti-inflammatory, cholagogue
- Antispasmodic used for biliary colic, intestinal spasms, gallbladder spasms
- Dysmenorrhea with nausea; ovarian pain
- Antiemetic used for morning sickness, biliousness, nausea, and vomiting
- Used along with fringe tree and celandine to pass small gallstones
- Mild anti-inflammatory for symptomatic relief of arthritis pain

Current Use

- It is an excellent herb for hepatic or intestinal spasms: IBS, biliary colic, diverticulitis, intestinal colic, painful flatulence, and biliousness. Use with chamomile, kudzu, huang qin, or catnip (Hoffmann, 2003; Winston, 2006).

- Can be useful for dysmenorrhea with nausea (Brinker, 1997) along with black haw, ginger, or cyperus (Winston, 2006).

Available Forms, Dosage, and Administration Guidelines

Preparations: Dried root, tea, capsules, tincture

Typical Dosage

- *Dried root:* 2 to 4 g a day
- *Tea:* 1 tsp dried cut/sifted root to 1 cup water, decoct 15 to 20 minutes, steep half-hour; take up to two cups a day
- *Capsules:* Two 500-mg capsules three times a day
- *Tincture* (1:2, 35% alcohol): 40 to 80 gtt (2–4 mL) three times a day

Pharmacokinetics—If Available (form or route when known): Not known

Toxicity: Overdose may cause nausea, vomiting, diarrhea, and headache.

Contraindications: None known

Side Effects: In overdose, nausea, vomiting, diarrhea, headache

Long-Term Safety: No adverse effects expected with normal therapeutic doses (Anonymous, 2004)

Use in Pregnancy/Lactation/Children: Small amounts have traditionally been used in formulas for morning sickness. No adverse effects are known. Very little research has been done on this plant. One study suggests that wild yam appeared to suppress progesterone synthesis, but no direct effect on estrogen or progesterone receptors was found (Der Marderosian & Beutler, 2004). Use with caution.

Drug/Herb Interactions and Rationale (if known): None known

Special Notes: Wild yam has been the subject of numerous myths. Some marketers and publications state that it contains natural progesterone or that natural progesterone can be synthesized in vivo from its steroidal saponin, diosgenin. Other equally inaccurate claims suggest that it contains DHEA or stimulates the body's production of DHEA. The last of these rumors is that wild yam can be used as a "natural" form of birth control. This seems to be based on the fact that progesterone was originally synthesized from diosgenin extracted from the Mexican species. All of these claims are totally false and spurred by ignorance and/or avarice (Zava et al., 1998).

Many topical wild yam creams are marketed as natural hormone replacement therapy. There are two types of products on the market: those containing actual pharmaceutical progesterone and those that contain wild yam without added progesterone. Only the creams containing pharmaceutical progesterone (the source of which is unimportant) are clinically useful for relieving hot flashes, formication, and vaginal dryness (Komesaroff et al, 2001).

BIBLIOGRAPHY

Anonymous. (2004). Final report of the amended safety assessment of *Dioscorea villosa* (wild yam) root extract. *International Journal of Toxicology*. 23[Suppl. 2]:49–54.

Bone K. (1997). Progesterogenic herbs? *Modern Phytotherapist*. 3(2):14–16.

Brinker F. (1997). A comparative review of eclectic female regulators. *British Journal of Phytotherapy*. 4(3):123–145.

Der Marderosian A, Beutler J. [Eds.]. (2004). *The review of Natural Products*. St. Louis, MO: Facts and Comparisons.

Hoffmann D. (2003). *Medical Herbalism* (p. 543). Rochester, VT: Inner Traditions.

Integrative Medicine Access. (2000). *Wild Yam*. Newton, MA: Integrative Medicine Communications.

Komesaroff PA, et al. (2001). Effects of wild yam extract on menopausal symptoms, lipids and sex hormones in healthy menopausal women. *Climacteric*. Jun;4(2):144–150.

Winston D. (2006). *Winston's Botanic Materia Medica*. Washington, NJ: DWCHS.

Zava D, et al. (1998). Estrogen and progestin bioactivity of foods, herbs, and spices. *Proceedings of the Society for Experimental Biology and Medicine*. 217(3):369–378.

 NAME: Willow (*Salix* spp.)

Common Names: Bay willow (*S. daphnoides*), crack willow (*S. fragilis*), purple willow (*S. purpurea*), white willow (*S. alba*)

Family: *Salicaceae*

Description of Plant
- Willow trees thrive in moist areas and often grow along river banks.
- Bark is harvested in early spring or autumn from 2- to 3-year-old branches.

Medicinal Part: Dried bark

Constituents and Action (if known)
- Phenolic glycosides (2.5%–11.0%)
  ○ Salicin, salicortin, tremulacin, populin (Wichtl & Bisset, 1994): anti-inflammatory activity (ESCOP, 2003; Mills et al., 1996)
- Tannins (8%–20%): catechins, gallotannins
- Flavonoids (isoquercitrin, naringenin) (Wichtl & Bisset, 1994)

Other Actions: Has very mild effect on platelet function (Krivoy et al., 2001)

Nutritional Ingredients: None known

Traditional Use
- Anti-inflammatory, analgesic, antipyretic, antirheumatic, astringent
- Internally: to reduce fevers, muscle aches, arthritic pains, headaches, and inflammation
- Externally: as a wash for wounds, a poultice or bath for sore joints and muscle pain

Current Use
- Mild pain reliever (analgesic); can be used for arthritic and back pain (see next bullet point) as well as mild headaches, gout, fevers, and aches associated with influenza and colds
- Anti-inflammatory and analgesic for arthralgias, lumbago, low back pain, tendonitis, bursitis, and sprains. According to the *British Herbal Pharmacopoeia* (1996), willow combines well with guaiac, black cohosh, and celery seed for rheumatoid arthritis. Several studies have shown willow bark is effective for relieving the inflammation and pain of osteoarthritis (Schmid et al., 2001) and low back pain (Chrubasik et al., 2000; Chrubasik et al., 2001). A more recent study found that a willow bark extract was not effective for relieving pain caused by osteo- or rheumatoid arthritis (Biegert et al., 2004).
- Can be useful for mild diarrhea with cramps

Available Forms, Dosage, and Administration Guidelines

Preparations: Dried bark, capsules, tea, tincture. European products are standardized to 1% salicin.

Typical Dosage

- Unless otherwise prescribed: liquid and solid preparations for internal use with an average daily dosage corresponding to 60 to 120 mg total salicin (Blumenthal, 2000), which is equivalent to 6 to 12 g dried bark (Schilcher, 1997)
- *Dried bark:* 1 to 3 g three times daily (Newall et al., 1996)
- *Decoction:* 1 to 2 tsp finely chopped or coarsely powdered bark in 8 oz cold water, bring to a boil and simmer for 10 minutes, steep half-hour; take 8 oz three times a day (Meyer-Buchtela, 1999; Wichtl & Bisset, 1994)
- *Tincture* (1:5, 30% alcohol): 80–120 gtt (4–6 mL) three times daily
- *Spray-dried extract:* Standardized to contain 20 to 40 mg total salicin three times daily

Pharmacokinetics—If Available (form or route when known): In a human study, 86% of orally administered salacin was excreted in the urine as metabolites (mainly salicyluric acid) over several hours, showing a more prolonged effect than acetylsalicylic acid (Upton, 1999). The half-life is 2.5 hours.

Toxicity: None known

Contraindications: There is a concern that salicin may cause a response in patients with allergies to ASA based on a possible willow bark–induced case of anaphylaxis (Boullata et al., 2003). Although they have similar activity, salicin is metabolized differently and does not provoke many of the adverse responses associated with ASA (reduced clotting, Reye's syndrome, gastric irritation, and allergic reaction).

Side Effects: Mild GI irritation from tannins

Long-Term Safety: No adverse effects expected with appropriate dosage

Use in Pregnancy/Lactation/Children: No restriction known; use with caution

Drug/Herb Interactions and Rationale (if known): Use cautiously with nonsteroidal anti-inflammatories: may increase likelihood of GI irritation and bleeding due to tannins. Willow bark has been shown to have a very mild inhibitory effect on platelet aggregation (Krivoy et al., 2001). It is unclear whether it can interact with blood-thinning medication. Use together cautiously.

Special Notes: There are few clinical trials, but extensive empirical and ethnobotanical use clearly shows the benefits of willow bark. More research would be useful to clarify the differences between willow bark and pure acetylsalicylic acid and to put to rest fears concerning adverse reactions.

BIBLIOGRAPHY

Biegert C, et al. (2004). Efficacy and safety of willow bark extract in the treatment of osteoarthritis and rheumatoid arthritis: Results of 2 randomized double-blind controlled trials. *Journal of Rheumatology.* Nov;31(11):2121–2130.

Blumenthal M, et al. (2000). *Herbal Medicine, Expanded Commission E Monographs.* Austin, TX: American Botanical Council.

Boullata JI, et al. (2003). Anaphylactic reaction to a dietary supplement containing willow bark. *Annals of Pharmacotherapy.* 37(6):832–835.

Bradley PR. [Ed.]. (1992). *British Herbal Compendium, Vol. I* (pp. 224–226). Bournemouth: British Herbal Medicine Association.

Bradley PR[Ed.]. (1996). *British Herbal Pharmacopoeia.* Exeter: British Herbal Medicine Association.

Bruneton J. (1999). *Pharmacognosy, Phytochemistry, Medicinal Plants* (2nd ed.; pp. 252–253). Paris: Lavoisier.

Chrubasik S, et al. (2000). Treatment of low back pain exacerbations with willow bark extract: A randomized double-blind study. *American Journal of Medicine.* 109:9–14.

Chrubasik S, et al. (2001). Potential economic impact of using a proprietary willow bark extract in outpatients treatment of low back pain: An open non-randomized study. *Phytomedicine.* 8(4):241–251.

European Scientific Cooperative on Phytotherapy.(2003). *ESCOP Monographs* (2nd ed.; pp. 445–449). New York: Thieme.

Krivoy N, et al. (2001). Effect of *Salicis cortex* extract on human platelet aggregation. *Planta Medica.* Apr;67(3):209–212.

Meyer-Buchtela E. (1999). *Tee-Rezepturen-Ein Handbuch fur Apotheker und Arzte.* Stuttgart: Deutscher Apotheker Verlag.

Mills SY, et al. (1996). Effect of a proprietary herbal medicine on the relief of chronic arthritic pain: A double-blind study. *British Journal of Rheumatology.* 35(9):874–878.

Schilcher H. (1997). *Phytotherapy in Paediatrics. Handbook for Physicians and Pharmacists* (pp. 134–135). Stuttgart: Medpharm.

Schmid B, et al. (2001). Efficacy and tolerability of a standardized willow bark extract in patients with osteoarthiritis: Randomized placebo-controlled, double blind clinical trial. *Phytotherapy Research.* 15(4):344–350.

Upton R. [Ed.]. (1999). *American Herbal Pharmacopoeia and Therapeutic Compendium—Willow Bark*. Santa Cruz, CA: AHP.

Wichtl M, Bisset NG. (1994). *Herbal Drugs and Phytopharmaceuticals* (pp. 437–439). Stuttgart: Medpharm.

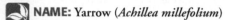

NAME: Yarrow (*Achillea millefolium*)

Common Names: Thousand-leaf, milfoil, woundwort

Family: *Asteraceae*

Description of Plant

- Hardy aromatic perennial, growing 2' to 3' tall; blooms June to October
- Native to Europe, Asia, and North America; common in fields and waste places
- There are numerous cultivars of yarrow that are not used medicinally.

Medicinal Part: Dried or fresh leaves and flowers

Constituents and Action (if known)

- EO (0.2%–1.0%): monoterpenes—linalool, camphor, borneol, eucalyptol: antimicrobial and antioxidant (Candan et al., 2003)
  - Sesquiterpenes (chamazulene): anti-inflammatory and antiallergenic properties (rat models) (Newall et al., 1996), beta-caryophyllene, sabinene, alpha- and beta-pinenes
- Flavonoids: apigenin, artemetin, casticin, luteolin, rutin
  - Antispasmodic activity (Newall et al., 1996)
  - Effective against diarrhea, flatulence, and cramping
- Sesquiterpene lactones: achillicin, achillin, leucodin, achillifolin, millefin—anti-inflammatory, digestive bitters

- Alkaloids: stachydrine, achilleine—hemostatic (Newall et al., 1996), digestive bitters
- Tannins (3%–4%)
- Coumarins

Other Actions

- Improves circulation and tones varicose veins (Chevallier, 1996)
- In animal studies, yarrow extracts had antiulcer (Cavalcanti et al., 2006), hepatoprotective, antispasmodic, and calcium channel blocking activity (Yaeesh et al., 2006).

Nutritional Ingredients: None

Traditional Use

- Antibacterial, antispasmodic, anti-inflammatory, bitter tonic, diuretic, diaphoretic, styptic, vulnerary, menstrual amphoteric, peripheral vasodilator
- Fresh leaf or flower can be applied topically as a poultice to stop bleeding from wounds (styptic).
- A bitter digestive tonic used for gas, nausea, poor fat digestion, and biliousness
- Reduces pain of toothache (fresh leaves, flowers, or roots, chewed)
- Helps regulate menstrual cycle (menorrhagia or amenorrhea)
- Used as a diaphoretic to increase sweating and lower fevers

Current Use

- Anti-inflammatory and antispasmodic activity, especially to GI tract; used for IBS, gastric ulcers with bleeding, mucous colitis, intestinal colic, enteritis, and diarrhea (Winston, 2006).
- Styptic: used topically for cuts and scratches hemorrhoids and episiotomy incisions (sitz bath; add 1–2 gtt lavender EO)
- It is also useful for minor internal bleeding: menorrhagia, hematuria, nosebleeds, and hemoptysis.
- Effective remedy for the early stages of influenza and fever management. Take as a hot tea with boneset or elderflower (Chevallier, 1996).
- A digestive tonic, useful for biliary dyskinesia, nervous dyspepsia, impaired fat digestion, and flatulence (Moore, 2003)

Available Forms, Dosage, and Administration Guidelines

Preparations: Dried herb, tea, tincture, succus (pressed juice from fresh herb); sitz baths

Typical Dosage

- *Infusion:* 1 tsp dried herb/flowers in 8 oz hot water, steep covered 20 to 30 minutes; take up to three cups a day
- *Succus:* 1 tsp (5 mL) three times daily between meals
- *Tincture* (1:5, 40% alcohol): 40 to 100 gtt (2–5 mL) three times a day
- *Sitz bath:* 4 oz dried yarrow in 1 gallon hot water, steep covered 40 minutes; add to just enough water to cover the hips with the knees up. Wrap upper body in towels, soak 10 to 20 minutes, rinse.

Pharmacokinetics—If Available (form or route when known): Not known

Toxicity: No acute or chronic toxicity known

Contraindications: Serious allergy to the aster family (ragweed, chamomile, chrysanthemum, etc.)

Side Effects: Contact dermatitis (rare)

Long-Term Safety: No adverse effects expected with normal therapeutic doses

Use in Pregnancy/Lactation/Children: Use cautiously during pregnancy; may have mild emmenagogue qualities. No adverse effects expected in lactating mothers or in children.

Drug/Herb Interactions and Rationale (if known): None known

Special Notes: Although there is little current research on yarrow, it has a long history of clinical use by herbalists and naturopathic and eclectic physicians. It also has extensive ethnobotanical use, and we have detailed knowledge of the herb's phytochemistry. This accumulated information gives adequate support for use of this herb.

BIBLIOGRAPHY

Bradley PR. (1992). *British Herbal Compendium, Vol. I* (pp. 227–229). Bournemouth: British Herbal Medicine Association.

Candan F, et al. (2003). Antioxidant and antimicrobial activity of the essential oil and methanol extracts of *Achillea millefolium* subsp. millefoium Afan. (Asteraceae). *Journal of Ethnopharmacology.* Aug:87(2–3):215–220.

Cavalcanti AM, et al. (2006). Safety and antiulcer efficacy studies of *Achillea millefolium* L. after chronic treatment in Wistar rats. *Journal of Ethnopharmacology.* Sep 19;107(2):277–284.

Chevallier A. (1996). *Encyclopedia of Medicinal Plants* (p. 54). New York: DK Publishing.

Hedley C. (1996). Yarrow: A monograph. *European Journal of Herbal Medicine.* 2(3):14–18.

Montanari T, et al. (1998). Antispermatogenic effect of *Achillea millefolium* L. in mice. *Contraception.* 58(5):309–313.

Moore M. (2003). *Medicinal Plants of the Mountain West* (pp. 269–270). Santa Fe: Museum of New Mexico Press.

Newall C, et al. (1996). *Herbal Medicines.* London: Pharmaceutical Press.

Skenderi G. (2003). *Herbal Vade Mecum* (p. 283). Rutherford, NJ: Herbacy Press.

Winston D. (2006). *Winston's Botanic Materia Medica.* Washington, NJ: DWCHS.

Yaeesh S, et al. (2006). Studies on hepatoprotective, antispasmodic and calcium antagonist activities of the aqueous-methanol extract of *Achillea millefolium. Phytotherapy Research.* Jul;20(7):546–551.

NAME: Yellow Dock Root (*Rumex crispus*)

Common Names: Curly dock, sour dock

Family: *Polygonaceae*

Description of Plant

- It is a common, weedy perennial that grows in waste places through the world's temperate regions.
- It has a yellow, bitter-tasting tap root and in its second year of growth sends up a flower stalk, which by late summer carries a heavy load of tiny, brown, buckwheat-like seeds.

Medicinal Part: The fresh or dried root

Constituents and Action (if known)

- Anthraquinone glycosides
  - Chysophanol: antifungal (Duke, 2006), antitumor (Bawadi et al., 2004), antiviral (Semple et al., 2001)

- ∘ Emodin: antibacterial, laxative (Duke, 2006), antiviral (Shuangsuo et al., 2006), antitumor (Olsen et al., 2006)
- ∘ Physcion: antibacterial, purgative (Duke, 2006)
- ∘ Nepodin: antifungal (Duke, 2006), antibacterial (Skenderi, 2003)
- Tannins: astringent (Skenderi, 2003), antioxidant, antibacterial, hepatoprotective, antidiarrheal (Duke, 2006)
- Oxalates: calcium oxalate can cause kidney stones and in larger quantities is irritating to the gastric mucosa

Nutritional Ingredients: The young leaves are cooked and eaten as a pot herb. The tiny seeds are rich in protein and rutin and have been used as a "wild" grain. The chaff surrounding the seed must be removed and then the seeds are toasted. The toasted seeds can be cooked as a "grain," and they taste like buckwheat.

Traditional Use
- Alterative, antibacterial, astringent, bitter tonic, cholagogue, mild laxative
- Yellow dock has a long history of use as an "alterative" for chronic degenerative diseases. It enhances liver and bowel function and is used for red, weeping skin conditions (eczema, psoriasis), arthritis, cancer, hypothyroidism, anemia, and constipation (Winston, 2006).
- The eclectic physicians found it especially useful for dry, irritive laryngeal or tracheal coughs (Felter & Lloyd, 1986), for wasting (cachexia) caused by cancer (Ellingwood, 1919), and for red, inflamed, oozing skin conditions (used orally and topically) with figwort and sarsaparilla.
- It has been used topically as a poultice or ointment for bedsores, mastitis, poison ivy, eczema, and psoriasis (Winston, 2006).

Current Use
- Little research has been done on this herb; it has a reputation of having significant levels of iron and is frequently used for iron-deficient anemia and low hemoglobin levels. In reality, its iron levels, while above average, are not unusually high. In clinical practice, giving small amounts of this herb along with an iron-rich diet [heme iron (red meat, molasses, dark green leafy vegetables)] enhances iron absorption. In one small, unpublished study (Burgess & Baillie, 2005), yellow dock mixed with molasses

dramatically improved hemoglobin, IBC ferritin, serum folate, and red blood cell folate levels in women over a 12-week time frame. The yellow dock or molasses by themselves did not have the same effect.

- Clinical herbalists use *Rumex* as a bitter tonic and cholagogue. It is useful for poor fat digestion, epigastric fullness, and biliary dyskinesia (Winston, 2006).
- Due to its tannin and anthraquinone content, this herb has both astringent and laxative effects. It is used for atonic constipation caused by chronic laxative abuse and diarrhea with a watery but painless discharge. Use it with chamomile, yarrow, and myrrh for the latter condition (Winston, 2006).

Available Forms, Dosage, and Administration Guidelines
Preparations: Tea, capsules, tincture
Typical Dosage
- *Tea:* 1 tsp dried root to 8 oz hot water, decoct 10 to 15 minutes, let steep 30 minutes; take 4 oz two to three times a day
- *Capsules:* One 00 (15 grains) capsule twice a day
- *Tincture* (1:2 or 1:5, 30% alcohol): 20 to 40 gtt (1–2 mL) three times a day. For dry coughs, 1 to 5 gtt up to six times a day.

Pharmacokinetics—If Available (form or route when known): Anthroquine glycosides are only minimally absorbed in the small intestine. Free anthroquines become available in the large intestine due to enzymatic hydrolysis of the glycosides. Because yellow dock does not contain large amounts of these compounds, the significant laxative effect found in senna or *Cascara sagrada* is much less likely to occur with normal doses of yellow dock.

Toxicity: There is one case in the medical literature of a man ingesting yellow dock and dying from hepatic necrosis. It is unclear whether he ate the leaves (which are much higher in oxalates) or the root, how much he consumed, and if there was a positive identification of the suspected plant. Overdoses of the root may cause diarrhea, nausea, vomiting, and polyuria (Der Marderosian & Beutler, 2006).

Contraindications: Hemachromatosis. Oxalates are contraindicated in patients with calcium oxalate kidney stones.

Side Effects: In sensitive people, it may exacerbate diarrhea or constipation.

Long-Term Safety: Probably best used in small amounts and for short periods of time

Use in Pregnancy/Lactation/Children: Yellow dock root is commonly used in small amounts with other nutritive or iron-rich herbs (nettles, dandelion leaf, ashwagandha, processed rehmannia) for low hemoglobin and hematocrit levels during pregnancy. Avoid using large quantities during pregnancy, lactation, or in small children.

Drug/Herb Interactions and Rationale (if known): None known

Special Notes: Alteratives are no longer used in orthodox Western medicine but are still commonly used in herbal and naturopathic practice to enhance the body's ability to eliminate wastes. Not only do "alterative" herbs promote normal eliminatory processes, many stimulate digestion, promote lymphatic drainage, enhance immune activity, and inhibit viruses, bacteria, and fungal pathogens.

BIBLIOGRAPHY

Bawadi HA, et al. (2004). Efficacy of rhubarb-derived chrysophanic acid on hypoxic and normoxic cancer cells. Retrieved October 30 2006, from http://ift.confex.com/ift/2004/techprogram/paper_24819.htm.

Brinker F. (2001). *Herb Contraindications & Drug Interactions* (3rd ed., pp. 218–220). Sandy, OR: Eclectic Medical Publications.

Burgess I, Baillie N. (2005). *Iron tonics—What really works?* Cambridge, NZ.

Der Marderosian A, Beutler J. [Eds.]. (2006). *The Review of Natural Products, Yellow Dock Monograph*. St. Louis, MO: Wolters Kluwer Health.

Duke J.(2006). Dr. Duke's Phytochemical and ethnobotanical databases. www.ars-grin.gov/duke/

Ellingwood F. (1919). *American Materia Medica, Therapeutics, and Pharmacognosy* (pp. 378–379). Evanston, IL: Ellingwood's Therapeutist.

Felter HW, Lloyd JU. (1986). *King's American Dispensatory* (19th ed.; pp. 1683–1685). Sandy, OR: Eclectic Medical Publications.

Olsen BB, et al. (2006). Emodin negatively affects the phosphoinositide 3-kinase/AKT signalling pathway: A study on its mechanism of action. *International Journal of Biochemistry and Cell Biology.* 39(1): 227–237.

Semple SJ, et al. (2001). In vitro antiviral activity of the anthraquinone chrysophanic acid against poliovirus. Mar;49(3):169–178.

Shuangsuo D, et al. (2006). Inhibition of the replication of hepatitis B virus in vitro by emodin. *Medical Science Monitor.* Aug 25;12(9):BR302–BR306.

Skenderi G. (2003). *Herbal Vade Mecum* (p. 133). Rutherford, NJ: Herbacy Press.

Winston D. (2006). *Winston's Botanic Materia Medica.* Washington, NJ: DWCHS.

Yildirim A, et al. (2001). Determination of antioxidant and antimicrobial activities of *Rumex Crispus* L. extracts. *Journal of Agricultural and Food Chemistry.* Aug;49(8):4083–4089.

 NAME: Yohimbe (*Pausinystalia yohimbe*)

Common Names: None

Family: *Rubiaceae*

Description of Plant: A tall evergreen tree native to West Africa (Nigeria, Cameroon, Gabon, and the Congo)

Medicinal Part: Dried bark

Constituents and Action (if known)
- Indole alkaloids (1%–6% total): yohimbine (10%–15%), coryanthine, pseudo-yohimbine, allo-yohimbine
- Yohimbe is a monoamine oxidase inhibitor (Leung & Foster, 1996) and a selective inhibitor of presynaptic alpha-2-adrenergic receptors, increasing sympathetic nervous system activity, norepinephrine release, and lipolysis. (Mitchel, 2003)
- Low doses are hypertensive and higher doses are hypotensive; it is a peripheral vasodilator (Bruneton, 1999).

Nutritional Ingredients: None

Traditional Use: Aphrodisiac, CNS stimulant, antidiuretic; used by tribal peoples in West Africa as an aphrodisiac for men with erectile dysfunction, as a stimulant, and for anginal pain and hypertension

Current Use

- The prescription drug yohimbine HCl is used for mild to moderate erectile dysfunction (ED) (Guay et al., 2002). A product combining yohimbine HCl and the amino acid argine glutamate was effective for treatment of mild to moderate ED (Lebret et al., 2002). This combination also mildly enhanced female libido (Meston & Worcel, 2002). This product did not cause hypertension in patients receiving IV nitroglycerin (Kernohan et al., 2005).
- Yohimbine HCl has also been used for orthostatic hypotension, chronic constipation, narcolepsy, and diabetic patients with incapacitating paresthesia of the lower limbs.
- Some practitioners are also using it for obesity, especially in the thighs and buttocks. It stimulates alpha-2-adrenergic receptors, which increases lipolysis of fat cells and inhibits hunger pangs (Mitchell, 2003).

Available Forms, Dosage, and Administration Guidelines

Preparations: Crude herb, tincture

Typical Dosage

- *Tincture* (1:5, 50% alcohol): 5 to 10 gtt (0.25–0.5 mL) twice a day
- *Yohimbine HCl* (prescription only): 5.4 to 6.0 mg three times a day; increased risk of adverse effects with doses of more than 10.0 mg

Pharmacokinetics—If Available (form or route when known): Most bioavailable if patient is fasting. Oral doses of 10-mg yohimbine HCl resulted in rapid absorption (absorption half-life of 0.17 ± 0.11 hours) and elimination (elimination half-life 0.60 ± 0.26 hours) (de Smet, 1997).

Toxicity: Use of yohimbe has been associated with a lupus-like syndrome, nausea, vomiting, tachycardia, hypertension, tremor, acute renal failure, psychiatric disorders (de Smet, 1997; Reichert, 1997). Long-term use of yohimbine HCl (more than 5 years at 5.4 mg three times a day) has been linked to agranulocytosis.

Contraindications: Hepatic insufficiency, liver disease, renal insufficiency, kidney disease, hypotension, hypertension (oral doses of 15–20 mg yohimbine HCl can increase blood pressure), depression, prostatitis, bipolar disorders (a dose of yohimbine HCl as low as 10 mg can trigger a manic episode in bipolar patients), schizophrenia, asthma, cardiac disease

Side Effects: Priapism, hypertension or hypotension depending on dosage, irritability, migraines, dizziness, tremors, bronchospasm, insomnia, tachycardia, nausea and vomiting

Long-Term Safety: Inappropriate for long-term use

Use in Pregnancy/Lactation/Children: Avoid in all

Drug/Herb Interactions and Rationale (if known):
Phenothiazines such as chlorpromazine increase yohimbe's toxicity; monoamine oxidase inhibitors; tricyclic antidepressants (12-mg yohimbine HCl elicited hypertensive crisis in patients taking these medications [de Smet, 1997]); antihypertensive medications (antagonizes effects of drugs such as clonidine). Yohimbe increases cravings in patients taking methadone (Stine et al., 2002).

Special Notes
- This herb's use should be restricted to trained clinicians.
- It has been suggested that yohimbe is effective for ED. There are no studies of the crude drug for this claim. Only yohimbine HCl has been tested, and results of studies on this alkaloid are contradictory.
- Yohimbine is also an active stimulant of the alpha-2-adrenergic receptors of adipocytes. This process is believed to increase lipolysis, but most trials using yohimbine HCl for weight loss have had negative results.
- Body builders tout yohimbe as a natural way to build muscle. Not only is this unproven, but it is potentially dangerous.
- Studies of commercial yohimbe products (crude herb) have often shown little or no yohimbe in the product. Yohimbine concentrations have ranged from less than 0.1 to 489.0 parts per million, compared with 7,089.0 parts per million in authentic material. Some of these products showed only

yohimbine HCl and none of the other indole alkaloids that should be present in the crude herb, suggesting that the product was "spiked" with minute amounts of the isolated alkaloid (Betz et al., 1995). With the problems of adulteration, possible drug/herb interactions, and toxicity, it is unwise for patients to self-medicate with this herb.

BIBLIOGRAPHY

Betz JM, et al. (1995). Gas chromatographic determination of yohimbine in commercial yohimbe products. *Journal of AOAC International.* 78(5):1189–1194.

Brinker F. (2001). *Herb Contraindications & Drug Interactions* (pp. 204–206). Sandy, OR: Eclectic Institute, Inc.

Bruneton J. (1999). *Pharmacognosy, Phytochemistry, Medicinal Plants* (2nd ed.; pp. 1015–1016). Paris: Lavoisier.

de Smet PA. (1997). Yohimbe alkaloids. In: de Smet et al. [Eds.]. *Adverse Effects of Herbal Drugs, Vol. 3.* (pp. 211–214). New York: Springer-Verlag.

de Smet PA, Oscar S. (1994). Potential risks of health food products containing yohimbe extracts. *British Medical Journal.* 309:958.

Ernst E, Pittler MH. (1998). Yohimbe for erectile dysfunction: A systematic review and meta-analysis of randomized clinical trials. *Journal of Urology.* 159(2):433–436.

Guay AT, et al. (2002). Yohimbine treatment of organic erectile dysfunction in a dose-escalation trial. *International Journal of Impotence Research.* Feb;14(1):25–31.

Kernohan AF, et al. (2005). An oral yohimbine/L-arginine combination (NMI 861) for the treatment of male erectile dysfunction: A pharmacokinetic, pharmacodynamic and interaction study with intravenous nitroglycerine in healthy male subjects. *British Journal of Clinical Pharmacology.* Jan;59(1):85–93.

Lebret T, et al. (2002). Efficacy and safety of a novel combination of L-arginine glutamate and yohimbine hydrochloride: A new oral therapy for erectile dysfunction. *European Urology.* Jan;41(6):608–613.

Leung A, Foster S. (1996). *Encyclopedia of Common Natural Ingredients* (2nd ed.; pp. 522–524). New York: John Wiley Sons.

Meston CM, Worcel M. (2002). The effects of yohimbine plus L-arginine glutamate on sexual arousal in postmenopausal women with sexual arousal disorder. *Archives of Sexual Behavior.* Aug;31(4):323–332.

Mitchell W. (2003). *Plant Medicine in Practice Using the Teachings of John Bastyr* (p. 247). St. Louis, MO: Churchill Livingstone.

Reichert R. (1997). Yohimbine pharmacokinetics. *Quarterly Review of Natural Medicine*. Spring:17–18.

Riley AJ. (1994). Yohimbine in the treatment of erectile disorder. *British Journal of Clinical Practice*. 48(3):133–136.

Stine SM, et al. (2002). Yohimbine-induced withdrawal and anxiety symptoms in opioid-dependent patients. *Biological Psychiatry*. Apr 15;51(8):642–651.

PART III

Nutritional Supplements

NAME: L-arginine

Common Names: Arginine

Description and Source: Semi-essential amino acid

Biologic Activity

- Substrate necessary for nitric oxide synthesis and maintenance of activity
- Nitric oxide acts as a vasodilator, reduces platelet aggregation, reduces monocyte/vessel wall interactions, and reduces smooth muscle cell proliferation (Boger & Ron, 2005). It also stimulates release of growth hormone, insulin-like growth factor 1, insulin, and prolactin and researchers are attempting to discover whether arginine via NO may actually promote or inhibit tumor growth (Lind, 2004).
- Improves blood flow and reduces total and very-low-density lipoproteins (Maxwell & Anderson, 1999)
- Carrier of nitrogen, which is important for ammonia detoxification

Nutritional Sources: Peanuts and peanut butter, brown rice, cashews, pecans, almonds, chocolate, sunflower seeds. Synthesized by the body from glutamine.

Current Use

- Improves coronary blood flow and endothelial function in persons with atherosclerosis (Yin et al., 2005) and MELAS (mitochondrial myopathy, encephalopathy, lactic acidosis, and stroke) (Koga et al., 2006) and in women with type II diabetes used along with vitamins C and E (Regensteiner et al., 2003)
- Improves walking distance in persons with intermittent claudication (Maxwell et al., 1999)
- Improves endothelium-dependent diabetes with significant hypercholesterolemia (7 g three times a day) (Clarkson et al., 1996; Yin et al., 2005). It also reduces LDL oxidation but may increase total cholesterol levels (Kumar et al., 2005).
- Improves blood flow and reduces chest pain in patients with nonobstructive coronary artery disease (Lerman et al., 1998). It did not benefit patients who had suffered an acute myocardial infarction (Schulman et al., 2006).

- May enhance penile engorgement in men and sexual function in women
- In a small study, L-arginine prolonged pregnancy and improved neonatal outcomes in women with pre-eclampsia (Rytlewski et al., 2006).
- Arginine alpha-ketoglutarate (AAKG) was given to athletically trained men, and it enhanced their exercise performance (Campbell et al., 2006).
- Patients with pressure ulcers received arginine, vitamin C, and zinc, which healed much quicker than in those taking a placebo (Desneves et al., 2005).
- May improve senile dementia (Ohtsuka & Nakaya, 2000)

Available Forms, Dosage, and Administration Guidelines: Dosages found to be effective for the treatment of cardiovascular disease range from 6 to 9 g a day. Sustained-release products maintain steadier blood levels.

Pharmacokinetics—If Available (form or route when known): Not known

Toxicity: None known

Contraindications: Persons susceptible to herpes: arginine activates herpesvirus replication

Side Effects: GI upset, may exacerbate GERD. It may also increase total cholesterol levels.

Long-Term Safety: Not known

Use in Pregnancy/Lactation/Children: Not known

Drug/Herb Interactions and Rationale (if known): Not known

Special Notes: Current studies are very short (6 months or less); long-term studies are necessary.

BIBLIOGRAPHY

Boger RH, Ron ES. (2005). L-arginine improves vascular function by overcoming deletevious effects of ADMA, a novel cardiovascular risk factor. *Alternative Medicine Review.* Nov;10(1):14–23.

Campbell B, et al. (2006). Pharmacokinetics, safety and effects on exercise performance of L-arginine alpha-ketoglutarate in trained adult men. *Nutrition.* Sep;22(9):872–881.

Clarkson P, et al. (1996). Oral L-arginine improves endothelium-dependent dilation in hypercholesterolemic young adults. *Journal of Clinical Investigation.* 97(8):1989–1994.

Desneves KJ, et al. (2005). Treatment with supplementary arginine, vitamin c, and zinc in patients with pressure ulcers: A randomised controlled trial. *Clinical Nutrition.* Dec;24(6):979–987.

Koga Y, et al. (2006). Endothelial dysfunction in MELAS improved by L-arginine supplementation. *Neurology.* Jun 13;66(11): 1766–1769.

Kumar P, et al. (2005). L-arginine supplementation increases serum cholesterol level. *Indian Journal of Pharmacology.* 37:183.

Lerman A, et al. (1998). Long-term L-arginine supplementation improves small-vessel coronary endothelial function in humans. *Circulation.* 97(21):2123–2128.

Lind DS. (2004). Arginine and cancer. *Journal of Nutrition.* Oct;134[10 Suppl.]:2837S–2841S; discussion 2853S.

Maxwell AJ, Anderson BA. (1999). A nutritional product designed to enhance nitric oxide activity restores endothelium-dependent function in hypercholesterolemia. *Journal of the American College of Cardiology.* 33:282A.

Maxwell AJ, et al. (1999). Improvement in walking distance and quality of life in peripheral arterial disease by a nutritional product designed to enhance nitric oxide activity. *Journal of the American College of Cardiology.* 33:277A.

Ohtsuka Y, Nakaya J. (2000). Effect of oral administration of L-arginine on senile dementia. *American Journal of Medicine.* Apr 1;108(5):439.

Regensteiner JG, et al. (2003). Oral L-arginine and vitamins E and C improve endothelial function in women with type 2 diabetes. *Vascular Medicine.* 8(3):169–175.

Rytlewski K, et al. (2006). Effects of L-arginine on the foetal condition and neonatal outcome in pre-eclampsia: A preliminary report. *Basic and Clinical Pharmacology and Toxicology.* Aug;99(2): 146–152.

Schulman SP, et al. (2006). L-arginine therapy in acute myocardial infarction: the Vascular Interaction With Age in Myocardial Infarction (VINTAGE MI) randomized clinical trial. *Journal of the American Medical Association.* Jan 4;295(1):58–64.

Swanson B, Keithly JK. (2002). A pilot study of the safety and efficacy of supplemental arginine to enhance immune function in persons with HIV/AIDS. *Nutrition.* Jul-Aug;18(708):688–690.

Yin WH, et al. (2005). L-arginine improves endothelial function and reduces LDL oxidation in patients with stable coronary artery disease. *Clinical Nutrition.* Dec;24(6):988–997.

🔖 NAME: L-carnitine

Common Names: L-carnitine (LC), acetyl-L-carnitine (ALC), l-propionylcarnitine (PLC)

Description and Source
- LC is an essential amino acid that is necessary for the conversion of fatty acids into energy for muscle activity. It is primarily stored in the muscles, including the heart.
- Three forms of carnitine are available
  - LC: the most common form; it has the most research and costs less than the other forms
  - ALC: effects are primarily directed toward cerebral function and memory
  - PLC: may have the most profound effect on the heart and its function
- Do not substitute one form of carnitine for another. D-carnitine competes with other forms of carnitine and can cause deficiency.

Biologic Activity
- Necessary for production of acetylcholine
- Antioxidant and O_2 free radical scavenger
- Facilitates transport of long chain fatty acids across cell membranes to be used in ATP production (Sinatra, 2005)
- ALC stimulates message transmission in brain cells, retards loss of receptors in brain cells (rats) (Castorina & Ferraros, 1994), and increases cerebral blood flow and enzyme activity in the brain.
- ALC is therapeutically active in hyperlipidemia, lowering LDL and very-low-density lipoprotein cholesterol and triglyceride levels (25%) and elevating HDL (63%). It is also indicated for preventing and treating atherosclerosis. LC has shown benefits for ischemic heart disease, CHF, angina pectoris, and mild arrhythmias (Stanley et al., 2005).
- Levels of LC may be low in patients with CFIDS; more research is necessary (Sinatra, 2005; Werbach, 2000).
- LC may play a role in reversing insulin resistance (Kelly, 2000).

Nutritional Sources: Red meats, and to a lesser degree poultry, fish, and dairy products

Current Use

- ALC may improve mental functioning in patients with mild Alzheimer's disease, senile dementia, chronic alcoholism, and Down syndrome (more research is necessary) (Pettegrew et al., 1995; Sano et al., 1992).
- ALC enhances behavioral performance and results on memory tests (Cucinotta et al., 1988; Salvioli & Neri, 1994).
- ALC can be used to prevent and treat ischemic heart disease (Singh et al., 1996; Sinatva, 2005).
- ALC has been shown to be a well-tolerated and effective treatment for paclitaxel, cisplatin, and antiretroviral-induced neuropathies (Maestri et al., 2005; Osio et al., 2006).
- ALC was effective in reversing and preventing symptoms of hyperthyroidism, and it showed benefit for enhancing bone density (Benvenga et al., 2001).
- ALC was more effective and safer than tamoxifen for treating acute and early Peyronie's disease (Biagiotti & Cavallini, 2001).
- Improves symptoms of neuropathy in diabetics (Fontana et al., 2006)
- Protects the heart from adriamycin toxicity (Pauly & Pepine, 2003)
- ALC is being given to AIDS patients (6 g a day) to reduce the toxicity of AZT on the muscle cells, thus reducing muscle fatigue and pain.
- ALC should be considered in treating hyperlipidemia and atherosclerosis.
- ALC has shown benefits in reducing muscle pain and fatigue associated with CFS/fibromyalgia (Plioplys & Plioplys, 1997). It also improved muscle tone and exercise endurance in thalassemic patients (El-Beshlawy et al., 2007).
- Increases sperm motility in men who are infertile (Isidori et al., 2006)

Available Forms, Dosage, and Administration
Guidelines: 1 to 3 g a day, divided into two or three doses

Pharmacokinetics—If Available (form or route when known): Eliminated in urine: PLC—½ to 1½ hours; LC—½ to 15 hours

Toxicity: None known

Contraindications: Seizure activity, bipolar disorders, liver or kidney disease

Side Effects: Diarrhea, nausea, vomiting with 4 g or more a day; fishy body odor

Long-Term Safety: Unknown; additional research needed

Drug/Herb Interactions and Rationale (if known):
Co-Q10 seems to enhance ALC's effects but may increase anticoagulation effects. Do not take when on dialysis or in hypothyroidism. Monitor carefully with antiseizure medications.

BIBLIOGRAPHY

Benvenga S, et al. (2001). Usefulness of L-carnitine, a naturally occurring peripheral antagonist of thyroid hormone action, in iatrogenic hyperthyroidism: A randomized, double-blind, placebo-controlled clinical trial. *Journal of Clinical Endocrinology and Metabolism.* Aug;86(8):3579–3594.

Biagiotti G, Cavallini G. (2001). Acetyl- L-carnitine vs. tamoxifen in the oral therapy of Peyronie's disease: A preliminary report. *BJU International.* Jul;88(1):63–67.

Castorina M, Ferraros L. (1994). Acetyl- L-carnitine affects aged brain receptorial system in rodents. *Life Science.* 54:1205–1214.

El-Beshlawy A, et al. (2007). Effect of L-carnitine on the physical fitness of thalassemic patients. *Annals of Hematology.* Jan;86(1): 31–34.

Ferrari R, et al. (2004). Therapeutic effects of L-carnitine and propionyl- L-carnitine on cardiovascular diseases: A review. *Annals of the New York Academy of Sciences.* Nov;1033:79–91.

Fontana G, et al. (2006). Nitrogenous compounds of interest in clinical nutrition. *Nurtrición Hospitalaria.* May;21(Suppl. 2):14–27; 15–29.

Isidori AM, et al. (2006). Medical treatment to improve sperm quality. *Reproductive Biomedicine Online.* Jun;12(6):704–714.

Kelly GS. (1998). L-carnitine: Therapeutic applications of a conditionally essential amino acid. *Alternative Medicine Review.* 3(5):345–360.

Maestri A, et al. (2005). A pilot study on the effect of acetyl-L-carnitine in paclitaxel- and cisplatin-induced peripheral neuropathy. *Tumori.* Mar-Apr;91(2):135–138.

Osio M, et al. (2006). Acetyl-L-carnitine in the treatment of painful antiretroviral toxic neuropathy in human immunodeficiency virus patients: An open label study. *Journal of the Peripheral Nervous System.* Mar;11(1):72–76.

Pauly DF, Pepine CJ. (2003). The role of carnitine in myocardial dysfunction. *American Journal of Kidney Disease.* Apr;41[4 Suppl. 4]:S35–S43.

Pettegrew JW, et al. (1995). Clinical and neurochemical effects of acetyl-L-carnitine in Alzheimer's disease. *Neurobiology of Aging.* 16:1–4.

Plioplys AV, Plioplys S. (1997). Amantadine and L-carnitine treatment of chronic fatigue syndrome. *Neuropsychology.* 35(1):16–23.

Salvioli G, Neri M. (1994). L-acetyl-carnitine treatment of mental decline in the elderly. *Drugs: Experimental and Clinical Research.* 20:169–176.

Sano M, et al. (1992). Double-blind parallel design pilot study of acetyl levo-carnitine in patients with Alzheimer's disease. *Archives of Neurology.* 49:1137–1141.

Sinatra ST, et al. (2005). *The Sinatra Solution: Metabolic Cardiology.* New Jersey: Basic Health Publications.

Singh RB, et al. (1996). A randomized, double-blind, placebo-controlled trial of L-carnitine in suspected acute myocardial infarction. *Postgraduate Medicine.* 72:45–50.

Stanley WC, et al. (2005). Metabolic therapies for heart disease: Fish for prevention and treatment of cardiac failure? *Cardiovascular Research.* Nov 1;68(2):175–177.

Tamamogullari N, et al. (1999). L-carnitine deficiency in diabetes mellitus complications. *Journal of Diabetes Complications.* 13(5–6):251–253.

Werbach MR. (2000). Nutritional strategies for treating chronic fatigue syndrome. *Alternative Medicine Review.* 5(2):93–108.

 NAME: Chondroitin

Common Names: Chondroitin sulfate

Description and Source

- A high-viscosity mucopolysaccharide (glycosaminoglycan)
- Can be extracted from natural sources (bovine, porcine, avian) or synthesized in the laboratory
- Is a flexible connecting matrix between proteins and filaments in cartilage

- May replace proteoglycans, a substance that forms cartilage (Morreale et al., 1996)

Biologic Activity

- Helps and attracts essential fluid into proteoglycan molecules, "water magnets" that act as shock absorbers, and moves nutrients into cartilage (Lamari et al., 2006)
- Stimulates chondrocyte activity. Chondrocytes must get their nutrition from the synovial fluid because there is no vasculature to nourish them. During inflammation, chondrocyte activity is disturbed (Volpi, 2006).
- May inhibit human leukocyte elastase and hyaluronidase, which are found in high concentrations in persons with rheumatoid disease
- Chondroitin sulfate B inhibits venous thrombosis; antithrombolytic and may decrease heparin requirements

Nutritional Sources: None

Current Use

- Several studies show that chondroitin has some benefit for treating osteoarthritis of the hands and knees (Rovetta et al., 2004; Uebelhart et al., 2004).
- Patients taking chondroitin sulfate for osteoarthritis had significant improvement in existing psoriasis (Verges et al., 2005).

Available Forms, Dosage, and Administration

Guidelines: Follow manufacturer directions. Usually combined with glucosamine sulfate. Dosage is based on weight.

<120 lb: 800 mg
120 to 200 lb: 1,200 mg
>200 lb: 1,600 mg

Divide into two to four smaller doses and take with food

Pharmacokinetics—If Available (form or route when known): Absorption, 0% to 13%; very large molecule size

Toxicity: None known; long-term clinical trials needed

Contraindications: Bleeding disorders

Side Effects: GI upset (dyspepsia, nausea), headache

Long-Term Safety: Unknown

Use in Pregnancy/Lactation/Children: Unknown; do not use

Drug/Herb Interactions and Rationale (if known): Do not take with anticoagulants: may potentiate bleeding.

Special Notes: In clinical practice, the effects of chondroitin seem marginal, especially compared with those of glucosamine sulfate. Purity is a problem with chondroitin. There is a significant variability with different products.

BIBLIOGRAPHY

Lamari FN, et al. (2006). Metabolism and biochemical/physiological roles of chondroitin sulfates: Analysis of endogenous and supplemental chondroitin sulfates in blood circulation. *Biomedical Chromatography.* Jun;20(607):539–540.

McCarty MF, et al. (2000). Sulfated glycosaminoglycans and glucosamine may synergize in promoting synovial hyaluronic acid synthesis. *Medical Hypotheses.* 54(5):798–802.

Morreale P, et al. (1996). Comparison of the anti-inflammatory efficacy of chondroitin sulfate and diclofenac sodium in patients with knee osteoarthritis. *Journal of Rheumatology.* 23:1385–1391.

Rovetta G, et al. (2004). A two-year study of chondroitin sulfate in erosive osteoarthritis of the hands: Behavior of erosions, osteophytes, pain and hand dysfunction. *Drugs Under Experimental and Clinical Research.* 30(10):11–16.

Uebelhart D, et al. (2004). Intermittent treatment of knee osteoarthritis with oral chondroitin sulfate: A one-year, randomized, double-blind, multicenter study versus placebo. *Osteoarthritis and Cartilage.* Apr;12(4):269–276.

Verges J, et al. (2005). Clinical and histopathological improvement of psoriasis with oral chondroitin sulfate: A serendipitous finding. *Dermatology Online Journal.* Mar 1;11(1):31.

Volpi N. (2006). Advances in chondroitin sulfate analysis: Application in physiological and pathological states of connective tissue and during pharmacological treatment of osteoarthritis. *Current Pharmaceutical Design.* 12(5):639–658.

NAME: Chromium

Common Names: None

Description and Source
- Naturally occurring trace element
- The organic form found in natural foods appears to be absorbed better than the inorganic form.

Biologic Activity
- Required for normal glucose metabolism (Keszthelyi et al., 2004; Mita et al., 2005)
- Glucose tolerance factor chromium increases HDL after 2 months in patients taking beta-blockers (Yang et al., 2005)
- May exert anabolic effect by enhancing the effect of insulin and increasing the uptake of amino acids into muscle cells (Rabinovitz et al., 2004)

Nutritional Sources: Brewer's yeast, liver, lean meats, whole grains, and cheese. Cooking with stainless-steel cookware increases the chromium content of foods (Integrative Medicine Access, 2000).

Current Use
- Low chromium levels may contribute to hypoglycemia, cardiovascular disease, glaucoma, and osteoporosis.
- Chromium promotes a normal insulin activity in persons with diabetes (enhances insulin use) (Yang et al., 2005). A combination of chromium picolinate (600 mg) and biotin (2 mg) improved glucose control and triglycerides in patients taking oral antihyperglycemic medication (Singer & Geohas, 2006).
- May benefit insulin resistance (metabolic syndrome)

Available Forms, Dosage, and Administration Guidelines
Preparations: Capsules, tablets. Several forms of chromium are available in the marketplace, including chromium polynicotinate and chromium picolinate (the best forms to use), chromium-enriched yeast, and chromium chloride.

Typical Dosage: 50 to 500 mcg a day; diabetics: 500 mcg BID; hypoglycemia: 200 mcg a day

Pharmacokinetics—If Available (form or route when known): Eliminated through the kidney

Toxicity: Irritation of GI tract (nausea, vomiting, ulcers) at high doses. Hexavalent (industrial) chromium is a heavy metal and causes kidney, liver, and lung damage.

Contraindications: Not known

Side Effects: Rare, but headache, irritability, and insomnia have been reported

Long-Term Safety: Safe

Use in Pregnancy/Lactation/Children: Safe

Drug/Herb Interactions and Rationale (if known): Calcium carbonate and antacids reduce chromium absorption.

Special Notes
- Adequate intake of chromium
  - Males (14–50): 35 mcg a day
  - Females (19–50): 30 mcg a day
  - Pregnancy: 30 mcg a day
- Although rare, chromium deficiency (e.g., peripheral neuropathy or encephalopathy, increased glucose use during pregnancy) may play a role in the development of adult diabetes.
- Chromium deficiency leads to impaired lipid and glucose metabolism and may put the person at risk for cardiovascular disease (Keszthelyi et al., 2004).
- Several studies have not found a correlation between chromium levels and diabetes (Gunton et al., 2005; Komorowski & Juturu, 2005).

BIBLIOGRAPHY

Aghdassi E, et al. (2006). Is chromium an important element in HIV-positive patients with metabolic abnormalities? An hypothesis generating pilot study. *Journal of the American College of Nutrition.* Feb;25(1):56–63.

Cerulli J, et al. (1998). Chromium picolinate toxicity. *Annals of Pharmacotherapy.* 32:428–431.

Gunton JE, et al. (2005). Chromium supplementation does not improve glucose tolerance, insulin sensitivity, or lipid profile: A randomized, placebo-controlled, double-blind trial of supplementation in subjects with impaired glucose tolerance. *Diabetes Care.* Mar;28(3):712-e.

Integrative Medicine Access. (2000). *Chromium.* Newton, MA: Integrative Medicine Communications.

Keszthelyi Z, et al. (2004). The central effect of chromium on glucose metabolism. *Pharmacopsychiatry.* Sep;37(5):242.

Komorowski J, Juturu V. (2005). Chromium supplementation does not improve glucose tolerance, insulin sensitivity, or lipid profile: A randomized, placebo controlled, double-blind trial of supplementation in subjects with impaired glucose tolerance. Response to Gunton et al. *Diabetes Care.* Jul;28(7):1841–1842, author reply 1842–1843.

Mita Y, et al. (2005). Supplementation with chromium picolinate recovers renal Cr centration and improves carbohydrate metabolism and renal function in type 2 diabetic mice. *Biological Trace Element Research.* Summer;105(1–3):229–248.

Rabinovitz H, et al. (2004). Effect of chromium supplementation on blood glucose and lipid levels in type 2 diabetes mellitus elderly patients. *International Journal for Vitamin and Nutrition Research.* May;74(3):178–182.

Shara M, et al. (2005). Safety and toxicological evaluation of a novel niacin-bound chromium (III) complex. *Journal of Inorganic Biochemistry.* Nov;99(11):2161–2183.

Singer GM, Geohas J. (2006). The effect of chromium picolinate and biotin supplementation on glycemic control in poorly controlled patients with type 2 diabetes mellitus: A placebo-controlled, double-blinded, randomized trial. *Diabetes Technology and Therapeutics.* Dec;8(6):636–643.

Yang X, et al. (2005). A newly synthetic chromium complex-chromium(phenylalanine)3 improves insulin responsiveness and reduces whole body glucose tolerance. *FEBS Letters.* Feb 28;579(6): 1458–1464.

Yang X, et al. (2006). Insulin-sensitizing and cholestrol-lowering effects of chromium (d-phenylalanine) (3). *Journal of Organic Biochemistry.* Jul;100(7):1187–1193.

NAME: Coenzyme Q10

Common Names: Vitamin Q, ubiquinone, Co-Q10

Description and Source: Naturally occurring antioxidant. Lipid-soluble benzoquinones, similar in structure to vitamin K. They are found in almost all aerobic organisms in the mitochondria. The Q10 structure is unique to humans.

Biologic Activity
- Powerful lipophilic antioxidant present in all tissue (Kontush et al., 1997)
- Membrane-stabilizing properties (Britt, 2005)
- Improves stroke volume and cardiac output in patients with CHF (Soja & Mortensen, 1997)
- Improves ejection fraction (Sinatra, 2005)
- Inhibits platelet vitronectin receptor to reduce thrombotic complications (Serebruany et al., 1997)
- Works with other enzymes to bring about its effects (Sinatra, 2005)
- Precursor to energy production in mitochondria (adenosine triphosphate)
- Oxygen free radical scavenger
- Regenerates vitamin E from its oxidized form (Ernster et al., 1995)

Nutritional Sources: Small amounts in meat and seafood

Current Use
- Improves CHF. Research suggests that patients with New York Hospital Association class III and IV disease with Co-Q10 deficiencies can become class I and II with treatment (Morisco et al., 1993). Co-Q10 improved systolic function in patients with chronic heart failure, but treatment with ACE inhibitors seems to reduce its benefits (Sander et al., 2006). Twenty-seven patients awaiting heart transplants were given Co-Q10. While their echocardiograms did not change, there was improvement in functional status, clinical symptoms, and quality of life (Berman et al., 2004).
- Benefits cardiomyopathies caused by ischemia and toxins: angina, cardiotoxicity caused by doxorubicin (adriamycin)

- Slows progression of breast cancer (Lockwood et al., 1994) and enhances immune response
- Improves tissue health and healing in gingivitis (Integrative Medicine Access, 2000)
- May improve survival after MI if administered within 3 days (120 mg a day) (Singh et al., 1998; Singh & Niaz, 1999)
- Decreases blood pressure (Singh et al., 1999): 39% of patients with hypertension have a Co-Q10 deficiency. Four to 12 weeks of supplementation showed benefit (Integrative Medicine Access, 2000).
- Improves tissue reperfusion after cross clamping during cardiac bypass surgery (Chillo et al., 1996; Nibori et al., 1998)
- May improve mitral valve prolapse (use with hawthorn), arrhythmias, diabetes, migraines, asthenozoospermia, and age-related macular degeneration
- Patients with bronchial asthma were able to reduce dosage of corticosteroids when taking Co-Q10 and vitamins E and C (Gvozdjakova et al., 2005).
- Neuroprotective, Co-Q10 slows the degeneration of neurons in patients with Frederick's ataxia and Parkinson's disease (Littarru & Tiano, 2005; Shults, 2005).
- A combination of Co-Q10, omega 3 fatty acids, and acetyl-L-carnitine prevented further degeneration in patients with early age-related macular degeneration (Feher et al., 2005).
- Reduces migraines by 50% (Modi & Lowder, 2006).

Available Forms, Dosage, and Administration Guidelines: Varies with condition; take 50 mg a day as baseline. Use oil-based soft gel for better absorption. Take with food. Take with piperine (Bioperine) (black pepper) for increased absorption (by 30%). Doses over 100 mg a day should be divided. For patients with Parkinson's disease, take 300 to 1200 mg a day. For hypertension, take 100 to 150 mg a day. For HIV/AIDS, take 200 mg a day. Avoid suddenly stopping taking Co-Q10, as symptoms of heart disease or Parkinson's may worsen (Bhagavan & Chopra, 2006).

Pharmacokinetics—If Available (form or route when known): Not known

Toxicity: None known

Contraindications: None known

Side Effects: Loss of appetite (rare), nausea, diarrhea (rare)

Long-Term Safety: Not known

Use in Pregnancy/Lactation/Children: Unknown; do not use

Drug/Herb Interactions and Rationale (if known)

- Warfarin is possibly less effective; monitor INR carefully (Landbo & Almdal, 1998). Interaction unlikely.
- HMG-CoA reductase or statin drugs (lovastatin [Mevacor], simvastatin [Zocor]) decrease absorption of Co-Q10. Supplement with 60 to 90 mg a day as a replacement dose (Levy & Kohlhaas, 2006; Palomaki et al., 1998; Vercelli et al., 2006).
- ACE inhibitors seem to reduce effectiveness of Co-Q10 in patients with chronic heart failure (Sander et al., 2006).

Special Notes: Mixed research exists. There are more positive results than negative (Watson et al., 1999), but further research is needed. The number in Co-Q10 refers to the number of isoprene units of the terpenoid side chain. Serum levels decline with age and illness (Sinatra, 2005).

BIBLIOGRAPHY

Berman M, et al. (2004). Coenzyme Q10 in patients with end stage heart failure awaiting cardiac transplantation: A randomized, placebo-controlled study. *Clinical Cardiology.* May;27(5): 295–299.

Bhagavan HM, Chopra RK. (2006). Coenzyme Q10: Absorption, tissue uptake, metabolism and pharmacokinetics. *Free Radical Research.* May;40(5):445–453.

Chillo M, et al. (1996). Protection by coenzyme Q10 of tissue reperfusion injury during abdominal aortic cross-clamping. *Journal of Cardiovascular Surgery (Torino).* 37(3):229–235.

Feher J, et al. (2005). Improvement of visual functions and fundus alterations in early age-related macular degeneration treated with a combination of acetyl-L-carnitine, n-3 fatty acids, and coenzyme Q10. *Opththalmologica.* May-Jun;219(3):154–166.

Gvozdjakova A, et al. (2005). Coenzyme Q10 supplementation reduces corticosteroids dosage in patients with bronchial asthma. *Biofactors.* 25(1–4):235–240.

Hirano M, et al. (2006). Restoring balance to ataxia with coenzyme Q10 deficiency. *Journal of Neurosurgical Sciences.* Jul 15;246(1–2): 11–12.

Integrative Medicine Access. (2000). *Co-enzyme Q10.* Newton, MA: Integrative Medicine Communications.

Kontush A, et al. (1997). Plasma ubiquinol-10 is decreased in patients with hyperlipidaemia. *Atherosclerosis.* 28;129(1):119–126.

Landbo C, Almdal TP. (1998). Interaction between warfarin and coenzyme Q10. *Ugeskrift for Laeger.* 160(22):3226–3227.

Langsjoem PH. (1994). *Introduction to Coenzyme Q10.* Tyler, TX: Research Reports.

Levy HB, Kohlhaas HK. (2006). Considerations for supplementing with coenzyme Q10 during statin therapy. *Annals of Pharmacotherapy.* Feb;40(2):290–294.

Littarru GP, Tiano L. (2005). Clinical aspects of coenzyme Q10: An update. *Current Opinion in Clinical Nutrition and Metabolic Care.* Nov;8(6):641–646.

Lockwood K, et al. (1994). Apparent partial remission of breast cancer in high risk patients supplemented with nutritional antioxidants, essential fatty acids and coenzyme Q10. *Molecular Aspects of Medicine.* 15[Suppl.]:S231–S240.

Modi S, Lowder DM. (2006). Medications for migraine prophylaxis. *American Family Physician.* Jan 1;73(1):72–78.

Morisco C, et al. (1993). Effect of coenzyme Q10 therapy in patients with congestive heart failure: A long-term multicenter randomized study. *Clinical Investigations.* 71[8 Suppl.]:S134–S136.

Mortensen SA, et al. (1997). Dose-related decrease of serum coenzyme Q10 during treatment with HMG-CoA reductase inhibitors. *Molecular Aspects of Medicine.* 18[Suppl.]:S137–S144.

Nibori K, et al. (1998). Acute administration of liposomal coenzyme Q10 increases myocardial tissue levels and improves tolerance to ischemia reperfusion injury. *Journal of Surgical Research.* 79(2):141.

Palomaki A, et al. (1998). Ubiquinone supplementation during lovastatin treatment: Effect on LDL oxidation ex vivo. *Journal of Lipid Research.* 39(7):1430–1437.

Sander S, et al. (2006). The impact of coenzyme Q10 on systolic function in patients with chronic heart failure. *Journal of Cardiac Failure.* Aug;12(6):464–472.

Serebruany UL, et al. (1997). Could coenzyme Q10 affect hemostasis by inhibiting platelet vitronectin (CD51/CD61) receptor? *Molecular Aspects of Medicine.* 18[Suppl.]:S189–S194.

Shults CW. (2005). Therapeutic role of coenzyme Q[10] in Parkinson's disease. *Pharmacology and Therapeutics.* Jul;107(1):120–130.

Sinatra ST. (2005). *The Sinatra Solution: Metabolic Cardiology.* New Jersey: Basic Health Publications.

Singh RB, et al. (1998). Randomized, double-blind placebo-controlled trial of coenzyme Q10 in patients with acute myocardial infarction. *Cardiovascular Drugs and Therapy.* 12(4):347–353.

Singh RB, et al. (1999). Effect of hydrosoluble coenzyme Q10 on blood pressures and insulin resistance in hypertensive patients with coronary artery disease. *Journal of Human Hypertension.* 13(3):203–208.

Singh RB, Niaz MA. (1999). Serum concentration of lipoprotein(a) decreases on treatment with hydrosoluble coenzyme Q10 in patients with coronary artery disease: Discovery of a new role. *International Journal of Cardiology.* 68(1):23–29.

Soja AM, Mortensen SA. (1997). Treatment of congestive heart failure with coenzyme Q10 illuminated by meta-analyses of clinical trials. *Molecular Aspects of Medicine.* 18[Suppl.]:S159–S168.

Vercelli L, et al. (2006). Chinese red rice depletes muscle coenzyme Q10 and maintains muscle damage after discontinuation of statin treatment. *Journal of the American Geriatrics Society.* Apr;54(4):718–720.

Watson PS, et al. (1999). Lack of effect of coenzyme Q on left ventricular function in patients with congestive heart failure. *Journal of the American College of Cardiology.* 33(6):1549–1552.

NAME: Fish Oils

Common Name: Fish oil, fatty marine oils, PUFA, W-3 fatty acids, omega-3 fatty acids, N-3 fatty acids

Description and Source:

- Fish oils come from marine fish, with mackerel, halibut, salmon, blue fish, mullet, sable fish, anchovy, herring, lake trout, coho, and sardines being the best sources. Each of the above-mentioned fish provides 1 g or more of omega-3 fish oil per 100 g or 3.5 oz of fish.
- Fish oils from the fatty fish are comprised of eicosa-pentaenoic acid (EPA) and docosahexaenoic acid (DHA). In fish, the EPA to DHA ratio is 1:5 to 1. In humans, DHA can be converted to EPA. DHA is most important for neurotransmitter production and cell wall production in the brain. The brain is the largest consumer of DHA.

DHA is currently being added to infant formulas (Vidaihet, 2007; Cunnane et al., 2000).
- Recent evaluations of many different fish oils suggest a very low level of mercury and other contaminates. For a review of individual products, visit www.consumerlab.com.

Biological Activity:
- Anti-inflammatory effect
  - Likely due to inhibition of leukotriene synthesis (Navarro et al., 2000)
  - Compete with arachidonic acid in the cyclooxygenase and lipoxygenase pathways (de Souza et al., 2006; Tjonahen et al., 2006; Massaro et al., 2006)
- Decrease production of VLDL and improve VLDL clearance (Simopoulos, 2006)
- Improve hepatic uptake of triglycerides
- Decrease cholesterol absorption and synthesis
- Improve HDL production (Simopoulos, 2006)
- Antithrombotic activity results from prostacyclin syntheses effect and a reduction of thromboxane 2
- Anticarcinogenic effect in colon, protects against colon cancer (Kimura, 2006; Larsen, 2006)
- Restores lipid profiles in bone marrow secondary to statins (Pritchett, 2007)
- Fatty acids are required to synthesize dopamine and may improve symptoms of schizophrenia (O'Hara, 2006)
- Improves low levels of long-chain omega-3 fatty acids in adults with ADD (Young et al, 2005)

Nutritional Sources: Fatty fish

Current Use:
- Reduces hypertriglyceridemia by 20% to 50%—reduction is very dose dependent (Qi et al., 2006)
- Reduces mortality after acute MI
- Reduces blood pressure—both systolic and diastolic—by about 4.4 mm Hg (Larsen, 2006)
- Improves depression by improving nerve signaling and serotonin levels; increases length of remission (Su et al., 2003; Marangell et al., 2003; Larsen, 2006).

- Decreases ventricular ectopy and risk of sudden death (Grundt et al., 2003; Rupp et al., 2004; Jabbar & Saldeen, 2006; Oh et al., 2006). However, one study found an increase in sudden death in persons with implanted defibrillators.
- May help reduce cyclosporine-induced nephrotoxicity
- Reduces inflammation in rheumatoid arthritis (EPA is decreased in total plasma fatty acids and both EPA and DHA are decreased in synovial fluid), and reduces need for NSAIDs.
  - Eskimos have a very low incidence of RA and psoriasis and have a very high intake of fish oils in their diet (Larsen, 2006)
- Decreases blood viscosity and increases red blood cell deformability
- Has antithrombotic activity due to vasodilation, platelet adhesiveness reduction, platelet count reduction and prolonged bleeding time (Pedersen et al, 2003)
- In Type 2 diabetes, may improve arterial compliance (Pedersen et al., 2003)
- Improves lipid composition of bone marrow and joints (Pritchett, 2007)
- Improves phosphatidylcholine docosahexaenoic acid in brain—may decrease risk of Alzheimer's and dementia (Schaefer et al., 2006; Morris, 2006; de Ladoucette, 2006; Freund-Levi et al., 2006)
- Protects against ischemia, light, oxygen, inflammatory and age-associated pathology of the vascular and neural retinae (SanGiovanni & Chew, 2005)
- Decreases disease activity in ankylosing spondylitis (Sundstrom et al., 2006); hypertriglyceridemia reduced by 20% to 50%—reduction very dose dependent (Qi et al., 2006)

Available Forms, Dosage, and Administration Guidelines: Generally available as 1 g capsules.
- Adult dose: 1 to 10 g/day/divided
  - Read the label carefully. The best product is like the fatty fish (EPA 1.5 to DHA 1), so EPA 180:DHA 120, or EPA 300:DHA 200, etc. It is permissible to have

omega 9 (olive, canola, or peanut oil) in the fish oil, but omega 6 should NEVER be added. Omega 3 and 9 are both anti-inflammatory oils. Omega 6 (vegetable oils such as corn, sunflower, safflower, etc.) is an inflammatory oil.

° Fish oil is highly unstable and begins to oxidize after extraction from the fish and exposure to light, heat, and metals. Fish oils become rancid easily, so there should be an antioxidant in the capsule (rosemary or vitamin E [d-alpha, NOT dL]).

° To eliminate "fishy burps," put fish oil capsules in freezer (good-quality fish oil should not freeze solid) and take out of freezer and swallow with water. It is best when consumed with food. When buying fish oils, it is a good idea to actually chew a capsule from the bottle. If it tastes "terrible" it is probably rancid and will actually create more O_2 radicals in the body, and may increase the risk of ASHD.

Pharmakinetics—If Available (form or route when known):
Absorbed: Easily absorbed
Distributed: Transported to liver
Metabolized: Liver—majority of fatty acids are oxidized to meet energy requirements

Toxicity: None

Contraindications: In persons demonstrating hypersensitivity to fish

Side Effects: Dyspepsia and eructation of fishy taste. Heartburn, nosebleeds, nausea, loose stools

Use in Pregnancy/Lactation/Children: No data suggests toxicity, but studies are unavailable. Long-chain fatty acids are required during pregnancy and lactation (Jensen et al., 2005; Makrides & Gibson, 2000)

Drug/Herb Interactions and Rationale (if known):
• Fish oils may increase the anticoagulant effect and therefore bleeding risk in patients taking Warfarin (Buckley, 2004).

Patients taking Warfarin need to advise their practitioners, and their INRs must be evaluated carefully.
- May induce activity of the cytochrome P450 enzymatic system in the liver; needs further study
- Theoretical concern with concurrent vitamin E, gingko, angelica, *Panax ginseng*, horse chestnut, and willow (these herbs are believed to have a blood-thinning effect)

Special Notes:

- In 2006, the pharmaceutical industry released a prescription fish oil, omega-3 acid ethyl esters (Omacor). Omacor has an unreal EPA:DHA ratio (EPA—460 mg: DHA—300 mg)
- Omacor is indicated for hypertriglyceride level >500 mg/dL (ideal level <150 mg/dL) and prevention of myocardial infarction
- Omacor has soy as an excipient, so it should be avoided by anyone with soy allergy
- Cod liver oil, extracted from cod liver, is an excellent source of vitamins A and D, but has very small amounts of EPA and DHA

BIBLIOGRAPHY

Buckley MS, et al. (2004). Fish oil interaction with warfarin. *Annals of Pharmacotherapy*. Jan;38(1):50–52.

Cunnane SC, et al. (2000). Breast-fed infants achieve a higher rate of brain and whole body docosahexaenoate accumulation than formula-fed infants not consuming dietary docosahexaenoate. *Lipids*. Jan;35(1):105–111.

de Ladoucette O. (2006). New therapeutic approaches to Alzheimer's disease (In French). *Soins. Gérontolie*. Sept–Oct; (61):11–13.

de Souza PM, et al. (2006). Targeting lipoxygenases with care. *Chemistry & Biology*. Nov;13(11):1121–1122.

Freund-Levi Y, et al. (2006). Omega-3 fatty acid treatment in 174 patients with mild to moderate Alzheimer disease: OmegAD study: a randomized double-blind trial. *Archives of Neurology*. Oct;63(10):1402–1408.

Grundt H, et al. (2003). Increased lipid peroxidation during long-term intervention with high doses of n-3 fatty acids (PUFAs) following an acute myocardial infarction. *European Journal of Clinical Nutrition*. Jun;57(6):793–800.

Jabbar R, Saldeen T. (2006). A new predictor of risk for sudden cardiac death. *Upsala Journal of Medical Sciences.* 111(2): 169–177.

Jensen CL, et al. (2005). Effect of docosahexaenoic acid supplementation of lactating women on the fatty acid composition of breast milk lipids and maternal and infant plasma phospholipids. *American Journal of Clinical Nutrition.* Jul;82(1):125–132.

Kimura Y. (2006). Fish, n-3 polyunsaturated fatty acid and colorectal cancer prevention: a review of experimental and epidemiological studies (In Japanese). *Nippon Koshu Eisei Zasshi.* Oct;53(10): 735–748.

Larsen HR. (2006). Fish oils: the essential nutrients. Retrieved Dec 20, 2006, from www.pinc.com/healthnews/fishoils.html.

Makrides M, Gibson RA. (2000). Long-chain polyunsaturated fatty acid requirements during pregnancy and lactation. *American Journal of Clinical Nutrition.* Jan;71(1 Suppl):307S–311S.

Marangell LB, et al. (2003). A double-blind, placebo-controlled study of the omega-3 fatty acid docosahexaenoic acid in the treatment of major depression. *American Journal of Psychiatry.* 160(5):996–998.

Massaro M, et al. (2006). The omega-3 fatty acid docosa-hexaenoate attenuates endothelial cyclooxygenase-2 induction through both NADP(H) oxidase and PKC epsilon inhibition. *Proceedings of the National Academy of Science U S A.* Oct;103 (41):15184–15189.

Morris MC. (2006). Docosahexaenoic acid and Alzheimer disease. *Archives of Neurology.* Nov;63(11):1527–1528.

Navarro E, et al. (2000). Abnormal fatty acid pattern in rheumatoid arthritis. A rationale for treatment with marine and botanical lipids. *Journal of Rheumatology.* Feb;27(2):298–303.

Oh RC, et al. (2006). The fish in secondary prevention of heart disease (FISH) survey–primary care physicians and omega3 fatty acid prescribing behaviors. *Journal of the American Board of Family Medicine.* Sep–Oct;19(5):459–467.

Ohara K. (2006). The n-3 fatty acid/dopamine hypothesis in schizophrenia (In Japanese). *Nihon Shinkei Seishin Yakurigaku Zasshi.* Aug;26(4):149–153.

Pedersen H, et al. (2003). Influence of fish oil supplementation on in vivo and in vitro oxidation resistance of low-density lipoprotein in type 2 diabetes. *European Journal of Clinical Nutrition.* May;57(5):713–720.

Pritchett JW. (2007). Statins and dietary fish oils improve lipid composition in bone marrow and joints. *Clinical Orthopaedics and Related Research.* Mar;456:233–237.

Qi K, et al. (2006). Triglycerides in fish oil affect the blood clearance of lipid emulsions containing long- and medium-chain triglycerides in mice. *Journal of Nutrition.* Nov;136(11):2766–2772.

Rupp H, et al. (2004). Risk stratification by the "EPA+DHA level" and the "EPA/AA ratio" focus on anti-inflammatory and antiarrhythmogenic effects of long-chain omega-3 fatty acids. *Herz.* Nov;29(7):673–685. Review. Erratum in: *Herz.* Dec;29(8):805.

SanGiovanni JP, Chew EY. (2005). The role of omega-3 long-chain polyunsaturated fatty acids in health and disease of the retina. *Progress in Retinal and Eye Research.* Jan;24(1):87–138.

Schaefer EJ, et al. (2006). Plasma phosphatidylcholine docosahexaenoic acid content and risk of dementia and Alzheimer disease: the Framingham Heart Study. *Archives of Neurology.* Nov;63(11):1545–1550.

Simopoulos AP. (2006). Evolutionary aspects of diet, the omega-6/omega-3 ratio and genetic variation: nutritional implications for chronic diseases. *Biomedicine & Pharmacotherapy.* Nov;60(9): 502–507.

Su KP, et al. (2003). Omega-3 fatty acids in major depressive disorder. A preliminary double-blind, placebo-controlled trial. *European Neuropsychopharmacology.* Aug;13(4):267–271; Erratum in: *European Neuropsychopharmacology.* 2004 Mar;14(2):173.

Sundstrom B, et al. (2006). Supplementation of omega-3 fatty acids in patients with ankylosing spondylitis. *Scandinavian Journal of Rheumatology.* Sep–Oct;35(5):359–362.

Tjonahen E, et al. (2006). Resolvin E2: identification and anti-inflammatory actions: pivotal role of human 5-lipoxygenase in resolvin E series biosynthesis. *Chemistry & Biology.* Nov;13(11):1193–1202.

Vidailhet M. (2007). Omega 3: is there a situation of deficiency in young children? (In French). *Archives de Pédiatrie.* Jan;14(1):116–123.

Young GS, et al. (2005). Effect of randomized supplementation with high dose olive, flax or fish oil on serum phospholipid fatty acid levels in adults with attention deficit hyperactivity disorder. *Reproduction, Nutrition, Development.* Sep–Oct;45(5):549–558.

NAME: Glucosamine Sulfate (2-amino 2-deoxyglucose; glucosamine HCl)

Common Names: GS, chitosamine

Description and Source: A simple molecule composed of glucose, an amine (nitrogen and hydrogen), and sulfur.

Glucosamine is a fundamental building block of cartilage
glycosaminoglycan (GAG) and is a natural substance found in
mucopolysaccharides, mucoproteins, and chiten. Glucosamine
sulfate is manufactured. Sulfate is the preferred form. Sulfur is
an essential nutrient for joint tissue that stabilizes the
connective tissue matrix of cartilage.

Biologic Activity
• Glucosamine is formed from the glycolytic intermediate
  fructose-6-phosphate via amination, with glutamine acting as
  the donor, yielding glucosamine-6-phosphate, which is
  acetylated and/or converted to galactosamine for
  incorporation into the growing GAG (Reginster et al., 2006).
• Stimulates the manufacture of cartilage components and
  promotes the incorporation of sulfur into cartilage (Kelly, 1998)
• Stimulates joint repair; some people lose the ability to
  manufacture glucosamine and therefore cannot repair joints
  (Barclay et al., 1998; Da Camara & Dowless, 1998)
• Allows cartilage to act as a shock absorber (Verbruggen, 2006)
• Reduces tenderness and improves mobility (Qiu et al., 1998)

Nutritional Sources: None known

Current Use: Antiarthritic for osteoarthritis; prevents joint
space narrowing. May stimulate hyaluronic acid, which is anti-
inflammatory and an analgesic. Glucosamine is as effective as
nonsteroidal anti-inflammatories in improving mobility and
decreasing the pain of osteoarthritis without irritating the
gastric mucosa (Poolsup et al., 2005; Reginster et al., 2006).

Available Forms, Dosage, and Administration Guidelines
Preparations: Capsules, tablets
Typical Dosage: Divide the total dosage into three or four
doses a day and take with food. As improvement occurs,
reduce the dose to the lowest effective dose. European studies
suggest that people who are very obese or are taking diuretics
may need higher doses (McCarty, 1994; Qiu et al., 1998).
Take product for 3 months to determine efficacy.

Pharmacokinetics—If Available (form or route when known): Ninety percent is absorbed with oral administration,

but substantial amounts are metabolized by the liver, and only 26% reaches the blood.

Toxicity: None known

Contraindications: Patients with type 2 diabetes should monitor blood sugar levels. It has been reported that patients with insulin resistance might find that glucosamine worsens their symptoms (elevated triglycerides, obesity, carbohydrate cravings). A recent study found no increase of insulin resistance or endothelial dysfunction with glucosamine usage (Muniyappa et al., 2006).

Side Effects: Mild GI upset and irritation, diarrhea, and flatulence; drowsiness, skin reactions, headaches. Some studies suggested glucosamine might increase blood suger levels but more recent research found no effect on blood glucose (StumpF & Lin, 2006).

Long-Term Safety: Short-term studies suggest safety, but no long-term studies are available.

Use in Pregnancy/Lactation/Children: Not known; do not use

Drug/Herb Interactions and Rationale (if known): None known

Special Notes: Chronic use of nonsteroidal anti-inflammatories has been shown to prevent joint repair. Glucosamine sulfate has been shown to reduce pain and inflammation and allows the joint to heal. Many glucosamine products are derived from crab shells. People with shellfish allergies should avoid these products and use glucosamine derived from corn.

BIBLIOGRAPHY

Barclay TS, et al. (1998). Glucosamine. *Annals of Pharmacotherapy*. 32(4):574–579.

Da Camara CC, Dowless GV. (1998). Glucosamine sulfate for osteoarthritis. *Annals of Pharmacotherapy*. 32(5):580–587.

Kelly GS. (1998). The role of glucosamine sulfate and chondroitin sulfates in the treatment of degenerative joint disease. *Alternative Medicine Review*. 3(1):27–39.

McAlindon TE, et al. (2000). Glucosamine and chondroitin for treatment of osteoarthritis: A systematic quality assessment and meta-analysis. *Journal of the American Medical Association.* 283(11):1469–1475.

Muniyappa R, et al. (2006). Oral glucosamine for 6 weeks at standard doses does not cause or worsen insulin resistance or endothelial dysfunction in lean or obese subjects. *Diabetes.* Nov;55(11):3142–3150.

Poolsup N, et al. (2005). Glucosamine long-term treatment and the progression of knee osteoarthritis: Systematic review of randomized controlled trials. *Annals of Pharmacotherapy.* Jun;39(6):1080–1087.

Qiu GX, et al. (1998). Efficacy and safety of glucosamine sulfate versus ibuprofen in patients with knee osteoarthritis. *Arzneimittelforschung.* 48(5):469–474.

Reginster JY, et al. (2006). Glucosamine as a pain-modifying drug in osteoarthritis. What's new in 2006? *Revue Medicale de Liege.* Mar;61(3):169–172.

Rindone JP, et al. (2000). Randomized, controlled trial of glucosamine for treating osteoarthritis of the knee. *Western Journal of Medicine.* 172(2):91–94.

Rovati LC. (1994). A large randomized, placebo-controlled, double-blind study of glucosamine sulfate vs. piroxicam and vs. their association, on the kinetics of the symptomatic effect in knee osteoarthritis. *Osteoarthritis and Cartilage.* 2[Suppl. 1]:56.

Rozendaal RM, et al. (2005). The effect of glucosamine sulphate on osteoarthritis: Design of a long-term randomised clinical trial (ISRCTN54513166). *BMC Musculoskeletal Disorders.* Apr 26;6(1):20.

StumpF JL, Lin SW. (2006). Effect of glucosamine on glucose control. *Annals of Pharmacotherapy.* Apr;40(4):694–698.

Verbruggen G. (2006). Chondroprotective drugs in degenerative joint diseases. *Rheumatology (Oxford).* Feb;45(2):129–139.

NAME: Lipoic Acid

Common Names: Alpha lipoic acid, thioctic acid, thioctacid, acetate replacing factor

Description and Source: Fat- and water-soluble, sulfur-containing antioxidant that can be synthesized in the body

Biologic Activity
- May be the most powerful antioxidant made by the body (Ley, 1996)

- Boosts levels and can recycle glutathione by 30%
- Recycles other antioxidants, vitamins A and C
- Turns off "bad" genes (aging, cancer)
- Enhances immune function
- Protects neurotransmitters
- Functions as a coenzyme with pyrophosphatase in carbohydrate metabolism
- Oxygen free radical scavenger inside and outside cell

Nutritional Sources: Yeast, liver, and spinach are fairly good sources; broccoli, kidney, heart, and potatoes contain small amounts of lipoic acid

Current Use
- May benefit patients with HIV and prevent cancer
- Prevents cataracts and other degenerative eye diseases
- Decreases stroke-related injuries
- Treats hepatotoxicity caused by poisonous mushroom ingestion, so initial evidence suggests that it may protect the liver in cirrhosis and hepatitis B and C (Berkson, 1999)
- Decreases complications in diabetes (diabetic retinopathy, cataracts, neuropathy) (Ziegler et al., 1997), prescribed in Germany for diabetic neuropathy (Hahm et al., 2004), improves blood sugar metabolism, improves burning mouth syndrome (Femiano & Scully, 2002)
- A pilot study found that children with severe kwashiokor had improved survival rates and recovery when alpha lipoid acid, reduced glutathione, or N-acetylcysteine was added to their diets (Becker et al., 2005).

Available Forms, Dosage, and Administration Guidelines: 500 to 600 mg a day divided into two doses

Pharmacokinetics—If Available (form or route when known): Not known

Toxicity: None known. A two-year animal study found no toxicity or histopathological changes (Cremer et al., 2006).

Contraindications: None known

Side Effects: Rarely, skin rash

Long-Term Safety: Unknown

Use in Pregnancy/Lactation/Children: No data suggests toxicity. Pregnant and lactating women should consult with their physician.

Drug/Herb Interactions and Rationale (if known): If taken with insulin and antidiabetic drugs, dosage of medications may need to be reduced. Monitor blood sugar levels closely. ALA may reduce toxicity of gentamicin and cisplatin when given concurrently.

Special Notes: Recent research suggests that lipoic acid does not change current symptoms but may decrease overall complications associated with diabetic neuropathy. More research is needed (Ziegler et al., 1999a, 1999b).

BIBLIOGRAPHY

Becker K, et al. (2005). Effects of antioxidants on glutathione levels and clinical recovery from the malnutrition syndrome kwashiorkor—A pilot study. *Redox Report.* 10(4):215–226.

Berkson BM. (1999). A conservative triple antioxidant approach to the treatment of hepatitis C. Combination of alpha-lipoic acid (thioctic acid), silymarin, and selenium: Three case histories. *Medizinsiche Klinikum.* 94[Suppl. 3]:84–89.

Cremer DR, et al. (2006). Long-term safety of alpha-lipoic acid (ALA) consumption: A 2-year study. *Regulatory Toxicology and Pharmacology.* Dec;46(3):193–201.

Femiano F, Scully C. (2002). Burning mouth syndrome (BMS): Double-blind controlled study of alpha-lipoic acid (thioctic acid) therapy. *Journal of Oral Pathology and Medicine.* May;31(5):267–269.

Gleiter CH, et al. (1999). Lack of interaction between thioctic acid, glibenclamide and acarbose. *British Journal of Clinical Pharmacology.* 48(6):819–825.

Hahm JR, et al. (2004). Clinical experience with thioctacid (thioctic acid) in the treatment of distal symmetric polyneuropathy in Korean diabetic patients. *Journal of Diabetes and Its Complications.* Mar-Apr;18(2):79–85.

Henricksen EJ. Exercise training and the antioxidant alpha-lipoic acid in the treatment of insulin resistance and type 2 diabetes. *Free Radical Biology and Medicine.* Jan 1;40(1):3–12.

Marangon K, Devaraj S. (1999). Comparison of the effect of alpha-lipoic acid and alpha-tocopherol supplementation on measures of oxidative stress. *Free Radicals Biology in Medicine.* 27(9–10): 1114–1121.

Ruhnau KJ, et al. (1999). Effects of 3-week oral treatment with the antioxidant thioctic acid (alpha-lipoic acid) in symptomatic diabetic polyneuropathy. *Diabetes Medicine.* 16(12):1050–1053.

Ziegler D, et al. (1997). Effects of treatment with the antioxidant alpha-lipoic acid on cardiac autonomic neuropathy in NIDDM patients. A 4-month randomized controlled multicenter trial. *Diabetes Care.* 20:369–373.

Ziegler D, et al. (1999a). Alpha-lipoic acid in the treatment of diabetic polyneuropathy in Germany: Current evidence from clinical trials. *Experimental and Clinical Endocrinology and Diabetes.* 107(7):421–430.

Ziegler D, et al. (1999b). Treatment of symptomatic diabetic polyneuropathy with the antioxidant alpha-lipoic acid: A 7-month multicenter randomized controlled trial. *Diabetes Care.* 22(8):1296–1301.

 NAME: Lycopene

Common Names: None

Description and Source: A carotenoid that occurs in red and pink fruits

Biologic Activity

- Antioxidant: twice as effective as beta-carotene (Agarwal & Rao, 1998; Hadley et al., 2003)
- Reduces activity of oxygen free radicals (Klebanov et al., 1998)
- Inhibits serum lipid peroxidation, decreases LDL cholesterol, and reduces risk of MI (Kohlmeier et al., 1997)
- Enhances immune function and cell-to-cell communication and inhibits tumor cell growth

Nutritional Sources: Red and pink fruits. Tomatoes are the best source, especially if cooked (increases the available lycopene; tomato paste, sauce, juice). Also watermelon, guava, pink grapefruit, strawberries, and apricots.

Current Use

- Lowers risk of prostate enlargement and prostate cancer, especially when combined with tocopherols (Amir et al., 1999; Gann et al., 1999; Fraser et al., 2005)

- Prevents macular degeneration, a leading cause of blindness in the elderly (Seddon et al., 1994); use with lutein, blueberry, and ginkgo for best results
- Lowers incidence of many cancers (stomach, pancreatic, prostate, colon, rectum, cervix) (Kantesky et al., 1998; Sengupta & Das, 1999)
- In a small study, lycopene (4 or 8 mg) was an effective treatment for oral leukoplakia (Zakrzewska, 2005).
- Pregnant women with pre-eclampsia or intrauterine growth retardation were given lycopene in a double-blind study. The women with pre-eclampsia had lower blood pressure than the placebo group, and it prevented uterine growth retardation (Sharma et al., 2003).
- Men with idiopathic male infertility had improved sperm concentration and motility when given lycopene (Gupta & Kumar, 2002).

Available Forms, Dosage, and Administration Guidelines: To enhance intestinal absorption of lycopene, consume oils or fats at the same time (Porrini et al., 1998). Intake goal is 10 half-cup servings of lycopene-rich food a week or one 10- to 15-mg gel cap a day. As a supplement, take 5 to 10 mg a day.

Pharmacokinetics—If Available (form or route when known): Not known

Toxicity: None known

Contraindications: None known

Side Effects: None known

Long-Term Safety: Safe in dietary quantities

Use in Pregnancy/Lactation/Children: Safe in dietary quantities; large amounts as an isolate, safety unknown

Drug/Herb Interactions and Rationale (if known): None known

Special Notes: Carotenoid mixtures, especially with lycopene and lutein, have a synergistic antioxidant and anticancer activity.

BIBLIOGRAPHY

Agarwal S, Rao AV. (1998). Tomato lycopene and low-density lipoprotein oxidation: A human dietary intervention study. *Lipids*. 33(10):981–984.

Amir H, et al. (1999). Lycopene and 1,25-dihydroxyvitamin D3 cooperate in the inhibition of cell cycle progression and induction of differentiation in HL-60 leukemic cells. *Nutrition and Cancer*. 33(1):105–112.

Ansari MS, et al. (2004). Lycopene: A novel drug therapy in hormone refractory metastatic prostate cancer. *Urologic Oncology*. Sep-Oct; 22(5):415–420.

Clinton S. (1998). Lycopene: Chemistry, biology, and implications for human health and disease. *Nutrition Review*. 56[2 Pt. 1]:35–51.

Engelhard YN, et al. (2006). Natural antioxidants from tomato extract reduce blood pressure in patient with grade-1 hypertension: A double-blind, placebo-controlled pilot study. *American Heart Journal*. Jan;151(1):100.

Fraser ML, et al. (2005). Lycopene and prostate cancer: emerging evidence. *Expert Review of Anticancer Therapy*. Oct;5(5): 847–854.

Gann PH, et al. (1999). Lower prostate cancer risk in men with elevated plasma lycopene levels: Results of a prospective analysis. *Cancer Research*. 59(6):1225–1230.

Gupta NP, Kumar R. (2002). Lycopene therapy in idiopathic male infertility—A preliminary report. *International Urology and Nephrology*. 34(3):369–372.

Hadley CW, et al. (2003). The consumption of processed tomato products enhances plasma lycopene concentrations in association with a reduced lipoprotein sensitivity to oxidative damage. *Journal of Nutrition*. Mar;133(3):727–732.

Kantesky P, et al. (1998). Dietary intake and blood levels of lycopene: Association with cervical dysplasia among non-Hispanic, black women. *Nutrition and Cancer*. 31(1):31–40.

Kirsh VA, et al. (2006). A prospective study of lycopene and tomato product intake and risk of prostate cancer. *Cancer Epidemiology, Biomarkers and Prevention*. Jan;15(1):92–98.

Klebanov GI, et al. (1998). The antioxidant properties of lycopene. *Membranes and Cell Biology*. 12(2):287–300.

Kohlmeier I, et al. (1997). Lycopene and myocardial infarction risk in the EURAMIC Study. *American Journal of Epidemiology*. 146(8):618–626.

Krinsky N. (1998). Overview of lycopene, carotenoids, and disease prevention. *Proceedings of the Society for Experimental Biology and Medicine*. 218(2):95–97.

Mohanty NK, et al. (2005). Lycopene as a chemopreventive agent in the treatment of high-grade prostate intraepithelial neoplasia. *Urologic Oncology.* Nov-Dec;23(6):383–385.

Porrini M, et al. (1998). Absorption of lycopene from single or daily portions of raw and processed tomato. *British Journal of Nutrition.* 80(4):353–361.

Sengupta A, Das S. (1999). The anti-carcinogenic role of lycopene, abundantly present in tomato. *European Journal of Cancer Prevention.* 8(4):325–330.

Sharma JB, et al. (2003). Effect of lycopene on pre-eclampsia and intra-uterine growth retardation in primigravidas. *International Journal of Gynaecology and Obstetrics.* Jun;81(3):257–262.

Weisburger J. (1998). International symposium on the role of lycopene and tomato products in disease prevention. *Proceedings of the Society for Experimental Biology and Medicine.* 218(2):93–94.

Zakrzewska JM. (2005). Oral lycopene—An efficacious treatment for oral leukoplakia? *Evidence-Based Dentistry.* 6(1):17–18.

 NAME: Melatonin (*N*-acetyl-5-methoxytryptamine)

Common Names: Pineal hormone

Description and Source
- Melatonin is a hormone produced by the pineal gland during sleep. For melatonin to be produced, the pineal gland must perceive darkness; thus, people who work swing shifts and must sleep during the day make less melatonin and therefore have difficulty obtaining restful sleep and multiple REM cycles. Melatonin enhances REM cycles (Middleton, 2006).
- Melatonin production is highest in children and decreases with age.
- Natural or synthetically produced hormone
- Melatonin is produced from tryptophan → serotonin → melatonin.

Biologic Activity
- Enhances sleep (Zhdanova & Wurtman, 1997)
- Modulates circadian rhythm (Buscemi et al., 2006; Kunz et al., 2004; Zawilska & Nowak, 1999)
- Enhances immune system function (Lissoni et al., 2003)

- May decrease incidence of hormone-dependent cancers (e.g., breast, prostate cancers) (Erren & Piekarski, 1999; Lissoni et al., 2003; Reiter et al., 2002)
- May reduce stress (Kirby et al., 1999)
- Acts as an oxygen (hydroxyl) free radical scavenger (Reiter et al., 2002)

Nutritional Sources: Oats, sweet corn, and rice

Current Use
- May be useful for sleep disorders in children associated with autism, Down's syndrome, epilepsy, and cerebral palsy, and sleep latency
- Used to enhance sleep (blind persons, jet lag, insomnia, and the elderly) (Buscemi et al., 2006; Campos et al., 2004; Zhdanova et al., 1995). It also increased REM sleep in patients with neuropsychiatric sleep disorders (Kunz et al., 2004).
- Male patients with essential hypertension took 2.5 mg melatonin and had reduced nighttime blood pressure as well as enhanced sleep (Scheer et al., 2004).
- May be useful for seasonal affective disorder
- Stimulates the immune system: monocytes and NK cells
- Acts as an antioxidant, oxygen free radical scavenger
- Nightly supplement (10 mg) may improve cancer survival rates in persons with metastatic nonsmall—cell lung cancer, especially if combined with interferon or interleukin-2 therapy. It enhances their activity and reduces adverse effects.
- Melatonin and zinc, when used with or without metformin, improved fasting and postprandial glycemic control in type II diabetic patients (Hussain et al., 2006).

Available Forms, Dosage, and Administration Guidelines
- For sleep only: 0.1 to 0.3 mg (up to 1 mg) 1 hour before sleep
- For jet lag: start a day before travel (close to target bedtime at the destination). Then take every 24 hours for several days. Best dose is 0.1 to 0.5 mg. Larger doses are not as effective. Slow-release melatonin is not as effective as quick-release formulations. If dose is taken too early in the day, it may actually result in excessive daytime sleepiness and greater difficulty adapting to the destination time zone (Herxheimer et al., 2002).

- Slow-release melatonin, in 2-mg doses, may enhance sleep (Samuel, 1999).
- For children with developmental disorders: 5 mg a day
- For blind persons with sleep problems: 5 mg orally at bedtime
- For elderly persons with insomnia: 1 to 2 mg at bedtime (Haimov et al., 1995)
- Does not alter endogenous melatonin production
- Adjunctive therapy for cancer: 10–50 mg a day

Pharmacokinetics—If Available (form or route when known): Half-life, 20 to 50 minutes; metabolized in liver

Toxicity: No acute toxicity, but long-term potential for health problems unknown

Contraindications: Pregnancy and lactation, when trying to get pregnant, severe mental illness, autoimmune disease, cancers of the blood or bones, hepatic insufficiency from reduced clearance

Side Effects: Headache; vivid dreams, nightmares (Guardiola-Lemaitre, 1997); transient depression; morning lethargy; mood changes; drowsiness (use caution driving for 30 minutes after taking melatonin); unfavorable shifts in circadian rhythm

Long-Term Safety: No acute toxicity, but long-term safety issues are yet to be researched. In rats, long-term use inhibits uptake of T4 and T3.

Use in Pregnancy/Lactation/Children: Avoid in pregnant and lactating women; use in children under professional supervision only.

Drug/Herb Interactions and Rationale (if known)
- Antiseizure medication; research is mixed—may or may not affect seizure activity
- The following drugs may deplete melatonin: alcohol, antidepressants, anxiolytics, beta-blockers, Ca^{++} channel blockers, caffeine, nonsteroidal anti-inflammatories, steroids, tobacco, and immunosuppressive medications.

Special Notes
- There is no standardization for quality and purity among OTC products.

- May have some potential for use as contraceptive, but more research is needed
- Patient should be told that sleep disorders need a comprehensive program of behavior modification and counseling as well as pharmacologic agents.

BIBLIOGRAPHY

Benloucif S, et al. (1999). Nimodipine potentiates the light-induced suppression of melatonin. *Neuroscience Letters.* 272(1):67–71.

Blaicher W, et al. (2000). Melatonin in postmenopausal females. *Archives of Gynecology and Obstetrics.* 263(3):116–118.

Buscemi N, et al. (2006). Efficacy and safety of exogenous metatonin for secondary sleep disorders and sleep disorders accompanying sleep restrictions: meta-analysis. *British Medical Journal.* Feb 18;332(7538):385–393.

Campos FL, et al. (2004). Melatonin improves sleep in asthma: A randomized, double-blind, placebo-controlled study. *American Journal of Respiratory and Critical Care Medicine.* Nov 1;170(9):947–951.

Cardinali DP, et al. (2002). A double-blind placebo controlled study on metatonin efficacy to reduce anxislytic benzodiazepine use in the elderly. *Neuro Endocrinology Letteers.* Feb;23(1):55–60.

Chase JE, Gidal BE. (1997). Melatonin: Therapeutic use in sleep disorders. *Annals of Pharmacotherapy.* 31(10):1218–1226.

Citera G, et al. (2000). The effect of melatonin in patients with fibromyalgia: A pilot study. *Clinical Rheumatology.* 19(1):9–13.

Erren TC, Piekarski C. (1999). Does winter darkness in the Arctic protect against cancer? The melatonin hypothesis revisited. *Medical Hypotheses.* 53(1):1–5.

Garfinkel D, et al. (1995). Improvement of sleep quality in elderly people by controlled-release melatonin. *Lancet.* 346:541–544.

Guardiola-Lemaitre B. (1997). Toxicology of melatonin. *Journal of Biologic Rhythms.* 12(6):697–706.

Haimov I, et al. (1995). Melatonin replacement therapy of elderly insomniacs. *Sleep.* 18:598–603.

Herxheimer A, et al. (2002). Melatonin for the prevention and treatment of jet lag. *Cochrane Database of Systematic Reviews.* (2):CD001520.

Hussain SA, et al. (2006). Effects of melatonin and zinc on glycemic control in type 2 diabetic patients poorly controlled with metformin. *Saudi Medical Journal.* Oct;27(10):1483–1488.

Integrative Medicine Access. (2000). *Melatonin.* Newton, MA: Integrative Medicine Communications.

Kirby AW, et al. (1999). Melatonin and the reduction or alleviation of stress. *Journal of Pineal Research.* 27(2):78–85.

Kunz D, et al. (2004). Melatonin in patients with reduced REM sleep duration: Two randomized controlled trials. *Journal of Clinical Endocrinology and Metabolism.* Jan;89(1):128–134.

Lissoni P, et al. (1996). Is there a role for melatonin in the treatment of neoplastic cachexia? *European Journal of Cancer.* 32A:1340–1343.

Megwalu UC, et al. (2006). The effects of melatonin on tinnitus and sleep. *Otolaryngology—Head and Neck Surgery.* Feb;134(2):210–213.

Middleton B. (2006). Measurement of melatonin and 6-sulphatoxymelatonin. *Methods in Molecular Biology.* 324:235–254.

Nagtegaal JE, et al. (2000). Effects of melatonin on the quality of life in patients with delayed sleep phase syndrome. *Journal of Psychosomatic Research.* 48(1):45–50.

Ozbek E, et al. (2000). Melatonin administration prevents the nephrotoxicity induced by gentamicin. *BJU International.* 85(6):742–746.

Reiter RJ, et al. (2002). Melatonin reduces oxidant damage and promotes mitochondrial respiration: Implications for aging. *Annals of the New York Academy of Sciences.* Apr;959:238–250.

Rufo-Campos, M. (2002). Melatonin and epilepsy. *Review of Neurology.* Sep;35[Suppl. 1]:S51–S58.

Samuel A. (1999). Melatonin and jet-lag. *European Journal of Medical Research.* 4(9):385–388.

Scheer FA, et al. (2004). Daily nighttime melatonin reduces blood pressure in male patients with essential hypertension. *Hypertension.* Feb;43(2):192–197.

Zawilska JB, Nowak JZ. (1999). Melatonin: From biochemistry to therapeutic applications. *Polish Journal of Pharmacology.* 51(1):3–23.

Zhdanova IV, Wurtman RJ. (1997). Efficacy of melatonin as a sleep-promoting agent. *Journal of Biologic Rhythms.* 12(6):644–650.

 NAME: Methylsulfonylmethane (MSM)

Common Names: Crystalline $DMSO_2$

Description and Source

- MSM is a natural chemical found in green plants such as algae, fruit, vegetables, and grains.
- It occurs naturally in fresh food but is destroyed by heat, dehydration, and processing.

Biologic Activity

- MSM is the normal oxidation product of DMSO (dimethyl sulfoxide). It is odor-free and provides sulfur for methionine.

- May bind to surface receptors, preventing binding of parasite and host; therefore, it may prevent fungal and amebic infections (*Giardia lamblia, Trichomonas vaginalis*)
- May have chemopreventive action (in rats) (Ebisuzaki, 2003)
- Anti-inflammatory; may reduce fibroblast production

Nutritional Sources: Common in raw milk, uncooked grains, fruits, and vegetables

Current Use

- Clinical use to control GI upset, GERD, and Crohn's disease (Amemori et al., 2006)
- Relieves arthritis and musculoskeletal pain (bursitis, carpal tunnel syndrome, fibromyalgia, low back pain, tendinitis) (Kim & Axelrod, 2006; Lawrence, 1998)
- Oral administration of MSM ($DMSO_2$): in 15 patients with rheumatoid arthritis and amyloid A amyloidosis, half of those with early-stage renal dysfunction and proteinuria showed improvement. It also improved GI amyloidosis diarrhea and protein-losing gastroenteropathy (Amemori et al., 2006).
- May boost the immune system; it has delayed tumor growth in animals (Ebisuzaki, 2003)
- May benefit allergies and allergic asthma (Barrager & Schauss, 2003)
- Local application (intraurethral) has shown some effectiveness for reducing the inflammation and pain of interstitial cystitis (Childs, 1994).

Available Forms, Dosage, and Administration Guidelines

Preparations: Powder, capsules

Typical Dosage: Take 2 to 4 g a day with meals. Clinicians may recommend much higher doses. Follow manufacturer directions.

Pharmacokinetics—If Available (form or route when known): Not known

Toxicity: None known

Contraindications: None known

Side Effects: Occasional GI upset, diarrhea

Long-Term Safety: Unknown

Use in Pregnancy/Lactation/Children: Unknown; do not use

Drug/Herb Interactions and Rationale (if known): Use cautiously with ASA, heparin, or dicumarol: possible potentiation.

Special Notes: Additional research on this promising sulfur compound is needed to confirm its activity.

BIBLIOGRAPHY

Amemori S, et al. (2006). Oral dimethyl sulfoxide for systemic amyloid A amyloidosis complication in chronic inflammatory disease: A retrospective patient chart review. *Journal of Gastroenterology.* May;41(5):444–449.

Barrager E, Schauss AG. (2003). Methylsulfonylmethane as a treatment for seasonal allergic rhinitis: Additional data on pollen counts and symptom questionnaire. *Journal of Alternative and Complementary Medicine.* Feb;9(1):15–16.

Childs SJ. (1994). Dimethyl sulfone (DMSO$_2$) in the treatment of interstitial cystitis. *Urological Clinics of North America.* 21(1):85–88.

Der Marderosian A, Beutler J. [Eds.]. (2004). *The Review of Natural Products.* St. Louis, MO: Facts and Comparisons.

Ebisuzaki K. (2003). Aspirin and methylsuflonylmethane (MSM): A search for common mechanisms, with implications for cancer prevention. *Anticancer Research.* Jan-Feb;23(1A):453–458.

Jacob SW, et al. (1999). *The Miracle of MSM: The Natural Solution for Pain.* New York: GP Putnam's Sons.

Kim LS, Axelrod LJ. (2006). Efficacy of methylsulfonylmethane (MSM) in osteoarthritis pain of the knee: A pilot clinical trial. *Osteoarthritis and Cartilage.* Mar;14(3):286–294.

Lawrence RM. (1998). Methylsulfonylmethane (MSM): A double-blind study of its use in degenerative arthritis. *International Journal of Antiaging Medicine.* 1(1):50.

 NAME: Phosphatidylserine (PtdSer)

Common Names: PS

Description and Source
- Phospholipid present in all cell membranes but is most concentrated in brain cells
- Derived from soybeans (most research was originally performed on cow brain–derived PS)
- Similar to acetylcholine

Biologic Activity
- Memory rejuvenator, particularly in elderly
- Improves cognitive function and may reduce mental decline in as few as 3 months (Crook et al., 1992)
- Decreases apathy and withdrawal in elderly (Maggioni et al., 1990)
- Increases brain activity. It is necessary for cell signaling.
- Protects cell membranes from oxygen free radical damage, especially iron-mediated oxidation (Kingsley, 2006)
- May increase T-cell activity (Guarcello et al., 1990) and is necessary for apoptosis

Nutritional Sources: Soy (preferred source) and animal brains (not recommended)

Current Use
- Protects brain cells from oxygen free radical damage. May be useful to prevent ischemic damage after strokes. Boosts memory and cognitive function; may benefit patients with Alzheimer's and senile dementia (Cenacchi et al., 1993).
- Can be useful for geriatric depression (Maggioni et al., 1990) and menopausal cloudy thinking
- PS improved exercise capacity and endurance (Kingsley, 2006).

Available Forms, Dosage, and Administration Guidelines:
Take 100 to 300 mg three times a day with meals. After maximum effects are achieved, dose may be reduced to 100 mg a day. Action may persist for several months after stopping PS.

Pharmacokinetics—If Available (form or route when known): Not known

Toxicity: Not known

Contraindications: Not known

Side Effects: Nausea with large doses (more than 200 mg)

Long-Term Safety: Probably safe

Use in Pregnancy/Lactation/Children: Not known

Drug/Herb Interactions and Rationale (if known): May thin blood; caution with concurrent use of blood thinners

Special Notes: Positive studies have used animal-derived products. The effectiveness of vegetable-derived products have not been proven. Ninety-five percent of all PS is produced by Lucas Meyer in Decatur, Florida, under the trademark Leci-PS. It is packaged for many other companies.

BIBLIOGRAPHY

Cenacchi T, et al. (1993). Cognitive decline in the elderly: A double-blind, placebo-controlled multicenter study on efficacy of phosphatidylserine administration. *Aging (Milano)*. Apr;5(2):123–133.

Crook T, et al. (1992). Effects of phosphatidylserine in Alzheimer's disease. *Psychopharmacology Bulletin*. 28(1):61–66.

Guarcello V, et al. (1990). Phosphatidylserine counteracts physiological and pharmacological suppression of humoral immune response. *Immunopharmacology*. 19(3):185–195.

Kingsley M. (2006). Effects of phosphatidylserine supplementation on exercising humans. *Sports Medicine*. 36(8):657–669.

Maggioni M, et al. (1990). Effects of phosphatidylserine therapy in geriatric patients with depressive disorders. *Acta Psychiatrica Scandinavica*. 81(3):265–270.

 NAME: Red-Yeast Rice (*Monascus purpureus*)

Common Names: Cholestin (product name), *xue zhi kang* (Chinese), monascus, red rice yeast

Description and Source

- Red yeast fermented in cooked rice
- Red yeast is a natural source of at least 10 cholesterol-lowering chemicals known as HMG-CoA reductase inhibitors (the "statin" drugs).

Biologic Activity

- Monacolins (chemically similar to but a different compound from lovastatin): lowers cholesterol (Heber et al., 1999; Li et al., 2005)
- Inhibits HMG-CoA reductase, thus limiting cholesterol biosynthesis. Decreases LDL and very-low-density cholesterol and triglycerides, elevates HDL (Bliznakov, 2000; Heber, 1999; Journoud & Jones, 2004).

- Inhibits atherosclerotic plaque formation and improves endothelial function (Zhao et al., 2004)

Nutritional Sources: Used for centuries in China for making rice wine and Peking duck

Current Use
- To lower elevated total cholesterol caused by a high-fat diet, genetic factors, and HIV-related dyslipidemia (Journoud & Jones, 2004; Keithley et al., 2002)
- Protects preprandial and postprandial endothelial function in patients with coronary heart disease (Zhao et al., 2004)

Available Forms, Dosage, and Administration
Guidelines: A dosage of 600 mg twice a day with meals delivers 10 mg HMG-CoA reductase inhibitors daily. Do not take more than four capsules in 24 hours.

Pharmacokinetics—If Available (form or route when known): Not known

Toxicity: None found

Contraindications: Liver disease, intake of more than two alcoholic drinks a day, serious infection, recent surgery, yeast allergies

Side Effects: Mild and similar to those of HMG-CoA drugs: muscle pain, tenderness, weakness, gastric upset (Smith et al., 2003; Vercelli et al., 2006)

Long-Term Safety: Probably safe

Use in Pregnancy/Lactation/Children
- Pregnancy: do not take—cholesterol is needed for fetal development
- Lactation/children: do not take due to lack of safety data

Drug/Herb Interactions and Rationale (if known): Do not take with other cholesterol-lowering drugs (Heber et al., 1999) due to likely cumulative effects. Red-yeast rice, like statin drugs, inhibits Co-Q10 production. Take 30 to 60 mg of Co-Q10 a day to help prevent muscle pain. Taking CYP450 inhibitors while taking red-yeast rice may increase risk of muscle pain.

BIBLIOGRAPHY

Bliznakov EG. (2000). More on the Chinese red-yeast rice supplement and its cholesterol-lowering effect. *American Journal of Clinical Nutrition.* 71(1):152–154.

Heber D. (1999). Dietary supplement or drug? The case for cholestin. *American Journal of Clinical Nutrition.* 70(1):106–108.

Heber D, et al. (1999). Cholesterol-lowering effects of a proprietary Chinese red-yeast-rice dietary supplement. *American Journal of Clinical Nutrition.* 69(2):231–236.

Journoud M, Jones PJ. (2004). Red yeast rice: A new hypolipidemic drug. *Life Sciences.* Apr 15;74(22):2675–2683.

Keithley JK, et al. (2002). A pilot study of the safety and efficacy of cholestin in treating HIV-related dyslipidemia. *Nutrition.* Feb;18(2):201–204.

Li JJ, et al. (2005). Effects of xuezhikang, an extract of cholestin, on lipid profile and C-reactive protein: A short-term time course study in patients with stable angina. *Clinica Chimica Acta.* Feb;352(1–2):217–224.

Smith DJ, et al. (2003). Chinese red rice-induced myopathy. *Southern Medical Journal.* Dec;96(12):1265–1267.

Vercelli L, et al. (2006). Chinese red rice depletes muscle coenzyme Q10 and maintains muscle damage after discontinuation of statin treatment. *Journal of the American Geriatrics Society.* Apr;54(4):718–720.

Wigger-Alberti W, et al. (1999). Anaphylaxis due to *Monascus purpureus*-fermented rice (red-yeast rice). *Allergy.* 54(12):1330–1331.

Zhao SP, et al. (2004). Xuezhikang, an extract of cholestin, protects endothelial function through antinflammatory and lipid lowering mechanisms in patients with coronary heart disease. *Circulation.* Aug 24;110(8):915–920.

 NAME: SAMe (S-adenosylmethionine)

Common Names: "Sammy," ademetionine

Description and Source

- Synthesized naturally in the body from the amino acid methionine and adenosine triphosphate
- Necessary for mood-building neurotransmitters such as serotonin and dopamine (which it increases) by acting as a methyl donor for methylation reactions involving proteins,

phospholipids, catecholamines, and DNA; folic acid, vitamin B_{12} (cobalamin), and vitamin B_6 (pyridoxine) are also required for promoting serotonin and dopamine production. It also stabilizes norepinephrine levels.

• SAMe is grown in yeast before conversion to tablets

Biologic Activity

• Contributes to production of glutathione, a major antioxidant (Soeken et al., 2002)
• Generates taurine and cysteine in the body, essential amino acids (Brosnan & Brosnan, 2006)
• Lowers homocysteine levels, an amino acid associated with heart disease
• Improves nerve function and transmission time by increasing fat found in nerve cell membrane (Cestaro, 1994)
• Regenerates cartilage (Najm et al., 2004)
• Enhances liver health (Chavez, 2000)
• Enhances methylation, the process necessary for making neurotransmitters. SAMe is a methyl-group donor. When there is a shortage of methyl-donors, the risk of heart attack and stroke increases, and depression and memory loss occur. SAMe also promotes methylation of phospholipids, which is crucial to maintain the fluidity and responsiveness of nerve cell membranes. Vitamins B_6 and B_{12} and folic acid are also important for methylation (Bressa, 1994).

Nutritional Sources: Small quantities are found in foods, but not enough for therapeutic benefits.

Current Use

• Discovered in 1952; available in Europe since 1975 by prescription
• Numerous clinical studies have shown SAMe to be as effective or more effective than conventional antidepressants for mild to moderate depression (Bell et al., 1994; Bressa, 1994; Delle Chiaie et al., 2002; Williams et al., 2005). It also enhanced the effects of SSRIs or venlafaxine when given concurrently (Alpert et al., 2004).
• Arthritis has responded very well to SAMe. SAMe is as effective as nonsteroidal anti-inflammatories without the side effects, such as gastric irritation (Najm et al., 2004; Soeken et al., 2002).

- Slows progression of Parkinson's disease and side effects of medications
- Improves fatigue, depression, muscle pain, and morning stiffness in fibromyalgia (Integrative Medicine Access, 2000)
- Benefits liver disease with depletion of hepatic glutathione (alcohol-induced cirrhosis) (Barak et al., 1993) and intrahepatic cholestasis. It also protected against cancer chemotherapy-induced liver damage (Santini et al., 2003).

Available Forms, Dosage, and Administration Guidelines: SAMe is very unstable and easily absorbs moisture. Use only enteric-coated tablets in blister packs. Keep SAMe in its packaging until used. Do not take at night; may cause restlessness.

Typical Dosage
- *Arthritis:* 200 mg three times a day. Begins to reduce inflammation in 3 weeks; begins to build cartilage in about 3 months. Maintenance dose: 200 mg twice a day (Witte et al., 2002).
- *Mild depression:* 400 mg in the morning on an empty stomach and 400 mg before lunch. After 1 week, if depression is not improving, add another 400-mg dose 1 hour before dinner. Most European studies used 800 to 1,600 mg a day.
- *Fibromyalgia:* 800 mg a day
- *Liver disease:* 1,200 to 1,600 mg a day (Hardy et al., 2003)

Pharmacokinetics—If Available (form or route when known): None known

Toxicity: None known

Contraindications: Should not be used in bipolar conditions

Side Effects: Rare: heartburn, nausea, dry mouth, restlessness, diarrhea, headaches, may trigger manic phase in persons who are bipolar

Long-Term Safety: Very safe; no reports of toxicity in Europe

Use in Pregnancy/Lactation/Children: Unknown

Drug/Herb Interactions and Rationale (if known): Use cautiously with antidepressants, including supplements such as 5-HTP. Adjust dosages if necessary.

Special Notes: Short-term clinical use (3–4 weeks) in Europe suggests both efficacy and safety of SAMe. Most European studies have used intramuscular SAMe, which is unavailable in the United States. Most studies have been relatively short-term; longer human trials are needed. Most studies of depression used a dosage of 1,600 mg a day.

BIBLIOGRAPHY

Alpert JE, et al. (2004). S-adenosyl-L-methionine (SAMe) as an adjunct for resistant major depressive disorder: An open trial following partial or nonresponse to selective serotonin reuptake inhibitors or venlafaxine. *Journal of Clinical Psychopharmacology.* Dec;24(6):661–664.

Bell K, et al. (1994). S-adenosylmethionine blood levels in major depression: Changes with drug treatment. *Acta Neurologica Scandinavica.* 154:15–18.

Bottigueri T, et al. (1994). S-adenosylmethionine levels in psychiatric and neurological disorders: A review. *Acta Neurologica Scandinavica.* 154:19–26.

Bressa GM. (1994). SAMe (S-adenosyl-methionine) as antidepressant: Meta-analysis and clinical studies. *Acta Neurologica Scandinavica.* 89(154):7–14.

Brosnan JT, Brosnan ME. (2006). The sulfur-containing amino acids: an overview. *Journal of Nutrition.* Jun;136(6 Suppl.):1636S–1640S.

Cestaro B. (1994). Effects of arginine, S-adenosylmethionine and polyamines on nerve regeneration. *Acta Neurologica Scandinavica.* 154:32–41.

Chavez M. (2000). SAMe: S-Adenosylmethionine. *American Journal of Health Systems Pharmacy.* Jan 15;57(2):119–123.

Delle Chiaie R, et al. (2002). Efficacy and tolerability of oral and intramuscular S-adenosyl-L-methionine 1.4-butanedisulfonate (same) in the treatment of major depression: Comparison with imipramine in 2 multicenter studies. *American Journal of Clinical Nutrition.* Nov;76(5):S1172–S1176.

Hardy ML, et al. (2003). S-adenosyl-L-methionine for treatment of depression, osteoarthritis, and liver disease. *Evidence Report/Technology Assessment (Summary).* Aug;(64):1–3.

Integrative Medicine Access. (2000). *S-adenosylmethionine (SAMe).* Newton, MA: Integrative Medicine Communications.

Lesley D, et al. (1999). Brain S-adenosylmethionine levels are severely decreased in Alzheimer's disease. *Journal of Neurochemistry.* 67(3):1328.

Najm WI, et al. (2004). S-adenosyl methionine (SAMe) versus celecoxib for the treatment of osteoarthritis symptoms: A double-blind cross-over trial (ISRCTN36233495). *BMC Musculoskeletal Disorders*. Feb 26;5:6.

Santini D, et al. (2003). S-adenosylmenthionine (AdoMet) supplementation for treatment of chemotherapy-induced liver injury. *Anticancer Research*. Nov-Dec;23(6D):5173–5179.

Soeken KL, et al. (2002). Safety and efficacy of S-adenosylmethionine (SAMe) for osteoarthritis. *Journal of Family Practice*. May;51(5): 425–430.

Williams AL, et al. (2005). S-adenosylmenthionine (SAMe) as treatment for depression: A systematic review. *Clinical and Investigative Medicine*. Jun;28(3):132–139.

Witte S, et al. (2002). Meta-analysis of the efficacy of adenosylmethionine and oxaceprol in the treatment of osteoarthritis. *Orthopade*. Nov;31(11):1058–1065.

APPENDICES

Herbs Contraindicated During Pregnancy and Breast-Feeding

HERBS CONTRAINDICATED DURING PREGNANCY

Herb	Latin Name	Action
Andrographis herb	*Andrographis paniculata*	E, ?
Angelica root	*Angelica archangelica*	E, ?
Arnica flowers	*Arnica montana*	AT
Barberry root bark	*Berberis vulgaris*	US
Bethroot	*Trillium erectum*	E
Bitter melon	*Momordica charantia*	E
Black cohosh root	*Cimicifuga racemosa*	E, US
Blessed thistle herb	*Cnicus benedictus*	E
Bloodroot	*Sanguinaria canadensis*	AT, US
Blue cohosh	*Caulophyllum thalictroides*	A, E, T, US
Blue vervain	*Verbena hastate*	E, ?
Boldo herb	*Peumus boldus*	T
Borage herb	*Borago officinalis*	FH
Buchu herb	*Agathosma betulina*	E
Calamus root	*Acorus calamus*	E
Celandine herb	*Chelidonium majus*	US
Celery seed*	*Apium graveolens*	E, ?
Chamomile (Roman)	*Anthemis nobilis*	E, ?
Chaparral herb	*Larrea divaricata*	Possible FH
Chinese coptis	*Coptis teeta*	US
Chinese ligusticum	*Ligusticum chuanxiong*	E
Cinchona bark	*Cinchona* spp.	E, T
Coltsfoot leaves	*Tussilago farfara*	FH
Comfrey root or leaf	*Symphytum officinale*	FH
Cotton root	*Gossypium herbaceum*	A, E, US
Dan shen root	*Salvia miltiorrhiza*	US

(continued)

HERBS CONTRAINDICATED DURING PREGNANCY—cont'd

Herb	Latin Name	Action
Devil's claw root	*Harpagophytum procumbens*	US
Fenugreek seed*	*Trigonella foenum-graecum*	E, US, ?
Feverfew herb	*Tanacetum parthenium*	E, ?
Germander herb	*Teucrium* spp.	FH
Goldenseal root	*Hydrastatis canadensis*	US
Guarana seed	*Paullinia cupana*	S
Guggal gum resin	*Commiphora mukul*	E
Huang qin root	*Scutellaria baicalensis*	T, ?
Hyssop herb	*Hyssopus officinalis*	E, ?
Ipecac root	*Cephalis ipecacuanha*	US
Jamaica dogwood bark	*Piscidia erythrina*	AT
Juniper berries	*Juniperus communis*	E, US
Khella seed	*Amni visnaga*	E
Life root	*Senecio aureus*	FH
Lomatium root	*Lomatium disecctum*	E
Ma huang herb	*Ephedra sinica*	S, US
Male fern root	*Dryopteris filix-mas*	AT, E
Mayapple root/rhizome	*Podophyllum peltatum*	AT, T
Mistletoe herb	*Viscum album*	US
Motherwort herb	*Leonurus cardiaca*	E, ?
Mugwort herb	*Artemisia vulgaris*	E, ?
Mustard seed*	*Brassica nigra*	E
Myrrh gum	*Commiphora* spp.	E
Nutmeg seed*	*Myristica fragrans*	E
Oregon grape root	*Mahonia* spp.	US
Osha root	*Ligusticum porterii*	E
Parsley seed*	*Petroselinum crispus*	E
Pau d'arco	*Tabebuia avellanedae*	A,T
Pennyroyal herb/EO	*Hedeoma pulegioides, Mentha pulegium*	A, AT, E, US

(continued)

HERBS CONTRAINDICATED DURING PREGNANCY—cont'd

Herb	Latin Name	Action
Periwinkle herb	*Vinca rosea*	E, T
Petasites rhizome	*Petasites* spp.	H
Picrorrhiza root	*Picrorrhiza kurroa*	E
Pink root	*Spigelia marilandica*	AT
Pleurisy root	*Asclepias tuberosa*	E
Pokeweed root	*Phytolacca americana*	AT, SL, T
Pulsatilla herb	*Anemone pulsatilla*	AT
Quassia	*Picrasma excelsa*	US
Rauwolfia root	*Rauwolfia serpentaria*	AT
Rue herb	*Ruta graveolens*	A, E, US
Sandalwood	*Santalum album*	E
Shepherd's purse herb	*Capsella bursa-pastoris*	US, ?
Tansy herb	*Tanacetm vulgare*	A, E, US
Thuja	*Thuja occidentalis*	E
Thyme herb*	*Thymus vulgaris*	E, ?
Tienchi ginseng	*Panax pseudo-ginseng*	E
Tobacco leaves	*Nicotiana tabacum*	AT, T, US
Una de gato	*Uncaria tomentosa*	T
Uva-ursi herb	*Arctostyphlos uva-ursi*	US
Wild carrot seed	*Daucus carota*	E
Wild cherry bark	*Prunus serotina*	T, ?
Wild ginger rhizome	*Asarum canadense*	AT, E
Wild indigo	*Baptisia tinctoria*	AT
Wormseed	*Chenopodium ambrosioides*	AT, E
Wormwood	*Artemesia absinthium*	E
Yellow jasmine herb	*Gelsemium sempervirens*	AT
Yellow root	*Xanthorrhiza simplicissema*	US, ?
Yohimbe bark	*Pausinystalia yohimbe*	AT

*Small amounts for culinary use are safe.
E, emmenagogue; ?, possibly problematic, inadequate data; AT, acute toxin; US, uterine stimulant; A, abortifacient; T, teratogenic; FH, fetal hepatotoxin; S, CNS stimulant; H, hepatotoxic; SL, stimulant laxative.

HERBS TO USE ONLY UNDER PROFESSIONAL GUIDANCE DURING PREGNANCY

Black horehound	Kava
Chaste tree	Lobelia
Dong quai	Prickly ash

STIMULANT LAXATIVES (CONTRAINDICATED DURING PREGNANCY BECAUSE THEY CAN STIMULATE CONTRACTIONS)

Herb	Latin Name
Aloe latex	*Aloe* spp.
Blue flag rhizome	*Iris versicolor*
Buckthorn bark	*Rhamnus cathartica*
Cascara sagrada bark	*Rhamnus purshiana*
Castor oil	*Ricinus communus*
Culvers root	*Veronicastrum virginiana*
Rhubarb root	*Rheum palmatum*
Senna herb	*Cassia senna*

HERBS CONTRAINDICATED DURING BREAST-FEEDING

Herb	Latin Name	Action
Aloe latex	*Aloe* spp.	SL
Borage herb	*Borago officinalis*	H
Buckthorn bark	*Rhamnus cathartica*	SL
Cascara sagrada	*Rhamnus purshiana*	SL
Comfrey root and leaf	*Symphytum officinalis*	H
Life root	*Senecio aureus*	H
Ma huang (ephedra) herb	*Ephedra sinica*	S
Mayapple root	*Podophyllum peltatum*	SL, AT
Petasites root	*Petasites frigida*	H
Poke root	*Phytolacca americana*	SL, AT
Pulsatilla herb	*Amemone* spp.	AT
Rhubarb root	*Rheum palmatum*	SL
Rue herb	*Ruta gravelens*	E, US
Sage herb*	*Salvia officinalis*	*
Senna herb	*Cassia senna*	SL
Wild ginger root	*Asarum canadenis*	E, AT

*Small amounts for culinary use are safe.
SL, stimulant laxative; H, hepatotoxic; S, CNS stimulant; AT, acute toxin; E, emmenagogue; US, uterine stimulant; *, decreases milk flow.

BIBLIOGRAPHY

Brinker F. (1999). *Herb Contraindications and Drug Interactions* (2d ed.). Sandy, OR: Eclectic Institute, Inc.

De Smet PAGM, et al. [Eds.]. (1993). *Adverse Effects of Herbal Drugs, Vol. 2.* Berlin: Springer-Verlag.

De Smet PAGM, et al. [Eds.]. (1997). *Adverse Effects of Herbal Drugs, Vol. 3.* Berlin: Springer-Verlag.

Hobbs C, Keville K. (1998). *Women's Herbs, Women's Health.* Loveland, CO: Interweave Press, Inc.

McGuffin M, et al. [Eds.]. (1997). *Botanical Safety Handbook.* Boca Raton, FL: CRC Press.

Winston D. (2000). *Herbal Therapeutics, Specific Indications for Herbs and Herbal Formulas* (7th ed.). Washington, NJ: Herbal Therapeutics Research Library.

Condition/Disease and Possible Herbal/Supplemental Therapy

Condition/Disease	Possible Herbal/Supplemental Therapy
Achlorhydria	Angelica root, cayenne, gentian, ginger, orange peel (*Citris*)*
Adrenal exhaustion	American ginseng, Asian ginseng, cordyceps, holy basil, licorice, reishi, rhodiola schisandra, Siberian ginseng
AIDS	
Immune support	American ginseng, ashwagandha, Asian ginseng, astragalus, cartinine, cat's claw, cordyceps, holy basil, lipoic acid, maitake, reishi, rhodiola, SAMe, schisandra, shiitake, spirulina
Antivirals (supportive only)	Aloe (50:1) extract (oral), bitter melon, elderberry, garlic, hyssop, propolis rosemary, shiitake, St. John's wort, turmeric
Alcoholism	Fresh oat glycerite (*Avena*),* kudzu
Allergies	
Allergic rhinitis	Amla, bilberry/blueberry, eucalyptus, eyebright, huang qin, kudzu, licorice, ma huang, nettle leaf, reishi, sage, thyme

(continued)

Table Possible Herbal/Supplemental Therapy (Continued)

Condition/Disease	Possible Herbal/Supplemental Therapy
Allergic dermatitis	Borage seed oil, calendula (topical), evening primrose seed oil, flaxseed oil/omega-3 fatty acids, gotu kola, huang qin, sarsaparilla, turmeric
Alzheimer's disease	Acetyl-L-carnitine, ashwagandha, bacopa, ginkgo, holy basil, lemon balm, phosphatidylserine, rosemary, sage, Siberian ginseng
Anemia	Amla, ashwagandha, dong quai, nettles, parsley (*Petroselinum*),* spirulina, yellow dock,
Angina pectoris	Astragalus, cactus (*Selenicereus*),* cartinine, Co-Q10, dan shen, dong quai, hawthorn, kudzu, rhodiola
Ankylosing spondylitis	Ashwagandha, gotu kola, hawthorn, licorice, maitake (*Grifola*), picrorrhiza, reishi
Anorexia nervosa	Angelica root, artichoke leaf, dandelion root, fenugreek seed, saw palmetto, Siberian ginseng
Anxiety disorder	Ashwagandha, bacopa, blue vervain (*Verbena hastata*),* 5-HTP, gotu kola, kava, lavender, lemon balm, motherwort, passion flower, reishi, skullcap, valerian
Arrhythmias (mild)	Carnitine, Co-Q10, hawthorn, motherwort, reishi, rhodiola, Tienqi ginseng*
Arteriosclerosis/ atherosclerosis	Amla, cartinine, cayenne, dan shen, elderberry, flaxseed, garlic, ginkgo, grape seed extract, gum guggul, hawthorn, reishi, sage, turmeric
Asthma (allergic asthma)	Amla, angelica root, cordyceps, evening primrose oil, ginkgo, green tea, huang qin, khella (*Amni visnaga*),* licorice, lobelia, ma huang, MSM, picrorrhiza, propolis, reishi, schisandra, thyme
Athlete's foot	Lavender EO, myrrh, tea tree EO, thyme EO
Attention deficit disorder	Bacopa, hawthorn, holy basil, lemon balm, linden flower (*Tilea*),* rosemary, Siberian ginseng

Autoimmune disorders	*Artemisia annua*, cordyceps, dan shen, holy basil, flaxseed oil/omega-3 fatty acids, huang qin, licorice, maitake, picrorrhiza, reishi
Bacterial vaginosis	Garlic, goldenseal, propolis, usnea*
Bedwetting	Agrimony, ma huang, raspberry, St. John's wort
Benign prostatic hyperplasia	Agrimony (*Agrimonia*),* nettle root, pumpkinseed oil,* pygeum bark, rye pollen,* saw palmetto, soy, zinc*
Biliary dyskinesia	Angelica, artichoke leaf, barberry, blessed thistle, dandelion root, gentian, lavender, wild yam, yarrow, yellow dock
Blepharitis (topical application)	Calendula, flaxseed, goldenseal
Bronchitis	Black cohosh, boswellia, echinacea, fenugreek, garlic, huang qin, hyssop, licorice, plantain, red clover, saw palmetto, thyme
Buerger's disease	Co-Q10, dan shen, dong quai, hawthorn
Burns (topical application)	Aloe gel, calendula, echinacea, gotu kola, lavender EO, plantain, St. John's wort
Bursitis	Amla, black cohosh, boswellia, grape seed extract, meadowsweet, MSM, sarsaparilla, turmeric, willow
Cancer General preventive/ immune stimulation	Aloe (50:1) extract (oral), amla, ashwagandha, Asian ginseng, astragalus, bilberry/blueberry, burdock root, cat's claw, Co-Q10, cordyceps, flaxseed, garlic, grape seed extract, green tea, holy basil, kudzu, lipoic acid, lycopene, maitake, reishi, rhodiola, Siberian ginseng, turmeric, violet leaf (*Viola*)*

(continued)

Condition/Disease	Possible Herbal/Supplemental Therapy *(Continued)*
Breast cancer	American ginseng, *Artemisia annua*, flaxseed, green tea, melatonin, red clover, soy
Prostate cancer	Flaxseed, green tea, lycopene, nettle root, saw palmetto, soy
Candidiasis	Barberry, Chinese coptis (*Coptis teeta*),* echinacea, goldenseal, Oregon grape root, pau d'arco, propolis, sage, tea tree EO
Carpal tunnel syndrome	Ginger, sarsaparilla, St. John's wort, turmeric
Chronic fatigue syndrome	American ginseng, ashwagandha, Asian ginseng, astragalus, carnitine, cordyceps, gotu kola, holy basil, licorice, reishi, rhodiola, schisandra, shiitake, Siberian ginseng
Cirrhosis of the liver	Artichoke leaf, dong quai, licorice, lipoic acid, milk thistle, picrorrhiza, SAMe, schisandra, turmeric
Cold sores	Calendula, chamomile, goldenseal, lavender EO, lemon balm, myrrh, propolis
Colitis	Catnip, chamomile, flaxseed, kudzu, licorice, sarsaparilla, slippery elm, turmeric, yarrow
Common cold	Andrographis, catnip, echinacea, elderberry, ginger, hyssop, meadowsweet, propolis, sage, thyme, yarrow
Congestive heart failure (mild)	Astragalus, cactus (*Selenicereus*),* carnitine, Co-Q10, dan shen, dandelion leaf (edema), dong quai, hawthorn, kudzu
Conjunctivitis (eyewash)	Barberry, calendula, goldenseal, Oregon grape root
Constipation	Aloe gel (mild), artichoke, butternut bark (*Juglans cineraria*),* dandelion root, fenugreek, flaxseed, psyllium seed, senna, slippery elm

Coughs	
Dry	Coltsfoot, fenugreek, flaxseed, licorice, marshmallow, saw palmetto, slippery elm
Wet	Eucalyptus, ginger, horehound (*Marrubium*),* propolis, sage, thyme, yerba santa (*Eriodictyon*)*
Spastic	Black cohosh, licorice, lobelia
Crohn's disease	Cat's claw, dan shen, kudzu, licorice, reishi, slippery elm, turmeric
Cystitis	Barberry root, cranberry, echinacea, meadowsweet, MSM, Oregon grape root, uva ursi
Depression (mild/moderate)	American ginseng, ashwagandha, bacopa, black cohosh (menopausal), 5-HTP, ginkgo, gotu kola, holy basil, lavender, lemon balm, melatonin, phosphatidyserine, rhodiola, rosemary, SAMe, schisandra, Siberian ginseng, St. John's wort
Diabetes (type 2)	Asian ginseng, astragalus, bitter melon, chromium, cinnamon, Co-Q10, evening primrose seed oil, fenugreek, grape seed extract, guggul, gymnema, holy basil, lipoic acid, maitake
Diabetic retinopathy	Amla, bilberry/blueberry, elderberry, ginkgo, grape seed extract, lipoic acid, lutein*
Diarrhea	Barberry, bilberry/blueberry, cat's claw, catnip, chamomile, cinnamon, flaxseed, garlic, ginger, goldenseal, huang qin, kudzu, meadowsweet, plantain, psyllium seed, raspberry leaf, sage, schisandra, slippery elm, willow, yarrow
Diverticulitis	Catnip, cat's claw, kudzu, licorice, plantain, sarsaparilla, slippery elm, turmeric, wild yam, yarrow
Dry skin	Burdock seed,* evening primrose seed oil, flaxseed oil/omega-3 fatty acids
Eczema	Borage seed oil, burdock seed, calendula (topical), chamomile (topical), echinacea (topical), evening primrose seed oil, flaxseed oil/omega-3 fatty acids, gotu kola, sarsaparilla, yellow dock
Edema	Dandelion leaf, gotu kola, green tea, hawthorn, nettle leaf, parsley*

(continued)

Condition/Disease	Possible Herbal/Supplemental Therapy *(Continued)*
Emphysema	Astragalus, prince seng *(Pseudostellaria)*,* thyme
Endometriosis	Black cohosh, blue cohosh (pain), chaste tree
Fatigue	Ashwagandha, American ginseng, Asian ginseng, cordyceps, gotu kola, guarana (stimulant), holy basil, L-cartinine, reishi, rhodiola, schisandra, Siberian ginseng, St. John's wort
Fibrocystic breast disease	Burdock root, chaste tree, red clover, red root *(Ceanothus)*,* violet leaf *(Viola)*,*
Fibroids, uterine	Chaste tree, cinnamon, dong quai, white ash bark *(Fraxinus)*,* white peony *(Peonia)*
Fibromyalgia syndrome	American ginseng, ashwagandha, black cohosh, carnitine, 5-HTP, kava, MSM, SAMe
Flatulence	Angelica, artichoke, blessed thistle, catnip, chamomile, cinnamon, dandelion root, fennel *(Foeniculum)*,* lavender, lemon balm, peppermint, rosemary, sage, thyme, yarrow
Gastric ulcers	Aloe gel, bilberry/blueberry, calendula, cinnamon, comfrey (PA-free), Co-Q10, garlic, goldenseal, grape seed extract, licorice, meadowsweet, pau d'arco, plantain, propolis, thyme, yarrow
Gastroenteritis	Chamomile, licorice, marshmallow, meadowsweet, plantain, yarrow
Gastroesophageal reflux disorder (GERD)	Chamomile, devil's claw, meadowsweet, MSM, slippery elm, wild yam
Gingivitis	Amla, calendula, Co-Q10, echinacea, goldenseal, myrrh, propolis, tea tree EO
Headache	
Migraine	Black cohosh, chaste tree (PMS migraine), evening primrose seed oil, feverfew, 5-http, ginger (nausea), guarana, kudzu, white peony *(Paeonia)*,*

Condition	Therapy
Stress-induced	Chamomile, hops, kava, lemon balm, meadowsweet, motherwort, passion flower, rosemary, skullcap, valerian, willow
Hemorrhoids	Aloe gel (topical), amla, bilberry/blueberry, collinsonia (*C. canadensis*),* figwort (*Scrophularia*),* horse chestnut, plantain (topical), yarrow
Hepatitis B and C	Amla, andrographis, artichoke leaf, bitter melon, dan shen, huang qin, licorice, lipoic acid, maitake, milk thistle, picrorrhiza, reishi, schisandra, shiitake, St. John's wort, turmeric
Herpes	
Simplex I & II	Bitter melon, hyssop, lemon balm, licorice, pau d'arco, propolis, reishi, rhubarb root,* sage, shiitake, St. John's wort
Zoster	Capsaicin cream (topical pain relief), lemon balm, licorice, St. John's wort
Hyperacidity (gastric)	Catnip, meadowsweet, marshmallow,* slippery elm*
Hyperinsulinemia (metabolic syndrome)	Artichoke leaf, Asian ginseng, carnitine, chromium, cinnamon, dandelion root, gentian, maitake
Hyperlipidemia	Artichoke leaf, cayenne, cordyceps, fenugreek, flaxseed, gentian, gum guggul, hawthorn, maitake, polycosonol/plant sterols,* psyllium seed, red yeast rice, reishi, shiitake, spirulina
Hypertension (mild/moderate)	Black haw, dandelion leaf, dan shen, evening primrose seed oil, garlic, grape seed extract, hawthorn, huang qin, kava, linden flower, melatonin, motherwort, olive leaf, reishi, spirulina

(continued)

Possible Herbal/Supplemental Therapy (Continued)

Condition/Disease	Possible Herbal/Supplemental Therapy (Continued)
Hyperthyroidism	Brassicas,* bugleweed (*Lycopus*),* lemon balm, motherwort
Hypoglycemia	American ginseng, dandelion root, licorice
Hypothyroidism	Ashwagandha, Asian ginseng, bacopa, gum guggul, rhodiola, schisandra
Immune deficiency	American ginseng, Asian ginseng, astragalus, cordyceps, holy basil, licorice, maitake, reishi, rhodiola, saw palmetto, schisandra, shiitake, Siberian ginseng
Impotence	Ashwagandha, cordyceps, epimedium,* ginkgo, muira-puama (*Liriosma*)*
Indigestion	Artichoke leaf, catnip, chamomile, dandelion root, devil's claw, gentian root, ginger, holy basil, lavender, meadowsweet, peppermint, thyme
Influenza	Andrographis, echinacea, elderberry, ginger, hyssop, pau d'arco, propolis, sage, St. John's wort, willow, yarrow
Insomnia	Ashwagandha, black cohosh (menopausal), chamomile, dan shen, 5-HTP, hops, kava, lavender, melatonin, passion flower, reishi, scullcap, valerian
Interstitial cystitis	Couch grass (*Elymus repens*),* kava (for pain), MSM, plantain, saw palmetto
Irritable bowel syndrome	Cat's claw, catnip, chamomile, evening primrose seed oil, hops, kudzu, licorice, meadowsweet, peppermint EO, sarsaparilla, slippery elm, wild yam, yarrow
Jaundice	Artichoke leaf, dan shen, huang qin, milk thistle, picrorrhiza, turmeric
Kidney disease	*Artemisia annua*, cordyceps, dan shen, nettle leaf, nettle seed
Macular degeneration	Amla, bilberry/blueberry, elderberry, grape seed extract, ginkgo, lutein,* lycopene

Memory problems	Acetyl-L-carnitine, ashwagandha, Asian ginseng, bacopa, ginkgo, gotu kola, holy basil, lavender, phosphatidyserine, reishi, rosemary, SAMe, schisandra
Ménière's disease	Bacopa, ginger, ginkgo, gastrodia (*G. elata*)*
Menopausal problems	
Anxiety, insomnia	Blue vervain (*Verbena hastata*),* chamomile, kava, lavender, motherwort, passion flower
Hot flashes, night sweats	Black cohosh, chaste tree, dong quai, flaxseed, isoflavones, motherwort, red clover, soy
Menstrual cramps	Angelica, black cohosh, black haw, chamomile, chaste tree, cyperus,* dong quai, motherwort
Morning sickness	Chamomile, ginger, raspberry leaf, wild yam
Muscle spasm	Ashwagandha, black cohosh root, black haw, kava, kudzu, lobelia, magnesium,* Roman chamomile, skullcap, valerian
Nausea/vomiting	Angelica, blessed thistle, catnip, chamomile, cinnamon, ginger, hyssop, lavender, lemon balm, peppermint, rosemary, thyme
Obesity	Ephedra, gum guggul (used with Triphila), gymnema, yohimbe(?)
Osteoarthritis	Amla, ashwagandha, black cohosh, boswellia, cayenne (capsaicin cream topically), chondroitin, dandelion root, devil's claw, feverfew, ginger, glucosamine sulfate, grape seed extract, gum guggul, meadowsweet, nettle leaf, SAMe, turmeric
Osteoporosis	Amla, black cohosh, boron,* calcium,* kudzu, red clover isoflavones, soy isoflavones
Otitis media	Echinacea, eyebright, garlic, goldenseal, kudzu, plantain, sage, thyme
Pancreatitis	Milk thistle, fringe tree (*Chionanthus*),* red root (*Ceanothus*)*

(continued)

Possible Herbal/Supplemental Therapy *(Continued)*

Condition/Disease	Possible Herbal/Supplemental Therapy *(Continued)*
Peripheral vascular disease	Alpha-lipoic acid, Amla, blueberry, cayenne, cinnamon, ginger, ginkgo, hawthorn, horse chestnut, L-carnitine, prickly ash (*Zanthoxylum*)*
Pneumonia	Andrographis, echinacea, elecampane (*Inula*),* garlic, huang qin, hyssop, sage, usnea*
Premenstrual syndrome	Black cohosh, black haw, borage seed oil, chaste tree, dong quai, evening primrose seed oil, flaxseed oil/omega-3 fatty acids, ginkgo, lavender, motherwort
Prostatitis	Chinese coptis,* echinacea, eucalyptus, pygeum bark
Psoriasis	Barberry, borage seed oil, burdock seed, evening primrose oil, flaxseed oil/omega-3 fatty acids, gotu kola, guggal, Oregon grape root, picrorrhiza, sarsaparilla
Pyelonephritis	Cranberry juice, huang qin, Oregon grape root, uva ursi
Raynaud's disease	Amla, bilberry/blueberry, cayenne, cinnamon, dong quai, ginger, ginkgo, horse chestnut
Rheumatoid arthritis	Amla, ashwagandha, borage seed oil, boswellia, flaxseed oil/omega-3 fatty acids, chondroitin, ginger, maitake, picrorrhiza, reishi, sarsaparilla, turmeric, willow
Seasonal affective disorder	Lavender, lemon balm, SAMe, St. John's wort
Sore throat	Burdock seed, cinnamon, echinacea, elderberry, eucalyptus, hyssop, licorice, myrrh, propolis, sage, thyme
Systemic lupus erythematosus	Ashwagandha, cordyceps, flaxseed oil/omega-3 fatty acids, gotu kola, huang qin, licorice, maitake, reishi

Tendinitis	Devil's claw, grape seed extract, hawthorn, sarsaparilla, St. John's wort, turmeric, omega-3 fatty acids
Tinnitus	Cordyceps, ginkgo, kudzu
Ulcerative colitis	Boswellia, calendula, catnip, chamomile, flaxseed, kudzu, licorice, plantain, sarsaparilla, slippery elm, turmeric, yarrow
Uterine prolapse	Raspberry leaf, ladies mantle,* partridge berry*
Vertigo	Ginger, ginkgo, gastrodia tuber,* kudzu
Vitiligo	Picrorrhiza, psorela seed (*Psoralea*)*
Warts	
Common (topical)	Celandine latex (*Chelidonium*),* dandelion latex, garlic
Venereal (topical)	Calendula, goldenseal, thuja (*T. occidentalis*)*

*Not covered in this text; see Appendix C.

An Annotated Guide to Recommended References

HERBAL MEDICINE

Brinker F. (2001). *Herb Contraindications & Drug Interactions*. Sandy, OR: Eclectic Medical Publications. One of the books containing the most accurate and available information on herb/drug interactions, safety, contraindications, and the like.

European Scientific Cooperative on Phytotherapy. (2003). *ESCOP Monographs*. New York: Thieme. Detailed monographs on plant drugs commonly used in European phytotherapy.

Hobbs C. (2003). *Medicinal Mushrooms* (New ed.). Santa Cruz, CA: Botanica Press. The most comprehensive guide to medicinal fungi, complete with research and clinical information.

Hoffmann D. (2003). *Medical Herbalism*. Rochester, VT: Inner Traditions. A textbook of practical clinical herbal medicine that includes therapeutics, phytochemistry, and materia medica.

Mills S, Bone K. (2000). *Principles and Practice of Phytotherapy*. Edinburgh: Churchill Livingstone. An exceptional work combining the knowledge of English herbal medicine and modern scientific research. The materia medica is small (only 40 herbs), but each plant is covered in a wonderfully detailed and accurate monograph. The section on therapeutics is one of the best in all of herbal literature.

Mills S, Bone K. (2005). *The Essential Guide to Herbal Safety*. St. Louis: Elsevier. One of the books containing the most accurate and available information on herb/drug interactions, safety, contraindications, and the like.

Moore M. (2003). *Medicinal Plants of the Pacific West* (2d ed.). Santa Fe, NM: Red Crane Books. Michael Moore is one of the most respected and talented American herbalists in the past 35 years. This title, as well as his study guide series, offers clear, insightful, humorous, and effective information on the use of herbs in clinical practice.

The following texts from Michael Moore's Southwest School of Botanical Medicine are available as free downloads from his website, *www.swsbm.com/manualsMM/mansMM.html*.

Moore M. (1990). *Herbal Repertory in Clinical Practice*. (3d ed.). A manual of differential therapeutics in 23 sections, with a cross index of symptoms. Dose and media are found in the herbal materia medica.

Moore M. (1991). *Herbal Repertory in Clinical Practice* (3d ed.).

Moore M. (1995). *Herbal-Medical Contraindications*.

Moore M. (1995). *Herbal Formulas for Clinic and Home*.

Moore M. (1995). *Herbal Materia Medica* (5th ed.).

Moore M. (1995). *Medical/Herbal Glossary*.

Moore M. (1995). *Herbal Tinctures in Clinical Practice* (3d ed.).

Moore M. (1995). *Herb-Medical Contraindications*.

Moore M. (1997). *Specific Indications in Clinical Practice* (2d ed.).

Skenderi G. (2003). *Herbal Vade Mecum*. Rutherford, NJ: Herbacy Press. A very useful desk reference on over 800 herbs and natural products with information on uses, constituents, cautions, herbal actions, and common/botanical names.

Trickey R. (1998). *Women, Hormones, and the Menstrual Cycle*. St. Leonards, Australia: Allen & Unwin. An exceptional work by an Australian medical herbalist; combines detailed knowledge of female physiology, gynecology, and the use of herbs to treat female reproductive problems.

Upton R. [Ed.]. *The American Herbal Pharmacopoeia and Therapeutic Compendium*. Santa Cruz, CA: AHP. An important scholarly project that brings together the most accurate information on each herb covered in this ongoing series. So far, monographs include ashwagandha, astragalus, black haw, chaste tree, cramp bark, cranberry, dang gui, echinacea, ginkgo, goldenseal, hawthorn berry, hawthorn flower and leaf, reishi, schisandra, St. John's wort, valerian, and willow bark. Each monograph includes the botany, history, pharmacognosy, clinical uses, and relevant research on the herb.

Weiss RF. (2001). *Weiss' Herbal Medicine-Classic Edition*. New York: Thieme. Weiss' text is a testament to 50 years of practice as an herbal physician (MD) in Germany. His book is full of clinical pearls that are left out of most texts. An exceptional guide for the physician who wants to include good herbal medicine into his or her practice.

Wynn S, Fougere B. (2007). *Veterinary Herbal Medicine*. St. Louis: Mosby. The first truly comprehensive text on the use of botanicals for treating animals. Both authors are veterinarians with extensive backgrounds in herbal and conventional practice. Highly recommended!

Yance D. (1999). *Herbal Medicine, Healing and Cancer*. Lincolnwood, IL: Keats Publishing. The author of this book specializes in the treatment of cancer. He is an herbalist who works closely with prominent oncologists and has won their respect and admiration for his knowledge, compassion, and clinical skills. This book shares many insights from his 20 years of clinical practice.

ECLECTIC AND PHYSIO-MEDICAL TEXTS

All of the following texts contain outdated terminology and medical concepts, but despite these limitations, they provide superb insights into the use of botanical medicine in daily clinical practice.

Cook W. (1985). *The Physio-Medical Dispensatory* (reprint of the 1869 ed.). Sandy, OR: Eclectic Medical Publications. The author was one of the foremost practitioners of physio-medical medicine. His practice was almost entirely herbal, without the more toxic remedies often used by the rival Eclectic physicians.

Ellingwood F. (1983). *The American Materia Medica, Therapeutics, and Pharmacognosy* (reprint of the 1919 2d ed.). Sandy, OR: Eclectic Medical Publications. Dr. Ellingwood was an excellent clinician, and his book provides a remarkable view into the use of botanical remedies. He includes specific indications for each medicine to help the clinician develop a clear understanding of the benefits of each herb.

Felter HW, Lloyd JU. (1986). *Kings American Dispensatory* (reprint of 1898 11th ed.). Sandy, OR: Eclectic Medical Publications. This huge two-volume reference contains the accumulated knowledge on the eclectic materia medica from thousands of physicians over a period of 90 years.

Felter HW. (1985). *The Eclectic Materia Medica, Pharmacology, and Therapeutics* (reprint of 1922 ed.). Sandy, OR: Eclectic Medical Publications. Another excellent reference to the use of the (mostly botanical) Eclectic remedies. Felter clearly notes the uses as well as the limitations of each herbal medicine.

Jones E. (2004a). *Cancer, Its Causes, Symptoms and Treatment* (reprint of 1911 ed.). India: Jain Publishing; available from Homeopathic Education Resources, Berkeley, CA. Dr. Eli Jones was the pre-eminent cancer specialist of his day. His therapies are not only of historical interest but also provide many valuable clinical insights for the botanical treatment of cancer today.

Jones E. (2004b). *Definite Medication* (reprint of 1919 ed.). New Delhi, India: B. Jain. Dr. Jones was perhaps the most eclectic of all Eclectic physicians. He was trained as an allopathic physician, an Eclectic, a homeopath, and a physiomedicalist. He practiced each of these unique forms of medicine for more than 50 years and combined the best of each into a system that he called *definite medication*.

CHINESE AND AYURVEDIC MEDICINE

Bensky D, Barolet R. (1990). *Chinese Herbal Medicine— Formulas and Strategies*. Seattle: Eastland Press. Rarely are Chinese herbs used as single herbs. This complete text reviews the major TCM formulas, how they are applied to illness, and how they can be altered to fit the patient.

Bensky D, et al (2003). *Chinese Herbal Medicine: Materia Medica* (3d ed.). Seattle: Eastland Press. An excellent Chinese materia medica that is very comprehensive. The individual medicines (herbs, minerals, animal parts) are discussed from a TCM perspective, with information on uses, actions, selected combinations, comparisons, toxicity, doses, and the like.

Bone K. (1996). *Clinical Applications of Ayurvedic and Chinese Herbs*. Queensland, Australia: Phytotherapy Press. A succinct materia medica of the best-known Chinese and Ayurvedic herbs. The focus is on Western medical uses of these Asian plants.

Caldecott T. (2006). *Ayurveda, the Divine Science of Life.*
Edinburgh: Mosby. Probably the best explanation of the
theories and practice of Ayurvedic medicine. It also includes
a materia medica of 50 of the most useful Indian medicinal
plants (with color photographs) and a formulary of
frequently used formulas.

Chen T, Chen T. (2003). *Chinese Medical Herbology and
Pharmacology.* City of Industry, CA: Art of Medicine Press.
A superb TCM materia medica with classic uses of
medicines as well as "off label uses" by experienced
clinicians. In my opinion, the best of all the English
language books on Chinese medicines.

Maccioca G. (1993). *Foundations of Chinese Medicine.*
Edinburgh: Churchill Livingstone. If you do not understand
the philosophy and theories of TCM, this book is the best
place to learn an entirely new way of perceiving health and
disease.

NUTRITION/COMPLEMENTARY ALTERNATIVE MEDICINE

Heber D, et al. (1999). *Nutritional Oncology.* San Diego:
Academic Press. An excellent clinical reference to diet and
nutrition as they relate to cancer.

Pizzorno J, Murray M. (2005). *Textbook of Natural Medicine*
(3d ed.). Edinburgh: Churchill Livingstone. Detailed text on
the practice of naturopathic medicine and naturopathic
therapies (nutrition, botanical medicine, hydrotherapy,
homeopathy, etc.).

Werbach M, Moss J. (1999). *Textbook of Nutritional Medicine.*
Tarzana, CA: Third Line Press. Two experienced clinicians
combined their knowledge and experience to create an
encyclopedia of nutritional therapies for treating disease.

RECOMMENDED JOURNALS FOR CLINICIANS

Alternative Medicine Review, Thorne Research, P. O. Box 25,
Dover, ID 83874, Website: *www.ithorne.com.*

HerbalGram, P. O. Box 144345, Austin, TX 78714-4345;
Website: *www.herbalgram.org.*

Journal of the American Herbalists Guild, AHG, 141 Nob Hill Rd., Cheshire, CT 06410; Website: *www.americanherbalistsguild.com*.

Journal of Medicinal Food, Mary Ann Liebert, Inc., Publishers, 140 Huguenot S., Third Floor, New Rochelle, NY 10801-5215; Website: *www.liebertpub.com*.

Medical Herbalism, P. O. Box 20512, Boulder, CO 80308; Website: *www.medherb.com*.

WEBSITES

American Botanical Counsel (*www.herbalgram.org*). A great assortment of information about herbs with an especially nice introduction for beginners and excellent links to other herbal sites.

David Winston's websites. Herbal Therapeutics, Inc. (*www.herbaltherapeutics.net*), and David Winston's Center for Herbal Studies (*www.herbalstudies.org*) are his forums for his 2-year education program (DWCHS) and his other activities—books by David; antiquarian books; free downloadable Eclectic, Thomsonian, and Physio-medical tests from the Herbal Therapeutics Research Library; lectures; and book reviews.

Henriette's Herbal Homepage (*www.henriettesherbal.com*). An eclectic assortment of good herb information with many downloadable texts and interesting links.

Herb Research Foundation (*www.herbs.org*). Good reviews of the most recent research in herbal medicine. Has many good links.

The Institute of Traditional Medicine (*www.itmonline.org*). Subhuti Dharmananda, PhD, has created a website with hundreds of clinically relevant, well-researched articles on the use of Chinese herbs, herb/drug interactions, TCM theory, phytochemistry, and much more.

Jonathan Treasure's website (*www.herbological.com*). Contains book reviews and many clinically relevant articles and downloads, especially on the many fallacies of herb/drug interactions, treatment of cancer with herbal/nutritional medicine, and his rather acerbic, funny, and accurate herb blog.

Michael Tierra's website (*www.planetherbs.com*). Full of excellent articles, an herb forum, and information about Michael's books, classes, and clinic.

Paul Bergner's website (*www.medherb.com*). Has downloadable back issues of his journal, *Medical Herbalism*, as well as books (*Physio-Medical Dispensatory*) and much more.

The Phytochemistry of Herbs website (*www.herbalchem.net*). A wealth of information on phytochemistry from beginning level to advanced and contains detailed articles (with illustrations) on phytoestrogens and human health.

Southwest School of Botanical Medicine (*www.swsbm.com*). Michael Moore's homepage. Includes great information on herbs and education, plus plant images and research reviews.

PROFESSIONAL ORGANIZATIONS

Clinical Herbalists

American Herbalists Guild, AHG, 141 Nob Hill Rd., Cheshire, CT 06410; Website: *www.americanherbalistsguild.com*.

Nutritionists

International & American Association of Clinical Nutritionists (IAACN), 16775 Addison Rd., Suite 102, Addison, TX 75001; Website: *www.iaacn.org*.

Glossary

Adaptogen: A substance that helps a living organism adapt to stress (environmental, physical, or psychological). According to the Soviet researcher I. I. Brekhman, who did most of the early research on adaptogens, these substances have very low toxicity, have little physiologic effect in healthy organisms, and improve endocrine, immune, and nervous system function in stressed subjects. Examples: Asian ginseng, Siberian ginseng.

Alterative: A substance that by increasing elimination helps to alter an unhealthy state into a healthier one; also known as a "blood purifier." Examples: burdock root, sarsaparilla.

Amphoteric: An herb that normalizes the function or activity of an organ or tissue. An immune amphoteric can either strengthen a deficient immune response or reduce excessive immune activity in allergies or autoimmune diseases. Examples: maitake, reishi.

Biliary dyskinesia: Improper bile flow associated with regulatory failure of the biliary system, pancreas, duodenum, and jejunum

Bitter tonic: A bitter-tasting herb that stimulates digestive, absorptive, and eliminatory functions. Bitters before or with meals increase gastric HCl production, bile secretion, pancreatic and small intestine juices, and bowel function. Examples: artichoke, gentian.

Borborygmus: Intestinal rumbling or gurgling, usually associated with flatulence and abdominal bloating

Carminative: An herb that relaxes the intestinal sphincters, relieving gas pain, and, as a result of high levels of volatile oils, reduces gas formation. Examples: chamomile, fennel.

Cholagogue: An herb that stimulates bile production. Examples: artichoke, dandelion root.

Choleretic: An herb that stimulates bile flow; usually considered interchangeable with the term *cholagogue*

Decoction: A method of making tea in which the plant material (usually bark or root) is gently simmered to increase the extraction of its constituents

Diaphoretic: A substance that gently increases body temperature and stimulates sweating to lower fevers. Examples: elderflower, yarrow.

Dysbiosis: Abnormal digestion and bowel flora causing flatulence, borborygmus, and belching

Emmenagogue: An herb that simulates menstrual flow. If taken during pregnancy, some emmenagogues may cause abortion. Examples: blue cohosh, pennyroyal.

Galactogogue: An herb that stimulates milk flow in breast-feeding mothers. Examples: fennel seed, milk thistle leaf.

Hepatoprotective: A substance that prevents liver damage and helps to improve liver function in hepatic disease caused by alcohol, solvents, and viruses. Examples: milk thistle, picrorrhiza, turmeric.

Hyperinsulinemia (metabolic syndrome): A cell-level insulin resistance with compensatory elevated insulin levels. Clinical manifestations include elevated triglyceride levels, decreased HDL choesterol, elevated cortisol levels, abdominal obesity, and a host of cardiovascular and systemic illnesses (atherosclerosis, hypertension, type 2 diabetes, PCOD). The causes of metabolic syndrome include excessive intake of calories, refined carbohydrates, and omega-6 fatty acids (relative to omega-3 fatty acids), mineral deficiencies (magnesium, chromium), and lack of exercise.

Infusion: A method of making tea in which the plant material (usually leaf or flower) is steeped. Heat-sensitive materials are best prepared by this method.

Nervine: An herb that tonifies the nervous system, producing a mild sense of relaxation. Examples: chamomile, lemon balm.

Rubefacient: A substance that acts as a counterirritant, causing increased localized blood flow and irritation. Examples: cayenne, ginger.

Solid extract: Also known as a native extract, this is a highly concentrated extract, usually in a glycerin or honey base. A good way to take medicinal fruits such as blueberries or hawthorn berries.

Tincture: A hydroalcoholic extract of an herb. Tinctures made with dry herbs are usually prepared in a ratio of 1 part herb to 5 parts menstruum (1:5). Fresh plant (green) tinctures are usually prepared in a ratio of 1 part fresh herb to 2 parts menstruum (1:2).

Trophorestorative: An herb that nourishes, strengthens, and tonifies a specific organ or function. Considered "food for the organ." Hawthorn, with its specificity for the heart and circulatory system, is a cardiovascular trophorestorative. Examples: fresh oat (nervous system), nettle seed (kidney).

Vulnerary: An old term for wound-healing plants. Vulneraries tend to have antibacterial, anti-inflammatory, and procicularization activities. They reduce healing time, prevent infection, increase granulation of tissue, and prevent scarring. Examples: calendula, plantain.

INDEX